Perinatal Brain Damage:
from Pathogenesis to Neuroprotection

Fondazione Pierfranco e Luisa Mariani ONLUS
viale Bianca Maria 28
20129 Milan, Italy

Telephone: +39 02 795458
Fax: +39 02 76009582
Publications coordinator: Valeria Basilico
e-mail: publications@fondazione-mariani.org
www.fondazione-mariani.org

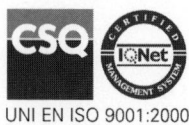

UNI EN ISO 9001:2000

Perinatal Brain Damage: from Pathogenesis to Neuroprotection

Edited by

Luca A. Ramenghi, Philippe Evrard
and Eugenio Mercuri

Mariani Foundation Paediatric Neurology Series: 19
Series Editor: Maria Majno

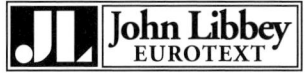

ISSN: 0969-0301
ISBN: 978-2-7420-0723-3

Cover illustration: drawing by Oreste Zevola for Fondazione Mariani elaborated by Nathalie Samson.

Technical and language editor: Oliver Brooke.

Published by

Éditions John Libbey Eurotext
127, avenue de la République, 92120 Montrouge, France
Tél.: 33 (0)1 46 73 06 60; Fax: 33 (0)1 40 84 09 99
e-mail: contact@jle.com
http//www.jle.com

© 2008 John Libbey Eurotext. All rights reserved.

Unauthorized duplication contravenes applicable laws.

It is prohibited to reproduce this work or any part of it without authorisation of the publisher or of the Centre Français d'Exploitation du Droit de Copie (CFC), 20, rue des Grands-Augustins, 75006 Paris.

Contents

Chapter 1	Neurotransmitters in the brain *Flaminio Cattabeni*	1
Chapter 2	Brain neuroreceptors: the molecular basis of drug action *Jean-Marie Maloteaux, Beryl Koener and Emmanuel Hermans*	9
Chapter 3	Multiple types of programmed cell death and their relevance to perinatal brain damage *Peter G. H. Clarke, Julien Puyal, Anne Vaslin, Vanessa Ginet and Anita Truttmann*	23
Chapter 4	Prenatal diffusion MRI characterization of fetal brain oedema *Andrea Righini, Cecilia Parazzini, Chiara Doneda, Laura Avagliano, Mariangela Rustico, Gaetano Bulfamante, Alessandra Kustermann, Roberto Fogliani, Umberto Nicolini and Fabio Triulzi*	37
Chapter 5	Intrauterine growth restriction and neurological damage *Enrico Ferrazzi and Serena Rigano*	41
Chapter 6	Fetal cytomegalovirus infection: the brain as a window in the establishment of prognosis *Gustavo Malinger and Tally Lerman-Sagie*	49
Chapter 7	Perinatal brain damage *Luca A. Ramenghi, Laura Bassi, Monica Fumagalli and Fabio Mosca*	55
Chapter 8	Is intensive care for all very immature babies justified? *Malcolm Levene*	65
Chapter 9	Twins and triplets: relative effect of plurality and prematurity on neurological outcome *Olivier Baud, Romain H. Fontaine, Gauthier Loron and Paul Olivier*	73

Chapter 10	Cerebral ischaemia: still a plausible pathway to white matter injury in the preterm infant? *Gorm Greisen*	81
Chapter 11	Oxidative stress in the developing brain *Giuseppe Buonocore, Serafina Perrone and Maria Carmela Muraca*	89
Chapter 12	Infection/inflammation – a complex hot topic in perinatal brain white matter damage aetiology *Olaf Dammann*	99
Chapter 13	White matter diseases of prematurity *Mary A. Rutherford*	103
Chapter 14	Maternal and infant characteristics associated with perinatal arterial stroke in the preterm infant *Manon Benders, Floris Groenendaal, Cuno Uiterwaal, Peter Nikkels, Hein Bruinse, Rutger-Jan Nievelstein, Linda de Vries*	113
Chapter 15	Neonatal arterial ischaemic stroke *Paul Govaert*	125
Chapter 16	Neonatal cerebral sinovenous thrombosis *Mahendranath Moharir and Gabrielle deVeber*	161
Chapter 17	The spectrum of visual disorders in children with perinatal brain lesions: long-term effects *Giovanni Cioni, Francesca Tinelli and Andrea Guzzetta*	181
Chapter 18	Early predictors of cognitive development in very low birth weight children *Roberto Militerni, Bianca Adinolfi, Luigi Falco, Alessandro Frolli and Guido Militerni*	197
Chapter 19	The Neuronal Group Selection Theory: a framework to understand typical and atypical motor development *Mijna Hadders-Algra*	205
Chapter 20	Brain plasticity in newborn infants with brain lesions: the role of brain MRI *Eugenio Mercuri, Daniela Ricci and Frances Cowan*	211
Chapter 21	Perinatal brain damage: from pathogenesis to neuroprotection *Géraldine Favrais, Luigi Titomanlio, Vincent Degos and Pierre Gressens*	219
Chapter 22	Caring for the preterm infant: earliest brain development and experience *Heidelise Als*	233

Chapter 23	Neonatal seizures: monitoring and treatment *Licia Lugli, Maria Pina Guerra, Maria Federica Roversi and Fabrizio Ferrari*	241
Chapter 24	Therapeutic approaches to psychomotor delay *Ermellina Fedrizzi and Elena Andreucci*	259

Chapter 1

Neurotransmitters in the brain

Flaminio Cattabeni

Centre of Excellence for Neurodegenerative Diseases, Department of Pharmacological Sciences, University of Milan, via Balzaretti 9, 20133 Milan, Italy
flaminio.cattabeni@unimi.it

Summary

Neurotransmitters are the key elements subserving the functioning of our brain. In the 70 years since their discovery, numerous examples have emerged. Their chemical structure ranges from simple molecules such as the monoamines to amino acids and fairly large peptides. All these molecules must fulfil strict criteria to be classified as neurotransmitters. Neurotransmitters are released from the synaptic terminals in a calcium-dependent fashion, impinge on their receptors located on postsynaptic neuronal cells, and are inactivated by metabolic processes or by reuptake mechanisms. Modern *in vivo* brain imaging techniques allow the visualization of these processes in humans under various pathophysiological conditions. The nature of the neurotransmitters synthesized by neurons (the phenotype) is not predetermined but is acquired during brain development. Brain development extends from the first trimester of pregnancy up to several years after birth and is susceptible to interference by genetic and epigenetic factors. Genetic factors affect brain development mainly in its early phases, whereas epigenetic factors are of importance in the later phases of development. Epigenetic factors can induce subtle and long-lasting effects on brain function, especially at a behavioural level.

Introduction

The concept of chemical transmission in the central nervous system originated in the early years of the twentieth century, when it was discovered that the functioning of the peripheral nervous system was dependent on the secretion of acetylcholine and noradrenaline. At this time, and based on the work of two Nobel laureates (whose Nobel lectures can be found at http://nobelprize.org) – Camillo Golgi from Italy and Santiago Ramon y Cajal from Spain – the 'neuron doctrine' was born. The physiologist Sherrington then proposed that nerve cells communicate with one another by liberating a neurotransmitter into the space called the 'synapse' (from the Greek συναπτο = to put in proximity, being in the vicinity of the nerve ending). For this discovery he received the Nobel Prize in 1932. Finally, Sir Bernard Katz, Ulf von Euler, and Julius Axelrod were awarded the Nobel Prize in 1970 for elucidating the nature of neurotransmitter actions, as discussed below. It must be emphasized that modern knowledge of neurotransmitters and their function in pathophysiology stems not only from the work of these distinguished researchers, but also from a large number of neuroscientists from all over the world who have dedicated their lives to unravelling how the brain works and what goes wrong in major neurological and psychiatric disorders. It should be borne in mind that, in terms of number of total disability-adjusted life years (DALYs) lost worldwide, brain-related disorders rank second only to infectious diseases (Hyman, 2000). Indeed, in most cases patients suffering from brain disorders (including brain ischaemia) live for decades with their disease, requiring health care and assistance and being unable to live a productive life. This is particularly true for perinatally-induced brain disorders.

Identified neurotransmitters

Chemicals suspected of acting as neurotransmitters must fulfil the following criteria.

1. The chemical must be produced within a neuron. This implies that the biochemical machinery to produce the neurotransmitter must be present within neurons.

2. The chemical must be found within a neuron and be stored within vesicles. These storage vesicles can be visualized by electron microscopy.

3. When a neuron is stimulated (depolarized), it must release the chemical in a calcium-dependent manner.

4. When a chemical is released, it must act on a postsynaptic receptor and cause a biological effect.

5. After a chemical is released, it must be inactivated. Inactivation can be through a reuptake mechanism and/or by an enzyme that stops the action of the chemical by transforming it into an inactive compound.

6. If the chemical is applied to the postsynaptic membrane, it should have the same effect as when it is released by a neuron.

The molecules that have been found in the last 50 years to fulfil these criteria are listed in Table 1.

Table 1. Identified neurotransmitters

Monoamines
   Acetylcholine
   Noradrenaline
   Dopamine
   Serotonin
   Histamine

Amino acids
   Glutamate
   γ-Amino butyric acid (GABA)
   Glycine
   Aspartate

Purines
   Adenosine
   Adenosine triphosphate (ATP)
   Uridine triphosphate (UTP)

Peptides   More than 100 peptides, usually composed of 3–30 amino acids: *e.g.*, encephalins (5 aa), somatostatin (14 or 28 aa), etc.

Monoamines were the first to be discovered in the 1950s, on the basis of work demonstrating their role in the peripheral nervous system. It is important to recall the seminal experiments of Otto Loewi who, in 1921, demonstrated chemical transmission by transferring the fluid bathing a stimulated frog heart onto a non-stimulated heart, showing that the effects of the nerve stimulus on the first heart were reproduced by the chemical activity of the solution flowing on the second and non-stimulated heart. The transmitter in question was than found to be acetylcholine. The other monoamines were then found to represent important neurotransmitters in the brain and their physiological and pathological role was established in the 1960s.

The discovery of γ-aminobutyric acid (GABA) as a neurotransmitter in the late 1960s opened the important amino acid chapter. Neurons utilizing GABA and glutamate as neurotransmitters are now known to represent the great majority (around 90 per cent) of active nerve cells in the CNS. GABA is the major inhibitory neurotransmitter and glutamate the major excitatory one. The great majority of drugs used in psychiatry and neurology today are derived from compounds acting upon these two classes of neurotransmitters. The only exceptions are the opiates, acting through the so-called peptidergic system.

Finally, it has been shown – particularly from the work of Geoffrey Burnstock from the United Kingdom – that purines play an important role in the CNS. Adenosine has major inhibitory functions, best exemplified by the stimulatory action of caffeine, an antagonist of adenosine receptors, while adenosine triphosphate (ATP) and uridine triphosphate (UTP) seem to serve stimulatory functions in selected brain areas (Burnstock, 2007).

Release of neurotransmitters

Depolarization of a neuron produces a concerted series of events leading to the release of neurotransmitters. The molecular processes involved have only recently been elucidated. In brief, the action potential arriving at the nerve terminal opens calcium channels. As the concentration of free calcium within the neuron is of the order of 10^{-9} M (which is about 10,000 times the outside concentration), calcium enters the presynaptic terminal and, by activating protein kinases, renders the vesicles capable of moving and docking onto the inner membrane of the terminal. Interactions between membrane-inserted proteins of the vesicles and the inner part of the nerve terminal lead to the process of exocytosis – that is, the vesicles fuse with the membrane of the terminal, liberating their content (neurotransmitters and other compounds, for example ATP) into the synaptic cleft. Once released, the neurotransmitter induces its physiological effects by interacting with the receptors (see chapter 2) and its action is then terminated in a matter of seconds by processes leading to its removal.

The elucidation of these molecular processes led to the discovery of the mechanism of action of the most potent toxins produced by bacteria belonging to the clostridial family: botulinum toxin and tetanus toxin. These toxins both act as proteolytic enzymes, their substrates being the proteins involved in docking of the vesicles at the terminal. This leads to a complete shut-down of the release of neurotransmitters. However, why should these two toxins – which both act through the same mechanism – have such different clinical effects, tetanus toxin producing muscular contractions and botulinum toxin inducing flaccid paralysis (Montecucco *et al.*, 2004)? The explanation lies in the fact that botulinum toxin blocks the release of neurotransmitters at the neuromuscular junction, whereas tetanus toxin, though taken up at the neuromuscular junction like botulinum toxin, exerts its proteolytic effects only after retrograde transport from the nerve ending to the cell body. On reaching the cell body, it is released and taken up by the terminals of the inhibitory neurons in the spinal cord, where the toxin exerts its proteolytic effect on the proteins involved in the release of glycine, the neurotransmitter that causes inhibition of motor neurons. This, in turn, results in a lack of inhibition of motor neurons and spastic contractions of muscles ensue (tetanus).

Synapse formation and related pathologies

Central to the correct functioning of the neurotransmitters is their release at the synapse, the basic structure responsible for the propagation of the information carried by the neurotransmitters. The two key elements in the synapse are the nerve terminal and the so-called postsynaptic element, containing the receptors for the neurotransmitter released in its proximity.

Synapses are formed in the last phases of CNS development (see below). It has been calculated that 10^6 synapses are formed every second in the fetus and newborn infant. The adult brain contains 10^{11} neurons and each neuron has 10^3 synapses, giving a total of 10^{14} synaptic contacts. As the majority of synapses are formed in the first two years of life, equivalent to 10^8 seconds, the number of synapses formed every second is $10^{14}/10^8$ ($= 10^6$).

Synapses fall into two categories: type I and type II. Type I synapses are termed non-symmetrical, while type II are termed symmetrical. Symmetry is determined by the thickness of the pre- and postsynaptic membranes, as seen in the electron microscope. When the thickness of the presynaptic membrane is similar to that of the postsynaptic membrane, the synapse is called symmetrical: this is the typical inhibitory GABAergic synapse. On the other hand, when the thickness of the postsynaptic element is much greater than that of the presynaptic element, the synapse is called asymmetrical: this is the case with the excitatory glutamatergic synapses. The reason for this enlargement of the postsynaptic element (postsynaptic densities, PSDs) is to be found in the great number of electron-dense proteins (nearly 400 different proteins) that can be classified on the basis of their function. These are as follows:
- plasma membrane proteins (that is, receptors, neuroligins);
- signalling proteins (protein kinases and other transducing enzymes);
- multimodular proteins or scaffolding proteins [that is, PSD-95 and other membrane associated guanylate kinases (MAGUKs)];
- cytoskeletal proteins (for example, actin).

Neuroligins are of the utmost importance because they serve to keep the postsynaptic elements in step with the presynaptic elements. Indeed, neuroligins are partners of neurexins, found on the presynaptic membrane. These two proteins keep the pre- and postsynaptic elements in close association. In humans, there are three neurexin and five neuroligin genes. Mutation of the DNA on one of these genes appears to be associated with an increased risk of autism. For instance, it has been shown that autistic individuals have a substantial loss of glutamatergic synapses in the cerebellar cortex, and this correlates with the severity of the disease (Autism Genome Project Consortium, 2007). It must be borne in mind that as autism is the prototypical pervasive developmental disorder, other diseases in this category (Rett syndrome, Asperger syndrome, fragile-X syndrome, tuberous sclerosis, and so on) are also linked to alterations in the DNA for neurexins and neuroligins.

Neurotransporters

Once the neurotransmitters have been released into the synaptic cleft, they act at their receptors and their action is then terminated by transformation to inactive metabolites or by reuptake, either into the nerve terminals from which they have been released or by uptake processes present in the glia surrounding the synapse (Table 2).

Table 2. Action of neurotransmitters at the synapse is terminated either by catabolism or by reuptake processes

Neurotransmitter	Catabolism	Reuptake
Acetylcholine	Acetylcholinesterases	No
Noradrenaline	COMT, MAO (after reuptake)	NET
Dopamine	COMT, MAO (after reuptake)	DAT
Serotonin	MAO (after reuptake)	SERT
GABA	GABA-transaminase (after uptake in glia)	GATs
Glycine	No	Gly-T
Glutamate	No	EAATs

COMT, catechol-*O*-methyl-transferase; DAT, dopamine transporter; EAAT, excitatory amino acid transporter; GABA, γ-amino butyric acid; GAT, GABA transporter; Gly-T, glycine transporter; MAO, monoamine oxidase; NET, norepinephrine (noradrenaline) transporter; SERT, serotonin transporter.

Acetylcholine is removed from the synapse only by catabolism: acetylcholinesterases rapidly remove acetylcholine by fission of the ester bond, introducing a molecule of water and forming choline and acetate.

Released catecholamines (noradrenaline and dopamine) are inactivated both through catabolism and through reuptake processes. Catabolism in the synaptic cleft is solely due to the activity of catechol-*O*-methyl-transferases (COMT) which methylate one of the hydroxyl groups in the aromatic ring. Once inside the nerve terminals after reuptake (which is the major means of inactivation, acting through norepinephrine transporter, NET, and dopamine transporter, DAT), catecholamines can be further catabolized by monoamine oxidases (MAO), converting the N-terminal amino group ($R-CH_2-NH_2$) to the corresponding aldehyde (R-CHO), and this in turn is either oxidized to the corresponding acid (R-COOH) or reduced to the corresponding alcohol ($R-CH_2OH$). Serotonin, however, is only taken up at nerve terminals by its transporter (serotonin transporter, SERT), and once inside the nerve terminals it is oxidized by MAO, in the same way as the catecholamines.

Reuptake processes represent the only means of inactivation for GABA, glycine, and glutamate. The reuptake of these amino acids is due to proteins inserted in the membrane of both nerve terminals and glial cells surrounding synapses.

For GABA, four transporters (GAT 1–3 and betaine/GABA transporter-1, BGT-1) have been identified and cloned in rat, mouse, and recently also in humans (Christiansen *et al.*, 2007). GAT-1 and GAT-3 are expressed exclusively in the brain (GAT-1 preferentially on neurons, GAT-3 in glia), whereas GAT-2 and BGT-1 are present both in brain and in the periphery.

For glutamate, five excitatory amino acid transporters (EAAT 1–5) have been cloned. EAAT 1 and 2 are expressed on glia, whereas EAAT 3 and 4 are expressed on nerve terminals and EAAT 5 in the neurons of the retina. It is important to note that glial EAAT show low affinity but high capacity, whereas neuronal EAAT show high affinity and low capacity. This is in accord with their proposed role: neuronal EAAT are involved mainly in the physiological role of glutamate as a fast excitatory neurotransmitter, whereas glial EAAT remove the excess of glutamate to avoid its neurotoxic actions. One of the explanations for ischaemic neuronal cell death is that the loss of ATP as the consequence of the interruption of blood supply to the brain suppresses the activity of glial EAAT, resulting in the accumulation of extrasynaptic glutamate, reaching neurotoxic concentrations (> 3 μmol/litre). Moreover, some forms of amyotrophic lateral sclerosis (ALS) seem to be due to mutations in the DNA of glial EAAT 2, with consequent motor neuron death in the cortex and spinal cord.

Neurotransporters are important from a pharmacological perspective, as several drugs acting on the CNS do so by blocking or activating these transporters. Inhibitors of NET, SERT, and DAT (either selective or non-selective) are major antidepressants. Cocaine is a selective inhibitor of DAT, whereas amphetamine seems to activate the transporter. Thus the resulting effect of both compounds is to increase the extrasynaptic levels of dopamine.

As many neurological (for example, epilepsy) and psychiatric disorders (anxiety, schizophrenia, drug addiction) seem to be caused by a reduction in the activity of the GABAergic system, inhibitors (non-subtype-specific) of GAT are used or have been proposed for these disorders. GAT-1 and GAT-3, being most exclusively expressed in brain, have attracted considerable attention as potential drug targets, with few side effects.

Imaging of neurotransmitter systems *in vivo*

One of the major advances in neuroscience has come from the possibility of visualizing the various components of neurotransmission in living human brain in physiological or pathological conditions. Today, positron emission tomography (PET) provides a powerful tool for investigating neurochemical variables in human subjects using methods originally developed for quantitative autoradiography. PET is based upon the use of radiolabelled tracers targeting the various components of the neurotransmitter system – neurotransporters, receptors, MAO, COMT, and so on. The only limitation stems from the availability of chemicals amenable to radiolabelling with positron emitting isotopes – that is, ^{18}F an ^{11}C – and targeting selectively the function to be studied. Neurotransmitter systems studied so far are the dopaminergic, noradrenergic, serotonergic, and GABAergic systems and, more recently, the glutamatergic system. These studies are important to establish the involvement of neurotransmitters in various neurological or psychiatric diseases. For instance, PET has been used to verify whether the dopamine transporter is affected in children with attention deficit/hyperactivity disorder (ADHD). Utilizing tracer amounts of an ^{11}C-labelled cocaine analogue it has been shown that there is an increase in the dopamine transporter (Spencer *et al.*, 2005). This is in line with pharmacological treatment using the amphetamine analogue methylphenidate, which, as discussed above, stimulates the activity of the transporter.

Another important means of imaging the CNS *in vivo* is magnetic resonance imaging (MRI). MRI allows visualization of brain areas that are activated when specific tasks are undertaken and is therefore an essential tool in mapping human brain function (Le Bihan *et al.*, 2006).

Stages of brain development

The extraordinary complexity of the human brain is well reflected by the time required for its formation – from the first trimester of gestation up to several years after birth. The major events and their peak time of occurrence are given in Table 3.

Table 3. Timetable of the major events in human brain development

Event	Peak time time of occurrence
Neural tube formation	3–4 weeks' gestation
Prosencephalic development	2–3 months' gestation
Neuronal proliferation	3–4 months' gestation
Neuronal migration	3–5 months' gestation
Organization	5 months' gestation to years after birth
Myelinization	At birth to years after birth

The first three events – neural tube formation, prosoencephalic development, and neuronal proliferation – are strictly under genetic control and the genes involved have been, at least in part, determined (Korzh, 1994). Mutations of these genes often result in severe brain abnormalities, which in some cases are incompatible with life (Volpe, 1995).

The later stages of development – that is, neuronal migration, organization, and myelinization – are on the other hand more susceptible to intrinsic and extrinsic environmental influences. Perturbation of these processes is often associated with neurological disorders that are compatible with life (for example, mental retardation, epilepsy, and so on), but will persist throughout the life of the affected individual. Several extrinsic factors may affect these processes: nutrition, exposure to chemicals, environmental stimuli or deprivation thereof have all been shown to affect brain development. What is most disturbing is that these effects are considered teratogenic in nature – that is, a short period of exposure can have long-lasting effects, persisting throughout life. For instance, exposure to methylmercury during gestation affects neuronal migration and layering of the cerebral cortex, causing neurological disorders in the newborn (epilepsy, ataxia, and mental retardation) (Choi et al., 1978).

Treatment of pregnant rats with an antimitotic agent, methylazoxy-methanol, on gestational day 15 alone results in a progeny showing cerebral heterotopias that share striking similarities with those observed in human periventricular nodular heterotopia (PNH), a cerebral dysgenesis frequently observed in human patients affected by drug-resistant focal epilepsy (Battaglia et al., 2003).

Another period of vulnerability which has not been sufficiently appreciated is that involving the establishment of neuronal connections, neurotransmitter activity, and receptor numbers. These processes are particularly sensitive to environmental influences, as neurons tend to establish their phenotype depending upon the milieu they find around them (Rodier, 2004). For instance, GABA, although the major inhibitory neurotransmitter in the mature CNS, has been shown to be excitatory to neurons in the developing hypothalamus (Gao & van den Pol, 2001).

Conclusions

The CNS is sensitive and vulnerable to both internal and external stimuli. What is most intriguing is that these stimuli, even though of short duration during development, have effects that persist throughout the life of the organism. Thus the final assembly of our brain, and its function, are strictly dependent upon the stimuli received from the environment and perceived through our sense organs in the first years of life.

References

Battaglia, G., Pagliardini, S., Saglietti, L., Cattabeni, F., Di Luca, M., Bassanini, S. and Setola, V. (2003): Neurogenesis in cerebral heterotopia induced in rats by prenatal methylazoxymethanol treatment. *Cereb. Cortex* **13**, 364–370.

Burnstock, G. (2007): Physiology and pathophysiology of purinergic neurotransmission. *Physiol. Rev.* **87**, 659–797.

Cattabeni, F., Gardoni, F. & DiLuca, M. (2004): Molecular biology of postsynaptic structures. In: *Molecular biology of the neuron*, 2nd edition, ed. R.W. Davies & B.J. Morris, pp. 165–181. Oxford: Oxford University Press.

Choi, B.H., Lapham, L.W., Amin-Zaki, L. & Saleem, T. (1978): Abnormal neuronal migration, deranged cerebral cortical organization, and diffuse white matter astrocytosis of human fetal brain: a major effect of methylmercury poisoning in utero. *J. Neuropathol. Exp. Neurol.* **37**, 719–733.

Christiansen, B., Meinild, A.-K., Jensen, A.A. & Brauner-Osborne, H. (2007): Cloning and characterization of a functional human gamma-aminobutyric acid (GABA) transporter, Human GAT-2. *J. Biol. Chem.* **282**, 19331–19341.

Gao, X.B. & van den Pol, A.N. (2001): GABA, not glutamate, a primary transmitter driving action potentials in developing hypothalamic neurons. *J. Neurophysiol.* **85**, 425–434.

Hyman, S. (2000): Mental illness: genetically complex disorders of neural circuitry and neural communication. *Neuron* **28**, 321–323.

Korzh, V.P. (1994): Genetic control of early neuronal development in vertebrates. *Curr. Opin. Neurobiol.* **4**, 21–28.

Le Bihan, D., Urayama, S., Aso, T., Hanakawa, T. & Fukuyama, H. (2006): Direct and fast detection of neuronal activation in the human brain with diffusion MRI. *Proc. Natl. Acad. Sci. USA* **103**, 8263–8268.

Montecucco, C., Rossetto, O. & Schiavo, G. (2004): Presynaptic receptor arrays for clostridial neurotoxins. *Trends Microbiol.* **12**, 442–446.

Rodier, P. (2004): Environmental causes of central nervous system maldevelopment. *Pediatrics* **113**, 1076–1083.

Spencer, T.J., Biederman, J., Madras, B.K., Faraone, S.V., Dougherty, D.D., Bonab, A.A. & Fischman, A.J. (2005): In vivo neuroreceptor imaging in attention-deficit/hyperactivity disorder: a focus on the dopamine transporter. *Biol. Psychiatry* **57**, 1293–1300.

Autism Genome Project Consortium, Szatmari, P., Paterson, A.D., Zwaigenbaum, L., Roberts, W., Brian, J., Liu, X.Q., Vincent, J.B., Skaug, J.L., Thompson, A.P., Senman, L., Feuk, L., Qian, C., Bryson, S.E., Jones, M.B., Marshall, C.R., Scherer, S.W., Vieland, V.J., Bartlett, C., Mangin, L.V., Goedken, R., Segre, A., Pericak-Vance, M.A., Cuccaro, M.L., Gilbert, J.R., Wright, H.H., Abramson, R.K., Betancur, C., Bourgeron, T., Gillberg, C., Leboyer, M., Buxbaum, J.D., Davis, K.L., Hollander, E., Silverman, J.M., Hallmayer, J., Lotspeich, L., Sutcliffe, J.S., Haines, J.L., Folstein, S.E., Piven, J., Wassink, T.H., Sheffield, V., Geschwind, D.H., Bucan, M., Brown, W.T., Cantor, R.M., Constantino, J.N., Gilliam, T.C., Herbert, M., Lajonchere, C., Ledbetter, D.H., Lese-Martin, C., Miller, J., Nelson, S., Samango-Sprouse, C.A., Spence, S., State, M., Tanzi, R.E., Coon, H., Dawson, G., Devlin, B., Estes, A., Flodman, P., Klei, L., McMahon, W.M., Minshew, N., Munson, J., Korvatska, E., Rodier, P.M., Schellenberg, G.D., Smith, M., Spence, M.A., Stodgell, C., Tepper, P.G., Wijsman, E.M., Yu, C.E., Rogé, B., Mantoulan, C., Wittemeyer, K., Poustka, A., Felder, B., Klauck, S.M., Schuster, C., Poustka, F., Bölte, S., Feineis-Matthews, S., Herbrecht, E., Schmötzer, G., Tsiantis, J., Papanikolaou, K., Maestrini, E., Bacchelli, E., Blasi, F., Carone, S., Toma, C., Van Engeland, H., de Jonge, M., Kemner, C., Koop, F., Langemeijer, M., Hijimans, C., Staal, W.G., Baird, G., Bolton, P.F., Rutter, M.L., Weisblatt, E., Green, J., Aldred, C., Wilkinson, J.A., Pickles, A., Le Couteur, A., Berney, T., McConachie, H., Bailey, A.J., Francis, K., Honeyman, G., Hutchinson, A., Parr, J.R., Wallace, S., Monaco, A.P., Barnby, G., Kobayashi, K., Lamb, J.A., Sousa, I., Sykes, N., Cook, E.H., Guter, S.J., Leventhal, B.L., Salt, J., Lord, C., Corsello, C., Hus, V., Weeks, D.E., Volkmar, F., Tauber, M., Fombonne, E. & Shih, A. (2007): Mapping autism risk loci using genetic linkage and chromosomal rearrangements. *Nat. Genet.* **207**, 319–328.

Volpe, J.J., ed. (1995): *Neurology of the newborn*, 3rd edition. Philadelphia: W.B. Saunders.

Chapter 2

Brain neuroreceptors: the molecular basis of drug action

Jean-Marie Maloteaux, Beryl Koener and Emmanuel Hermans

*Laboratoire de Pharmacologie Expérimentale, Université catholique de Louvain, 54.10, Av. Hippocrate 54,
B-1200 Brussels, Belgium*
jean-marie.maloteaux@uclouvain.be

Summary

Brain receptors and ion channels are classified into different families possessing specific ligands, and are therefore involved in cerebral physiology and pathology from the first developmental stages until neuronal cell death. Accordingly, they are the target of several drugs acting on the central nervous system. The receptors are not expressed to the same extent during development, maturity, and aging. Some may be transiently expressed during brain maturation, or under particular environmental conditions or during neurological disease progression.

Several receptor subtypes and ion channel subunits have been described, coupled with complex signal transduction mechanisms and interactions. Thus the assertion 'one transmitter – one receptor – one second messenger' is no longer valid.

This chapter describes the properties of receptors, their regulation mechanisms, their classification and their ontogeny, emphasizing their functions and therapeutic implications in nervous system diseases, including some receptor-mediated disorders. Though many receptors still have unknown tasks ('orphan receptors'), brain receptor study remains essential in the investigation of brain diseases and drug development.

Introduction – the receptor concept

Neuroreceptors and ion channels are involved in brain physiology from the first developmental stages until neuronal cell death. It is therefore not surprising that these cell surface proteins are among the most important target sites for a large variety of drugs. Receptors for growth factors and hormones also constitute key actors in the regulation of cell responses to changes in their environment, mainly during neuronal differentiation and the establishment of complex neuronal networks.

The term 'receptor' refers to signal-transducing proteins which, in the central nervous system, are involved in synaptic functions, neurotransmission, electrophysiological activity, and, at a higher level, with all primary and complex brain functions. The concept of receptor site was first proposed by Paul Ehrlich (1854–1915) and John Newport Langley (1852–1925). In 1878, Langley, working at Cambridge University, explained that the functional antagonism observed between atropine and pilocarpine was reflecting the competition of these drugs for a specific substance in the nerves or gland cells. In the same year, Ehrlich (from the University of Leipzig and later the University of Berlin) developed the 'side chain concept', in which the protoplasm was envisaged as a giant molecule consisting of a chemical nucleus with attached chemical side chains. The side chains were thought to be involved in different processes such as nutrition or neutralization of bacterial toxins. Later, Ehrlich suggested that some toxins might interact with side chains that are normally involved in some physiological activities, leading to the blockade of cell functions. According to Ehrlich, the consequence of such blockade was an increased production of side chains, which were released into the blood stream and were able to neutralize the toxin molecules by combining with them (what we now describe as antibodies or antitoxins). Ehrlich sometimes referred to the side chains as 'receptors'.

It took Ehrlich about 10 years to apply his side chain concept to the mechanism of drug action. By June 1906, he stated that some chemically defined substances were attached to the cell by atom groupings that were analogous to toxin receptors, and he distinguished these atom groupings from the toxin receptors by defining them as chemoreceptors. At the same time, Langley, studying the antagonism between nicotine and curare, returned to his suggestion of 1878, arguing that the two drugs had to compete for the same 'receptive substance'. He suggested that the function of this receptive substance was to transmit a stimulus from the nerve to the muscle, and that different cells possess different types of receptive substances. The impact of these two investigators' receptor theory on pharmacology was very limited in their lifetimes and it took several decades (up to the 1950s) before the receptor theory became a major area of research in pharmacology.

The characterization of receptor sites has been greatly facilitated by the development of simple and sensitive techniques to measure the binding of radioactive drugs or neurotransmitter molecules to brain membranes. A first binding experiment was reported in 1965 by Paton and Rang, aimed at monitoring the uptake of radioactive atropine by intestinal muscle, which appeared to involve acetylcholine receptors. The strategy for measuring receptor binding was then applied to the study of the acetylcholine receptors in electric organs of fishes (Changeux *et al.*, 1970; Miledi *et al.*, 1971). In these organs, the receptors identified with toxins such as ^{125}I-α-bungarotoxin represent as much as 20 per cent of the membrane proteins. By contrasts, in the brain, neurotransmitter receptors represent about one millionth by weight of crude brain tissue. The detection of these minute densities of receptor sites was successfully achieved after developing rapid and extensive washing and filtration techniques and using selective ligands labelled at high specific activities. These techniques were applied first to opiate receptors in 1973 (Pert & Snyder 1973; Simon *et al.*, 1973; Terenius, 1973) and subsequently to a wide range of receptor sites. The main pitfall in this approach is related to the non-specific binding of the radioligand to other substrates than the target receptor or to sites devoid of any physiological or pharmacological role.

Receptor definition and characteristics

Affinity

Authentification of a putative receptor requires the binding of selective ligands with high affinity. Indeed, the affinity values largely depend on experimental conditions, but usually the affinity constant value (K_D) of ligands such as neurotransmitter antagonists, neuropeptides, growth factors, and potent toxins is measured in the nanomolar concentration range. Tetrodotoxin and saxitoxin bind to the sodium channels with a very high affinity (K_D value = 0.01 to

0.1 nM); growth factors have K_D values in the subnanomolar range; various pharmacological agents have K_D values in the 1 to 10 nM range. On the other hand, endogenous neuromediators and amino acid neurotransmitters, which are present in the synapse in relatively high concentrations, show lower affinities for their cognate receptors (0.1 to 10 µM) and are often less suitable for binding studies.

Saturation and reversibility

The specific binding to a receptor is saturable (the maximum binding capacity value of the ligand is expressed as the Bmax). The physical interaction of the ligand with its target receptor has to occur with reasonable speed (usually within a few minutes) and has to be reversible. Nevertheless, in some cases non-displaceable binding is observed, and this should correlate with non-reversible functional responses (for example, some toxins). Non-reversible ligands have limited interest for pharmacologists as such; their behaviour is commonly associated with toxicity or side effects. It is noteworthy that *in vivo* receptor occupancy also depends on pharmacokinetic variables such as drug metabolism and elimination rate. These pharmacokinetic variables must be taken into account when considering the time course of evolution of the pharmacological response. *In vitro*, few drugs display a very slow receptor dissociation kinetic. However, after *in vivo* administration, several compounds have a prolonged influence (lasting several hours) on receptor function, an effect which may be accentuated when drug metabolites bind with relevant affinity to the same receptor sites.

Stereoselectivity

The binding to a receptor is stereospecific: when stereospecific ligands are available, the biological isomer of the transmitter or the drug displays a much higher affinity for the receptor than the inactive or less active enantiomer.

Distribution

The tissue, regional, cellular, and subcellular localizations of the receptors may differ, especially in terms of species variation. As far as neuroreceptors are concerned, the sites are mainly localized in the synaptic membranes, allowing immediate modulation of neuronal cell response. Other receptors, such as those for steroid hormones, are localized both in the nuclear and the cytoplasmic compartments of the cells. Steroid hormones may induce changes in receptor conformation resulting in the binding of the receptor to specific chromosomal sites and the long-term regulation of gene expression. The regional distribution of receptors in the brain has been extensively studied *ex vivo* by autoradiographic analysis of radioligand binding on tissue sections. *In vivo* localization of receptors, including those in human brain, was made possible by the development of positron emission tomography (PET) techniques, using the same ligands as in *in vitro* studies (Wagner et al., 1983; Farde et al., 1998). Of interest, *in vivo* studies of receptor distribution in patients have enabled the determination of receptor changes associated with brain diseases. However, these changes often appear to be related to cell loss as a result of the disease progression. Changes in receptor distribution may also reflect adaptive mechanisms such as hypersensitivity due to neurotransmitter deficit or drug-induced receptor regulation. PET studies of high affinity ligand distribution also constitute a valuable approach to the quantitative evaluation of *in vivo* receptor occupancy or competition for the binding sites after selective drug administration. In that way, receptor studies have participated not only in pharmacodynamic studies but also in pharmacokinetic studies.

Transduction of the signal and cellular response

Besides the biochemical criteria, a receptor is defined by the existence of functional correlates. In most instances, complex behavioural responses are difficult to correlate with a single receptor activation or blockade. Therefore the physiological roles of a given receptor are often hypothesized from second messenger linkage, intracellular biochemical responses, or physiological effects on membranes. Indeed, one should always expect a correlation between the binding parameters of a drug and the related pharmacological activity (Creese et al., 1976).

Only a fraction of the whole population of neuroreceptors is involved in biological responses, and these receptors are thought to be localized at the synapses or at least at the cell surface, whereas other receptors are temporarily not involved in the biological response. Both functional and non-functional receptors are recognized by the ligands in tissue homogenates. Therefore the detection of specific binding of a ligand to receptors does not imply that all these receptors are efficiently linked to signalling cascades or are involved in the physiological or pharmacological responses. Besides, more sophisticated pharmacodynamic approaches have been proposed, focusing on functional receptors only (for example, guanylyl nucleotide binding, second messengers quantification).

The mechanisms by which neurotransmitter and neuropeptide receptors relay the incoming information from the cell surface towards intracellular targets are not fully understood, but several post-receptor transmembrane signalling pathways have been identified. Some receptors directly influence transmembrane ion fluxes such as the nicotinic acetylcholine receptor associated with a sodium channel or the type A γ-amino-butyric acid (GABA) receptor coupled with a chloride channel. Many other receptors (such as G-protein coupled receptor, GPCR) interact with a guanine-nucleotide-dependent binding protein (G-protein) leading to the control of ion channels or enzymes such as adenylyl cyclase activity or phospholipase C. A common feature of several intracellular signalling cascades associated with these receptors is their ability to modulate the phosphorylation of selected proteins that participate in the cell functions. Many subunits of the heterotrimeric G protein have been described which belong to the main subgroups of Gα, β, and γ subtypes. There is a substantial possibility of subunit combination, leading to complex interactions with ion channels or second messenger cascades. The activation of many receptors may lead to activation of the same G-protein, and cross-talk between receptors and effector systems has been shown in various experimental and physiological models (Bosier & Hermans, 2007).

At a molecular level, the actions of agonists on the receptor have been thoroughly investigated. In the case of GPCRs, intramolecular interactions are thought to constrain the receptor in an inactive form, which is released when agonist binding switches the protein to its active conformation. The multiple functional receptor conformations of GPCRs suggest the possibility of new ligands and drugs with functional selectivity.

The formation of dimers or heterodimers may be involved in the mode of action of some receptors like some tyrosine kinase receptors (Trk). Two different receptors may recognize neurotrophins: a Trk receptor, and also a $p75^{NTR}$ receptor of the tumour necrosis factor (TNF) receptor family, which recognizes neurotrophins with a lower affinity. Close interactions between Trk and $p75^{NTR}$ receptors lead to high affinity dimer sites. Neurotrophin-mediated activation of Trk receptors leads to a variety of biological responses, which include proliferation and survival, axonal and dendritic growth, remodelling and assembly of the cytoskeleton, membrane trafficking, and modifications of synaptic functions. Activation of $p75^{NTR}$ receptor may also be involved in apoptosis and neuronal death (Huang & Reichardt, 2003).

It is worth mentioning that binding experiments also allow one to identify 'acceptor sites' which may have most of the binding characteristics of receptors (high affinity ligand binding, saturability, regional distribution and so on) but which are not coupled to intracellular biochemical signals. Some acceptor sites may be involved in uptake processes, active transport mechanisms, and enzymatic reactions, but others are devoid of any physiological role. Some 'acceptor sites' possess all the properties of a receptor including the transmembrane structure and intracellular domain for G-protein binding. These receptor are classically referred to as 'orphan receptors' because their relevance in physiology is generally accepted while their natural ligand remains unknown.

In the past 50 years, molecular biological techniques have enabled receptors to be defined and have allowed the classification of their subtypes by identifying their structures and amino acid sequences. The recombinant proteins derived from the cloned sequences show the binding properties and biochemical characteristics of the native receptors, and human cloned receptors are now widely used for *in vitro* screening of new drugs.

Receptor regulation

The receptors are subject to various forms of regulation that allow their physiological responses to be modified appropriately according to the needs of the environmental state. Receptor regulation may lead to either an increase (hypersensitization) or a decrease (desensitization) of the response induced by the agonists. As with any other cell protein, receptors possess half-lives which depend on receptor synthesis and degradation rates. Several physiological regulatory mechanisms contributing to the modulation of receptor density and function have been described.

Receptor desensitization (or hypersensitization)

The agonist-induced receptor desensitization process is the tendency of responses to decrease progressively in intensity despite the continued presence of a constant stimulus. Desensitization is a common adaptive process, found throughout evolution from bacteria to higher eukaryotes, and is of fundamental physiological importance in hormonal, neurotransmitter, and sensory systems. The role of the desensitization process is to protect the cell, the tissue, or the organism from a 'sensory overload'. Desensitization was initially characterized in isolated organs. In 1898, Tigerstedt and Bergman described diminished pressure responses upon repeated renin administrations. In 1913, Dale observed desensitization in guinea pig smooth muscle, and since then numerous other examples have been described. Desensitization processes may be homologous or heterologous. In homologous desensitization, only responsiveness to the desensitizing agent is diminished whereas in heterologous desensitization, the cells become refractory to multiple classes of activators. This has been particularly well described in the case of the β-adrenergic receptor desensitization process. Desensitization also significantly limits the clinical use of many pharmacological agents and could play a role in the development of tolerance and dependence to several drugs such as opiates and benzodiazepines. However, the slow mechanism which leads to tolerance and dependence has to be distinguished from desensitization. Thus, most desensitization processes occur within seconds or minutes. Moreover, the downregulation of receptors (an agonist-induced decrease of the total receptor number) even occurs within a few hours, whereas sensitivity changes (tolerance) generally require weeks to reach their maximum, and disappear equally slowly when the stimulus is removed (Johnson & Fleming, 1989).

Receptor internalization (or recycling)

The functional receptors are thought to be located at the cell surface, ensuring a functional bridge between external stimuli and intracellular response. The cell trafficking of receptors toward the cell surface constitutes their 'externalization', and their disappearance from the surface corresponds to 'internalization'. In many experimental models, internalization has been shown to be strongly dependent on receptor activation, which is distinct from the 'constitutive internalization' which refers to the slow and non-modulated basal turnover. Receptor internalization is observed after activation by agonists which initially involve their clustering in coated pits and the formation of endocytic vesicles containing the receptors. Several synaptic proteins in the electron-dense material of post-synaptic membranes interact with receptors and participate in their regulation. This is the case for PSD95 proteins, a subfamily of the numerous proteins of the PSD (post-synaptic density) proteins which interact with many transmitters, receptors, or enzymes and function as a scaffold for larger molecular complexes. Post-synaptic scaffolding proteins, like 'SAPAP' (synapse-associated protein 90-postsynaptic density 95-associated protein) link receptors to the cytoskeleton and regulate the trafficking and the targeting of neuroreceptors like the glutamate or the cholinergic nicotinic receptors (Scannevin & Huganir 2000a; Scannevin & Huganir 2000b). The role of these proteins in the receptor regulation mechanisms is very important because the assembly-disassembly ratio of synaptic receptor clusters and neuroreceptors trafficking in the synaptic membranes is strongly regulated by neuronal activity (Carroll & Zukin, 2002; Wenthold et al., 2003).

The internalization of receptors may be followed either by their recycling or by their degradation. However, internalized receptors (or internalized ligand-receptor complexes) might also behave as intracellular messengers, involved in some delayed intracellular effects. This is the 'third messenger' system, where protein phosphorylation is likely to play a key role. Internalized receptors may move by retrograde axonal transport towards the cell body and perhaps the nucleus membrane. These receptors – for example, the nerve growth factor (NGF) receptor complexes – may be destroyed or could carry information that is useful for trophicity or plasticity of nerve cells.

Receptor downregulation (or upregulation)

Receptor downregulation results from receptor degradation and corresponds to a decrease in the number of receptors in the tissue. A downregulation of receptor mRNA has also been described after prolonged incubation in the presence of the agonist. Prolonged inhibition of receptors, obtained after sustained receptor occupancy by potent antagonists, may be followed by an upregulation of the receptor number, which is due to reduced degradation or increased synthesis rate. This is probably the mechanism underlying the neuroleptic-induced increase of dopamine receptors, which is associated with abnormal movements (tardive dyskinesia). Agonist-induced receptor regulation is a property shared by receptors for most transmitters and it has several physiological or pharmacological implications.

Several examples of interactions between receptors and neurotransmitter uptake sites (transporters) have recently been demonstrated, illustrating complex regulation processes affecting neuronal communication. Such interactions have been shown in the glutamatergic system where metabotropic glutamate receptors regulate the function of glutamate transporters (Vermeiren et al., 2005; Vermeiren et al., 2006). Another example of complex interaction is the regulation of the opioid receptor gene in dopamine transporter knock-out mice during development (Le Moine et al., 2002).

Chapter 2   Brain neuroreceptors: the molecular basis of drug action

Receptor classification

The classification of receptors has been established with respect to recognition by ligands from different chemical or pharmacological classes and their associated cellular responses. The recent cloning of genes encoding several receptor subtypes made us aware that the molecular structures of these proteins had to be considered in the receptor classification. Hence for decades this classification was subjected to a certain confusion, as illustrated by the complex nomenclature of dopamine, serotonin, opiate, or benzodiazepine receptor subtypes proposed in the early 1980s. Moreover, some 'acceptor sites' or drug-binding sites with unknown physiological roles, enzymes, and uptake sites involved in neurotransmission were sometimes included in the receptor classification. An international receptor nomenclature and classification was proposed by the International Union of Pharmacology (IUPHAR), where the criteria for qualification for the operational term 'receptor' are the functions of both recognition and transduction. A receptor must recognize a specific ligand (or a family of ligands) and must translate information in the cell (for example, the neuron) by a change in membrane permeability, activation of a second messenger cascade, or other intracellular reaction such as a change in DNA transcription or activation of protein kinases. The recognition of the binding site by the ligand has to fulfil several criteria, as described above (Kenakin *et al.*, 1992; Humphrey & Barnard 1998).

The existence of a natural ligand – an endogenous agonist – has not always been demonstrated. Several receptors are clearly the action sites of drugs, even if no mediators have been identified in the brain as yet. A typical example is the benzodiazepine receptors which are intimately coupled to the GABA receptors but where the most powerful ligands are the benzodiazepines, synthesized in the year 1970.

The modern pharmacological proposal for the classification of receptors (Fig. 1) is as follows:
- Ion channel receptors (activation of ion conductance);
- G-protein coupled receptors (activation of second messengers);
- Tyrosine kinase receptors (phosphorylation of tyrosine on key-signalling molecules);
- Nuclear receptors (activation of transcription and translation).

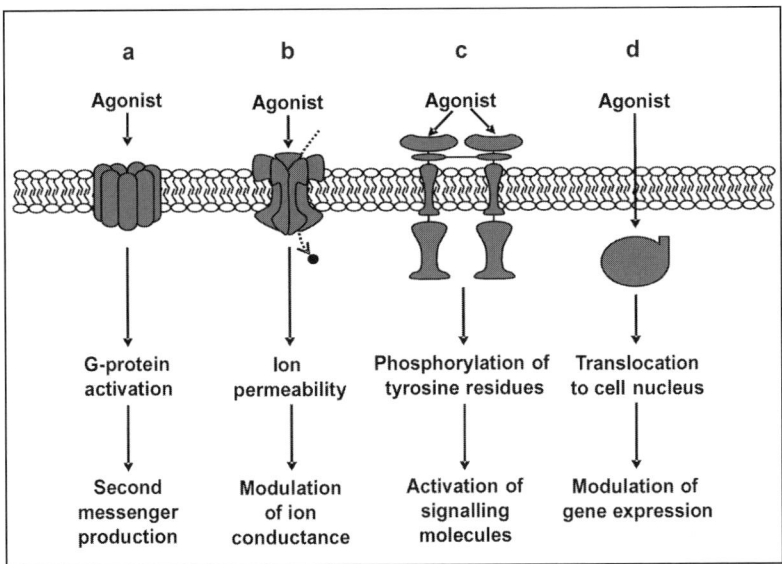

Fig. 1. The modern pharmacological proposal for the classification of receptors.

In the IUPHAR receptor code (Humphrey & Barnard, 1998), the endogenous agonist or a collective term (for example, cannabinoid) is used to define receptor families (M for muscarinic; D for dopamine; 5-HT for 5-hydroxytryptamine; NGF for nerve growth factor; PG for prostaglandins, and so on) and in each family, subtypes may be distinguished (such as D_1, D_2, D_3, D_4, and D_5 dopamine receptors). Three groups of GCPRs are distinguished: class A (rhodopsin-like) which contains adrenergic receptors, dopaminergic receptors, leucotriene receptors, platelet activating factors and so on; class B (secretin-like) which contains calcitonin, CGRP, corticotropin-releasing factor (CRF), glucagons, growth hormone releasing hormone (GHRH), secretin, vasoactive intestinal polypeptide (VIP) receptors, and others; and class C which includes metabotropic glutamate or $GABA_B$ receptors.

Receptor functions and therapeutic effects

Although binding studies constitute useful approaches in the study of drug/transmitter-receptor interaction, allowing affinities to be determined, these techniques fail to provide information about the potency and efficacy of ligands in a given system. Thus, beside affinity and receptor occupancy data, drug potency and intrinsic activity are key pharmacodynamic parameters that help one to predict the response to any pharmacologically active compound. Hence, the relative potency of agonists, partial agonists, and antagonists has to be measured in functional assays. It is worth mentioning that drugs acting as 'inverse agonists' were recently shown to modulate the basal activity associated with the presence of receptors. This property is of particular relevance for the development of therapeutic strategies of some diseases related to an increased receptor constitutive activity, as the latter should be effectively reduced by such 'inverse agonists'. In pathological conditions associated with a decreased availability of the endogenous mediator, administration of receptor agonists as substitutive therapeutic agents constitutes a trivial treatment. On the other hand, many therapeutic compounds behave as pure antagonists, some showing robust potency and a slow dissociation rate, resulting in genuinely prolonged activity. The trivial use of these drugs aims at reducing or interrupting a neurotransmission mechanism but often has compensatory effects, leading to side effects. As an example, prolonged dopamine transmission blockade by neuroleptics may lead to tardive dyskinesia as a consequence of dopamine receptor hypersensitivity.

There is therefore growing interest in more subtle modulation of neurotransmission, which can be achieved using less potent antagonists (for example, memantine in Alzheimer disease), fast dissociating drugs which allow some physiological stimulation of the system (such as quetiapine as an atypical neuroleptic), or partial agonists as therapeutic agents (for example, varenicline as a nicotinic substitutive agent or aripiprazole as a neuroleptic) (Burris et al., 2002). While the intrinsic activity of an agonist is a key variable in defining the amplitude of the pharmacological response associated with drug-receptor interactions, it also greatly influences the putative modifications of receptor sensitivity observed after prolonged administration. A partial agonist will allow a low physiological activity, whereas a potent antagonist will interrupt a pathway and lead to compensatory mechanisms, hypersensitivity, or erratic responses.

In some cases, modulation of neurotransmitter activity may appear more clinically effective than its inhibition. This has been demonstrated by the NMDA receptor antagonist memantine. NMDA receptor mediated transmission is of major importance for many physiological activities (such as learning and sensory functions). However, excessive NMDA receptor stimulation may lead to cell damage as a result of massive intracellular calcium mobilization (excitotoxicity). In several acute or chronic neurological diseases, inhibition of NMDA-glutamate transmission is thought to protect the neurons even if it is obvious that a strong and prolonged NMDA-glutamate inhibition is not compatible with physiological brain functioning. Memantine has NMDA-blocking properties, and has been approved for the treatment of some forms of Alzheimer disease, even though the benefits are small. A hypothesis to explain many neurodegenerative or chronic diseases (for example, Alzheimer disease, Parkinson disease, Huntington disease, and neuropathic pain) and acute nervous system lesions (stroke, seizures, and so on) is an overactivity of NMDA-glutamatergic transmission. Potent NMDA receptor antagonists like MK801, phencyclidine, or ketamine are toxic drugs and cannot be used as neuroprotective agents, but memantine must have a different mechanism of action. It acts as an open channel blocker (trapping blocker). The hypothesis is a blockade of the channel which only occurs after its opening, by competition with the Mg^{2+} binding site. Memantine should have a higher efficiency than Mg^{2+} when the neuron is depolarized. Under normal physiological conditions, Mg^{2+} concentration is high within the NMDA-receptor complexes and inhibits receptor function. As the receptor is not open, memantine has very few effects under physiological conditions. When depolarization occurs (in neurological diseases), it depletes Mg^{2+} from the sites and the binding and blocking effect of memantine can take place (Danysz et al., 2000). The beneficial effects of memantine on memory might be due to a reduction in the global NMDA-receptor mediated activity, allowing better discrimination of the essential stimuli.

The recent launch of partial agonists is another example of pharmaceutical neurotransmitter modulating activity. These agents reduce the activity of a neurotransmission system without blocking it completely. Three recent illustrations may underline the interest in partial agonists in therapeutics: buprenorphine (an agonist/antagonist of opiate receptors, a potent analgesic now also used for treatment of opiate drug addiction); aripiprazole (a new antipsychotic agent, a partial agonist of the dopaminergic receptors with an interesting pharmacological profile and fewer side effects); and varenicline (a nicotine receptor partial agonist, effective in the treatment of tobacco dependence and superior to bupropion in clinical trials). Partial agonists or weak antagonists might be more suitable than potent and long-acting antagonists for the treatment of some chronic nervous diseases.

Brain receptor ontogeny

It is well known that natural neuronal death occurs during the postnatal development of neurons and their projections. In several brain areas, there is a progressive decrease in the number of neurons in the postnatal period (Madalosso et al., 2005). One of the main roles of brain receptors is the refinement of topographical connections. The decrease in receptor number evolves in parallel with a decrease in receptor mRNA (Hermans et al., 1993). It probably corresponds to the postnatal destruction of neurons or synapses in order to reduce the imprecision of neuronal connections (Catsicas et al., 1987). Moreover, there may also be a transcription repression without cell death. Regressive events in neurogenesis have been clearly shown for several GPCRs like dopamine receptors (Brana et al., 1997). The ontogeny of functional receptors has also been studied by [^{35}S]GTPγS binding, an indicator of functional receptors coupled to G-proteins. The $GABA_B$ receptors were shown to be expressed and functional in the whole developing spinal cord of the rat, whereas in the adult, functional $GABA_B$ are mainly observed in the dorsal horn (Sands et al., 2003). Changes in functionality of opiate receptors have also been demonstrated during mouse brain development. Temporal and region-specific differences in the appearance and magnitude of functional activity in cell groups expressing μ or δ opioid receptors have been shown during development by studying opiate-receptor-induced [^{35}S]GTPγS binding (Nitsche et al., 2002).

Some receptors are of particular importance during development as they directly participate in the developmental mechanisms of neuronal projections. Ephrin receptors are crucial during development. This large tyrosine kinase receptor family (Tkrs) is made from more than 14 subtypes, the ligands of which are not soluble but membrane-bound. Gradients of receptor expression lead to axonal guides (Mancia & Shapiro, 2005). Developmental mechanisms underlying the thalamocortical projections largely depend on rostro-caudal and medio-lateral gradients of ephrin subtype in the brain (ephrin A5- EphAs, Ngn2, and so on) (Vanderhaeghen & Polleux, 2004). Differentiation in the cerebral cortex has been reported to be triggered by activation of phospholipase PLCβ1 by metabotropic glutamate receptors (mGLURs, mainly the $mGLUR_5$ subtype) (Hannan et al., 2001; Spires et al., 2005). Several transcription factors, such as NeuroD2, may be activated by PLCβ1 activation, protein kinase C, and Ca^{2+} generated influx. The NeuroD-mediated gene expression in cortical neurons regulates, by a retrograde signal, the thalamocortical axonal development and synapse formation (Ince-Dunn et al., 2006). As many other receptors – such as dopamine, 5-hydroxytryptamine ($5-HT_1$, $5-HT_{2A}$), neurotensin, and retinoids – are involved in specific signals during development, a toxic effect of drugs acting on these sites is understandable if drug exposure occurs at a critical point in brain development.

Receptors in neuronal growth and death

Developing neurons are dependent on trophic factors. The main neurotrophic factor families are: the neurotrophins, the glial-cell-derived neurotrophic factor (GDNF family), the neurotophic cytokines, and the HGF family.

The main neurotrophins are NGF, brain-derived neurotrophic factor (BDNF), and the neurotrophins 3 and 4 (NT3, NT4). The corresponding receptors are Trks (TrkA, B, C) and the low affinity site $p75^{NTR}$. Neurotrophins can bind to their specific receptors but also to a common $p75^{NTR}$ receptor (TNF receptor family) which has several functions including caspase activation and cell death. The low affinity site $p75^{NTR}$ receptors lack the tyrosine kinase domain, but enhance neurotrophin affinity for Trk receptors. Pro-neurotrophin, like NGF, has a higher affinity than neurotrophin for $p75^{NTR}$ and therefore a higher pro-apoptotic effect. The GDNF family is made up mainly of GDNF, neurturin, and artemin. The corresponding receptors are Ret and GFR subtypes. The principal neurotrophin cytokines are the ciliary neurotrophic factor (CNTF) and interleukin-6 (IL-6).

In the developing brain, cell differentiation may depend on specific trophic factors. For example, sympathetic neurons depend on NGF (Trk_A receptor expression) for their differentiation and survival.

Developing neurons may be sequentially dependent on different trophic factors during successive developmental stages. At the earliest stages of development, the growth of mouse trigeminal ganglion's neurons is independent of growth factors. Subsequently, these neurons are very sensitive to BDNF (Trk_B receptor) and NT3 but not NGF. A few days later, they become sensitive to NGF (Trk_A receptor) and less sensitive to BDNF. Later on and at birth, the same neurons are sensitive to MSP (Ron receptor) and less to NGF.

One or several trophic factors acting on their receptors may be necessary for neuronal development. On the other hand, other factors, like TNF, might promote neuronal cell death. As an example, NGF, neurotrophins, and their receptors regulate neuronal survival and death in many cell types of the developing nervous system, depending on the circumstances (Dechant et al., 1997; Davies, 2003).

Receptor-associated diseases

Receptors may be abnormal – for example, as a result of mutations or deletions in the coding gene – and this may lead to a true 'receptor-associated pathology'. Like the changes in enzyme function resulting from a genetic cause, a change in receptor sequence or conformation may lead to either a loss of function or, more surprisingly, an increase in function. A loss of performance may be caused by ineffective signal transmission and the consequence may be a pathological state. In some cases, a gain of function may occur: many examples of constitutive hyperactivation may result from constitutively active mutant receptors. Indeed, it is documented that several neurological disorders and muscle diseases may be related to inherited mutations affecting ion channel structures and function.

Multiple muscular diseases have been shown to result from receptors or ion channel abnormalities. These are called channelopathies and include: hyperkalaemic or hypokalaemic periodic paralysis; congenital paramyotonia and several myotonic disorders (SCN4A gene coding for a subunit of sodium channels); Andersen's syndrome; hypokalaemic periodic paralysis (KCNJ2 or KCNE3 gene coding for subunits of potassium channels); malignant hyperthermia (CACNA subunits of calcium channels); malignant hyperthermia and central core disease (RYR1 gene of ryanodine receptor of the sarcoplasmic calcium channels); congenital myotonia (CLCN1 gene of chloride channels in skeletal muscles); and congenital myasthenic syndromes (CHRN subunits of the nicotinic acetylcholine receptors in the skeletal muscles).

Many neurological diseases result from neuronal or glial channelopathies: some forms of generalized epilepsy, myoclonic epilepsy in childhood, episodic ataxia, benign neonatal convulsions, familial hemiplegic migraine, spinocerebellar ataxia, frontal lobe epilepsy, familial hyperplexia, X-linked Charcot-Marie-Tooth disease, and several forms of deafness or blindness (Kullmann & Hanna, 2002).

Thyrotropin receptors have been associated with various diseases such as adenomas and Grave's disease (Davies *et al.*, 2005). Many different thyroid stimulating hormone (TSH) receptor mutations have been reported to lead to hyperthyroidism by constitutive hyperactivation. Luteinizing hormone (LH) receptor mutations may induce precocious puberty, and various diseases are associated with mutations in receptors for follicle stimulating hormone (FSH), parathyroid hormone (PTH), and LH (Parnot *et al.*, 2002). Mutations in β-adrenergic receptors or angiotensin AT1 receptors may lead either to strong constitutive activity or, on the other hand, to weak receptor function. Various disorders have also been associated with mutations or deletions in neurotransmitter uptake site genes such as glutamate transporter genes (EAATs and GLUTs transporters). Mutations in dopamine or serotonin transporter genes may be involved in some psychiatric disorders (schizophrenia, paranoid psychosis).

Conclusions

Many specific receptors are involved in neurotransmission and consequently in brain physiology. The 'receptors' may be classified as intracellular receptors, recognized often as transcription modulators; tyrosine kinase receptors, especially involved in cellular differentiation and proliferation; ligand-gated ion channels, responsible for the control of transmembrane ion fluxes; and the large group of G-protein coupled receptors which induce intracellular signals through modulation of G-protein activity (GTP binding proteins). The ligand binds at the extracellular side of the receptor whereas the G-protein is linked to the intracellular domains. More than 1200 different G-protein-coupled receptors (including the subtypes) have been identified and one per cent of the genome encodes for them. All these GPCRs receptors have a structural similarity, with their seven hydrophobic transmembrane domains all interacting with guanylyl nucleotide binding proteins, but they do differ in their intracellular and extracellular loops and in their -NH_2 (external) and -COOH (internal) terminals. Brain receptors of the GPCR family belong mainly to the rhodopsin-like receptor group which contains receptors for classical transmitters (dopamine, serotonin, and so on), nucleotides, chemokines, neuropeptides, odorants, and others.

Most of the receptors are transmembrane proteins. Their task is to transduce an outside-cell message (often a ligand) into an intracellular signal. The ligands (neurotransmitters, neuropeptides) and specific drugs (agonists, partial agonists, or antagonists) bind with a high affinity to their specific receptors. However, a single ligand can match several receptor subtypes located on different cells, and induce various intracellular responses. Accordingly, the assertion 'one transmitter – one receptor – one second messenger' is no longer valid. Recent research revealed that there are many receptor subtypes and ion channel subunits, coupled with complex signal transduction mechanisms.

Receptors, like some other neuronal proteins, are synthesized in, brought to (axonal transport), recycled in, and finally destroyed in the nerve endings (synaptic recycling). This turnover participates in the sensitization and desensitization processes, and the receptors located on the cell surface are the effective ones. Receptors are not expressed at the same level during development, maturity, and aging. Some may be transiently expressed during brain maturation, or under other particular environmental conditions, or during neurological disease progression.

In conclusion, brain receptors are involved in cerebral physiology and pathologies, acting therefore as a target for many drugs active on the central nervous system. As the purpose of many of these receptors is still unknown ('orphan receptors'), their study remains a source of future knowledge in brain diseases and drug development.

Acknowledgments: B. Koener and E. Hermans are research assistant and Research Director of the Fonds National de la Recherche Scientifique (FNRS, Belgium).

References

Bosier & Hermans, E. (2007): Versatility of GPCR recognition by drugs: from biological implications to therapeutic relevance. *Trends Pharmacol. Sci.* **28**, 438–446.

Brana, C., Aubert, I., Charron, G., Pellevoisin, C. & Bloch, B. (1997): Ontogeny of the striatal neurons expressing the D2 dopamine receptor in humans: an in situ hybridization and receptor-binding study. *Brain Res. Mol. Brain Res.* **48**, 389–400.

Burris, K.D., Molski, T.F., Xu, C., Ryan, E., Tottori, K., Kikuchi, T., Yocca, F.D. & Molinoff, P.B. (2002): Aripiprazole, a novel antipsychotic, is a high-affinity partial agonist at human dopamine D2 receptors. *J. Pharmacol. Exp. Ther.* **302**, 381–389.

Carroll, R.C. & Zukin, R.S. (2002): NMDA-receptor trafficking and targeting: implications for synaptic transmission and plasticity. *Trends Neurosci.* **25**, 571–577.

Catsicas, S., Thanos, S. & Clarke, P.G. (1987): Major role for neuronal death during brain development: refinement of topographical connections. *Proc. Natl. Acad. Sci. U.S.A.* **84**, 8165–8168.

Changeux, J.P., Kasai, M., Huchet, M. & Meunier, J.C. (1970): [Extraction from electric tissue of gymnotus of a protein presenting several typical properties characteristic of the physiological receptor of acetylcholine]. *C. R. Acad. Sci. Hebd. Seances Acad. Sci. D.* **270**, 2864–2867.

Creese, I., Burt, D.R. & Snyder, S.H. (1976): Dopamine receptor binding predicts clinical and pharmacological potencies of antischizophrenic drugs. *Science* **192**, 481–483.

Danysz, W., Parsons, C.G., Mobius, H.J., Stoffler, A. & Quack, G. (2000): Neuroprotective and symptomatological action of memantine relevant for Alzheimer's disease – a unified glutamatergic hypothesis on the mechanism of action. *Neurotox. Res.* **2**, 85–97.

Davies, A.M. (2003): Regulation of neuronal survival and death by extracellular signals during development. *EMBO J.* **22**, 2537–2545.

Davies, T.F., Ando, T., Lin, R.Y., Tomer, Y. & Latif, R. (2005): Thyrotropin receptor-associated diseases: from adenomata to Graves disease. *J. Clin. Invest.* **115**, 1972–1983.

Dechant, G., Tsoulfas, P., Parada, L.F. & Barde, Y.A. (1997): The neurotrophin receptor p75 binds neurotrophin-3 on sympathetic neurons with high affinity and specificity. *J. Neurosci.* **17**, 5281–5287.

Farde, L., Ito, H., Swahn, C.G., Pike, V.W. & Halldin, C. (1998): Quantitative analyses of carbonyl-carbon-11-WAY-100635 binding to central 5-hydroxytryptamine-1A receptors in man, *J. Nucl. Med.* **39**, 1965–1971.

Hannan, A.J., Blakemore, C., Katsnelson, A., Vitalis, T., Huber, K.M., Bear, M., Roder, J., Kim, D., Shin, H.S. & Kind, P.C. (2001): PLC-beta1, activated via mGluRs, mediates activity-dependent differentiation in cerebral cortex. *Nat. Neurosci.* **4**, 282–288.

Hermans, E., Jeanjean, A.P., Laduron, P.M., Octave, J.N. & Maloteaux, J.M. (1993): Postnatal ontogeny of the rat brain neurotensin receptor mRNA. *Neurosci. Lett.* **157**, 45–48.

Huang, E.J. & Reichardt, L.F. (2003): Trk receptors: roles in neuronal signal transduction. *Annu. Rev. Biochem.* **72**, 609–642.

Humphrey, P.P. & Barnard, E.A. (1998): International Union of Pharmacology. XIX. The IUPHAR receptor code: a proposal for an alphanumeric classification system. *Pharmacol. Rev.* **50**, 271–277.

Ince-Dunn, G., Hall, B.J., Hu, S.C., Ripley, B., Huganir, R.L., Olson, J.M., Tapscott, S.J. & Ghosh, A. (2006): Regulation of thalamocortical patterning and synaptic maturation by NeuroD2. *Neuron* **49**, 683–695.

Johnson, S.M. & Fleming, W.W. (1989): Mechanisms of cellular adaptive sensitivity changes: applications to opioid tolerance and dependence. *Pharmacol. Rev.* **41**, 435–488.

Kenakin, T.P., Bond, R.A. & Bonner, T.I. (1992): Definition of pharmacological receptors. *Pharmacol. Rev.* **44**, 351–362.

Kullmann, D.M. & Hanna, M.G. (2002): Neurological disorders caused by inherited ion-channel mutations. *Lancet Neurol.* **1**, 157–166.

Le Moine, C., Fauchey, V. & Jaber, M. (2002): Opioid receptor gene expression in dopamine transporter knock-out mice in adult and during development. *Neuroscience* **112**, 131–139.

Madalosso, S.H., Perez-Villegas, E.M. & Armengol, J.A. (2005): Naturally occurring neuronal death during the postnatal development of Purkinje cells and their precerebellar afferent projections. *Brain Res. Brain Res. Rev.* **49**, 267–279.

Mancia, F. & Shapiro, L. (2005): ADAM and Eph: how Ephrin-signaling cells become detached. *Cell* **123**, 185–187.

Miledi, R., Molinoff, P. & Potter, L.T. (1971): Isolation of the cholinergic receptor protein of Torpedo electric tissue. *Nature* **229**, 554–557.

Nitsche, J.F., Schuller, A.G., King, M.A., Zengh, M., Pasternak, G.W. & Pintar, J.E. (2002): Genetic dissociation of opiate tolerance and physical dependence in delta-opioid receptor-1 and preproenkephalin knock-out mice. *J. Neurosci.* **22**, 10906–10913.

Parnot, C., Miserey-Lenkei, S., Bardin, S., Corvol, P. & Clauser, E. (2002): Lessons from constitutively active mutants of G protein-coupled receptors. *Trends Endocrinol. Metab.* **13**, 336–343.

Pert, C.B. & Snyder, S.H. (1973): Opiate receptor: demonstration in nervous tissue. *Science* **179**, 1011–1014.

Sands, S.A., Purisai, M.G., Chronwall, B.M. & Enna, S.J. (2003): Ontogeny of GABA(B) receptor subunit expression and function in the rat spinal cord. *Brain Res.* **972**, 197–206.

Scannevin, R.H. & Huganir, R.L. (2000a): Postsynaptic organization and regulation of excitatory synapses. *Nat. Rev. Neurosci.* **1**, 133–141.

Scannevin, R.H. & Huganir, R.L. (2000b): Postsynaptic organization and regulation of excitatory synapses. *Nat. Rev. Neurosci.* **1**, 133–141.

Simon, E.J., Hiller, J.M. & Edelman, I. (1973): Stereospecific binding of the potent narcotic analgesic (3H) etorphine to rat-brain homogenate. *Proc. Natl. Acad. Sci. U.S.A.* **70**, 1947–1949.

Spires, T.L., Molnar, Z., Kind, P.C., Cordery, P.M., Upton, A.L., Blakemore, C. & Hannan, A.J. (2005): Activity-dependent regulation of synapse and dendritic spine morphology in developing barrel cortex requires phospholipase C-beta1 signalling. *Cereb. Cortex* **15**, 385–393.

Terenius, L. (1973): Characteristics of the 'receptor' for narcotic analgesics in synaptic plasma membrane fraction from rat brain. *Acta Pharmacol. Toxicol. (Copenh.)* **33**, 377–384.

Vanderhaeghen, P. & Polleux, F. (2004): Developmental mechanisms patterning thalamocortical projections: intrinsic, extrinsic and in between. *Trends Neurosci.* **27,** 384–391.

Vermeiren, C., Najimi, M., Vanhoutte, N., Tilleux, S., de Hemptinne, I., Maloteaux, J.M. & Hermans, E. (2005): Acute up-regulation of glutamate uptake mediated by mGluR5a in reactive astrocytes. *J. Neurochem.* **94,** 405–416.

Vermeiren, C., Hemptinne, I., Vanhoutte, N., Tilleux, S., Maloteaux, J.M. & Hermans, E. (2006): Loss of metabotropic glutamate receptor-mediated regulation of glutamate transport in chemically activated astrocytes in a rat model of amyotrophic lateral sclerosis. *J. Neurochem.* **96,** 719–731.

Wagner, H.N., Burns, H.D., Dannals, R.F., Wong, D.F., Langstrom, B., Duelfer, T., Frost, J.J., Ravert, H.T., Links, J.M., Rosenbloom, S.B., Lukas, S.E., Kramer, A.V. & Kuhar, M.J. (1983): Imaging dopamine receptors in the human brain by positron tomography. *Science* **221,** 1264–1266.

Wenthold, R.J., Sans, N., Standley, S., Prybylowski, K. & Petralia, R.S. (2003): Early events in the trafficking of N-methyl-D-aspartate (NMDA) receptors. *Biochem. Soc. Trans.* **31,** 885–888.

Chapter 3

Multiple types of programmed cell death and their relevance to perinatal brain damage

Peter G. H. Clarke *, Julien Puyal *, Anne Vaslin *, Vanessa Ginet * °
and Anita Truttmann °

*Département de Biologie Cellulaire et de Morphologie (DBCM), University of Lausanne, rue du Bugnon 9, 1005 Lausanne, Switzerland;
° Division of Neonatology, Department of Paediatrics and Paediatric Surgery, University Hospital, 1011 Lausanne, Switzerland
Peter.Clarke@unil.ch

Summary

The well known apoptosis-necrosis dichotomy is being replaced by the recognition of at least three morphological types of programmed cell death. *Type 1, apoptosis* involves nuclear condensation and clumping of chromatin, moderate cytoplasmic condensation, and blebbing of the plasma membrane. Most apoptosis is mediated by caspases. *Type 2, autophagic cell death* involves intense (macro)autophagy. Although moderate autophagy occurs even in healthy cells and is generally protective, excessive autophagy can mediate death, as shown by the fact that inhibition of the autophagic pathway with RNA interference blocks autophagic cell death. The *type 3/necrosis subfamily* includes several cell death subtypes all characterized by 'empty' cytoplasmic vacuoles; we shall focus on type 3B ('cytoplasmic cell death' or 'paraapoptosis'), which has frequently been described *in vivo* during development. *Hybrid types of cell death* can occur, with multiple death pathways in a single cell, in which case blocking a single pathway may fail to prevent cell death. Each of the cell death types can occur in perinatal brain damage. In addition to reviewing the literature on different types of cell death, we present new evidence for the autophagic type in two neonatal rat models: focal cerebral ischaemia at P12, and cerebral hypoxia-ischaemia at P7.

Multiple mechanisms of cell death: basic principles

The fact that there are multiple mechanisms of cell death is of major importance for those who wish to control it. In some cases, such as the treatment of cancer, understanding the multiple death mechanisms provides the potential for inducing the death of cells that have become resistant to a particular death stimulus. But for the prevention of perinatal brain damage the aim is generally neuroprotection, and it is becoming increasingly accepted that the phenotypic diversity of the cell death mechanisms in conditions such as neonatal asphyxia or perinatal stroke will necessitate an inhibition of multiple death pathways – for example, by the use of a combination of anti-necrotic and anti-apoptotic agents (Northington *et al.*, 2005).

There is considerable evidence, however, that the dichotomy of apoptosis *versus* necrosis is too simple and does not provide an adequate framework for planning effective neuroprotection paradigms. During the last quarter of the 20th century, this rigid dichotomy became almost a dogma. Apoptosis was considered a clean and controlled way to die, which occurs in physiological or mildly pathological situations and involves destruction of the cell within its own membrane by 'active' mechanisms such as caspase activation, until finally the cell (or its membrane-bound fragments) was phagocytosed. This was contrasted with necrosis, which was considered to be the cellular equivalent of a squashed slug, dirty and uncontrolled, involving 'passive' mechanisms such as osmosis-induced swelling leading to membrane rupture and spillage of cytosol and organelles into the extracellular space, provoking an inflammatory reaction (Kerr *et al.*, 1972; Wyllie, 1987; Walker *et al.*, 1988). This view is still sometimes advocated (Higuchi *et al.*, 2007), but there is increasing agreement that this is too simple (Clarke, 1990; Clarke, 1999), and we will review evidence for at least three morphological types of cell death, all of which are 'programmed' in the sense that they involve cellular signalling pathways. Table 1 summarizes the different types of cell death that will be described.

Table 1. Summary of the three main types of cell death that occur in neurons (modified from Clarke (1990)

Designation(s)	Nucleus	Cell membrane	Cytoplasm
Type 1, apoptosis; shrinkage necrosis; nuclear type	Nuclear condensation, clumping of chromatin leading to pronounced pyknosis	Convoluted, forming blebs	Loss of ribosomes from RER and from polysomes; cytoplasm reduced in volume becoming electron-dense
Type 2, autophagic cell death	Pyknosis in some cases. Parts of nucleus may bleb or segregate	Endocytosis in some cases; blebbing may occur	Abundant autophagic vacuoles; Golgi often enlarged; ER and mitochondria sometimes dilated
Type3/necrosis family			
Necrosis	Swelling, increase in granularity of chromatin, then clumping of chromatin and pyknosis	May break	Swelling of entire cell; dilatation of organelles, forming 'empty' spaces that may fuse
Type 3B, cytoplasmic type; paraptosis	Late increase in granularity of chromatin	Rounding up of cell	Dilatation of ER, perinuclear space, Golgi and sometimes mitochondria, forming 'empty' spaces

ER, endoplasmic reticulum; RER, rough endoplasmic reticulum.

Type 1, apoptosis

Apoptosis was originally defined as involving nuclear condensation and clumping of chromatin, accompanied by more moderate shrinking of the cytoplasm and blebbing (outward budding) of the plasma membrane, and in some cases fragmentation of the cell into apoptotic bodies (Kerr *et al.*, 1972). An apoptotic-like dying neuron is shown in Fig. 1A. A vast amount of research on apoptosis has led to a very detailed understanding of the cellular pathways, and a full account would be beyond the scope of this chapter (for details see Kuwana & Newmeyer, 2003; van Gurp *et al.*, 2003). The essentials are summarized in Fig. 2. Apoptosis is triggered by two main pathways. The first is the extrinsic (death receptor) pathway, which is activated by ligands of the tumour necrosis factor receptor family, leading to the activation of caspase 8, and then of downstream 'effector' caspases 3, 6, or 7, and ultimately apoptosis. The second is the intrinsic (mitochondrial) pathway, which is activated by the release of various molecules from the intermembranous space of stressed or damaged mitochondria (Kuwana & Newmeyer, 2003). Cytochrome-C release activates the apoptosome, a complex involving cytochrome-C, Apaf-1, and the nucleosome dATP. Once formed, the apoptosome recruits and activates caspase-9, which in turn activates downstream caspases such as caspase-3. Other molecules released from mitochondria induce caspase-independent apoptotic mechanisms. These include AIF (apoptosis inducing factor) and endonuclease G (van Gurp et al., 2003).

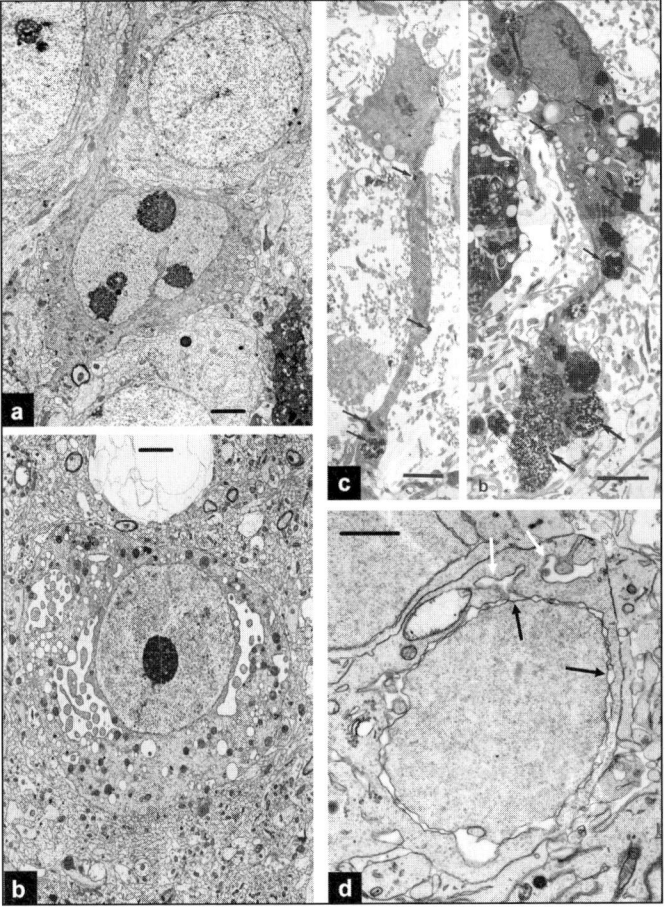

Fig. 1. Types of cell death. Apoptotic (a) and necrotic (b) neurons in the rat hippocampus following perforant path stimulation. From Sloviter et al. (1996). (c) Two type 2 (autophagic) dying neurons in the isthmo-optic nucleus of a 14-day-old chick embryo that had received an intravenous injection of horseradish peroxidase (to show endocytosis) 3 hours before fixation. The death of the neurons was provoked by blockade of axoplasmic transport in their axonal terminals. From Hornung et al. (1989). (d) Type 3B dying retinal ganglion cell in a chick embryo 24 hours after axotomy. From Borsello et al. (2002). Bars: 2 μm in each case. Reprinted with permission of Wiley-Liss, Inc., a subsidiary of John Wiley & Sons, Inc.

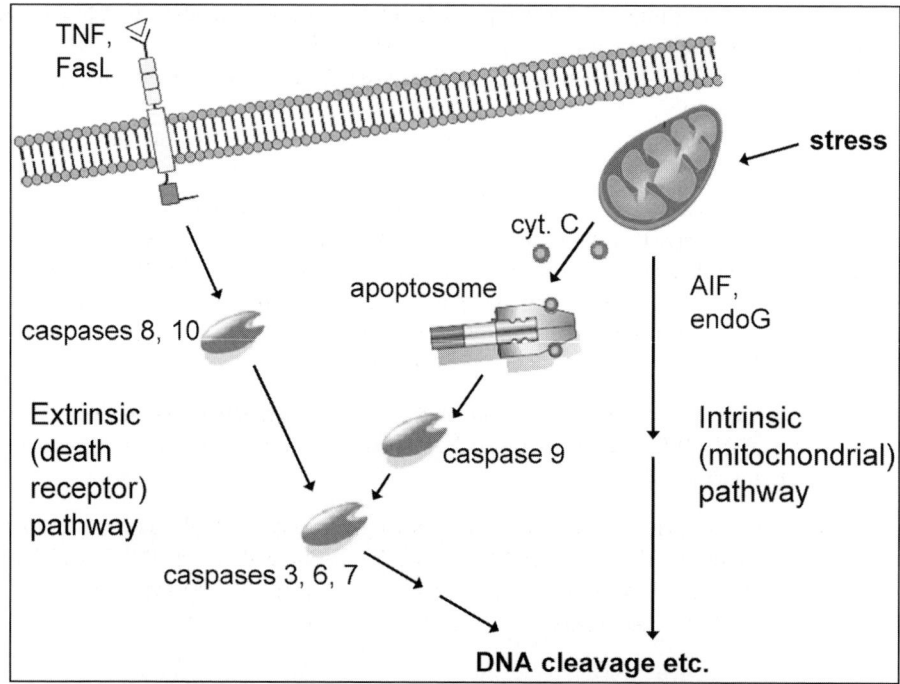

Fig. 2. The principal pathways of apoptosis. The extrinsic (or death receptor) pathway is triggered by the binding of ligands of the family of tumour necrosis factor (TNF) or Fas-ligand (FasL) to Fas or another member of the TNF superfamily of receptors. The intrinsic (or mitochondrial) pathway is triggered in one of two ways: caspase-9 is activated in the apoptosome following the release of cytochrome C (cyt. C); alternatively, caspase-independent pathways can be triggered by the release of a variety of molecules including apoptosis inducing factor (AIF) or endonuclease G (endoG). This figure is greatly simplified, ignoring the complex pathways that cause protein release from mitochondria as well as some of the released proteins (notably Smac/DIABLO and Omi/HtrA2, that counteract caspase inhibitor IAP).

Type 2, autophagic cell death

Autophagy is the mechanism by which cells degrade parts of their own cytoplasm using the lysosomal machinery. There are several types of autophagy, but the only type known to play a role in cell death is macroautophagy, which involves the engulfment of sizeable regions of cytoplasm, including organelles, in double-membrane vesicles called autophagosomes. Since the 1960s, numerous ultrastructural studies have revealed intense (macro)autophagy in dying cells with a non-apoptotic morphology (Clarke, 1990) (Fig. 1C), and it later became clear that the cell death was caspase-independent (reviewed by Guillon-Munos et al., 2005), but it was controversial whether the autophagy actually mediated the cell death. Opponents argued that moderate autophagy occurs even in healthy cells, and enhanced autophagy can be protective in many situations by providing nutrients or by degrading damaged organelles such as mitochondria which could activate cell death pathways. A death-mediating role was argued from the observation that most of the cytoplasm and even parts of the nucleus could be engulfed in autolysosomes (Hornung et al., 1989; Clarke, 1990). This has been supported by numerous reports since 1992 that inhibitors of autophagy such as 3-methyladenine protected cells against cell death with an autophagic morphology (for example, Sandvig & van Deurs, 1992; Xue et *al.*, 1999), although the inhibitors were not specific for autophagy. The inhibition of autophagy by 3-methyladenine reflects its ability to inhibit phosphoinositide 3-kinase (PI3-K) (Blommaart *et al.*, 1997), and more specific PI3-K inhibitors likewise inhibit autophagic cell death (Guillon-Munos *et al.*, 2005), but even these are not specific for autophagy. Conclusive evidence for a death-mediating role of the autophagy was finally provided in 2004 in two papers showing that inhibition of the autophagic pathway with RNA interference of autophagy genes (Atg 5, 6, or 7) blocked autophagy and the associated cell death in apoptosis-resistant cell lines (Shimizu *et al.*, 2004; Yu *et al.*, 2004). It is now almost universally accepted that (macro)autophagy can mediate autophagic cell death, at least in some cases, but how generally this is true is still debated. It is also uncertain how the autophagy kills the cells, but in one case this has been shown to involve the engulfment of peroxisomes and catalase degradation, leading to reduced resistance to reactive oxygen species (Yu *et al.*, 2006).

Autophagy has been reported in dying neurons in cerebral ischaemia (Nitatori *et al.*, 1995; Aggoun-Zouaoui *et al.*, 1998; Adhami *et al.*, 2006), but its role in perinatal brain damage has been neglected (Zhu *et al.*, 2005).

Strongly enhanced endocytosis has been shown to accompany several cases of autophagic neuronal death (Clarke, 1984; Clarke & Martin, 1985; Hornung *et al.*, 1989; Borsello *et al.*, 2003a) and we know of no exceptions, but enhanced endocytosis can also accompany non-autophagic neuronal death (Borsello *et al.*, 2003a).

The type 3/necrosis family of cell death subtypes

We group together type 3 cell death and necrosis because of their morphological similarities (Table 1). We focus here on type 3B rather than 3A, because 3B has been found frequently in neurons, especially during development, whereas 3A is rare and has never been found in neurons. In both type 3B and necrosis, the most striking morphological changes are in the cytoplasm (Fig. 1, panels B and D). Both show 'empty' cytoplasmic vacuoles that form primarily within organelles such as endoplasmic reticulum, Golgi, and mitochondria. The main differences are that the characteristics of type 3B are very constant, including dilatation of the perinuclear space, only minimal change in the nucleus (a slight increase in granularity), and no swelling, whereas necrosis is more variable, with pronounced swelling, chromatin clumping, and pyknosis in late stages, and sometimes disruption of the nuclear membrane. Whether these differences reflect a fundamental distinction at the level of mechanism is currently unclear.

Necrosis

The term *necrosis* has been used for two millennia to mean the mortification of tissue, and is still often used in this original sense, but in 1980 it was given a new and particular, cellular, sense corresponding to what pathologists had been calling 'coagulative necrosis' (Wyllie *et al.*, 1980). *Necrosis*, as thus defined, is characterized by cellular swelling and by dilatation of organelles and the formation of empty vacuoles in the cytoplasm (Fig. 1B). Understandably, some pathologists have objected to the kidnapping of a term already in use (Majno & Joris, 1995), but the alternative that they proposed, oncosis, suffers from the same objection, as it too already had a technical meaning (a morbid condition marked by the development of tumours). For better or worse, necrosis remains the standard term.

More serious than the terminology is the false assumption, still sometimes made (Higuchi et al., 2007), that necrosis is due merely to a 'passive' mechanism involving cell swelling and release of contents. The definitions of 'active' and 'passive' have varied over time. Initially, Kerr et al. (1972) stated that the morphological features of apoptosis suggested it was 'an active, inherently programmed phenomenon', and postulated that it might depend 'on expression of part of the genome, which is normally repressed in viable cells.' We now know that gene transcription is not essential to most cases of apoptosis, and the meanings of 'active' and 'programmed' have gradually shifted to denote organized cell signalling. But even the instigators of the apoptosis-necrosis dichotomy suggested that enzyme-controlled events activated by calcium (hence organized cell signalling) could be important in necrosis (Wyllie et al., 1980), and in the best studied example of necrosis (acute excitotoxicity) the cellular swelling is not a major contributor to cell death (Rothman, 1994). There is now abundant evidence that enzyme controlled pathways mediate various forms of necrosis (Arora et al., 1996; Yamashima, 2000; Arthur et al., 2007) in a manner analogous to the better understood pathways mediating apoptosis, so the active-passive distinction between apoptosis and necrosis would seem not to be valid (or perhaps valid only in some cases), and several investigators have started to use the term 'programmed necrosis' (Chan et al., 2003; Niquet et al., 2003). Despite our reservations, we do accept that apoptotic cells tend to be energy-rich and indeed require the energy for caspase activation (Nicotera et al., 2000), as is probably also the case for dying autophagic cells, as autophagy is likewise an energy-consuming event, whereas necrosis generally occurs in cells that are undergoing energy failure. One consequence of this is that necrosis must be associated with membrane depolarization and a resulting calcium influx. For this reason calpains are frequently attributed a role in necrosis, and calpain inhibitors are indeed neuroprotective against cerebral ischaemia (Ray, 2006) as well as neonatal hypoxia-ischaemia (Kawamura et al., 2005), but the subject is complicated because calpain activation can also lead to the activation of caspase-3 and apoptosis (Blomgren et al., 2001).

Type 3B ('cytoplasmic cell death' or 'paraptosis')

This cell death type is characterized by dilatation of the perinuclear space and organelles, with only minimal changes in the nucleus (Fig. 1D). Type 3B has often been described *in vivo* during development (reviewed by Clarke, 1999). In chick embryos subjected to a tectal lesion at E12, the resulting death of retinal ganglion cells is of this kind and does not involve activated caspase-3 (Borsello et al., 2002); studies involving the intraocular injection of various inhibitors indicate that the mediation of this cell death involves reactive oxygen species (Castagné & Clarke, 1996) and cyclin-dependent kinase-5 (Lefèvre et al., 2002). Mechanistic studies have been few, but cell death with a type 3B morphology has been found in two cell line models. In the first, involving the expression of EGF1 receptors in 293T cells or fibroblasts, caspase-9, MEK2, and JNK1 were implicated (Sperandio et al., 2000; Sperandio et al., 2004). The second involved the ceramide-induced death of differentiated PC12 cells (Muriel et al., 2000), where calcium levels decreased in the endoplasmic reticulum and increased in mitochondria by a process involving CDK5, the proapoptotic Bcl-2 family protein t-Bid (truncated Bid), and caspase-8 (Darios et al., 2003; Darios et al., 2005).

Hybrid types of cell death and mixed control mechanisms

The different pathways mediating cell death are summarized in Fig. 3. The fact that more than one of these pathways can occur in a single cell is a major problem for neuroprotection as it implies that blocking a single pathway may fail to prevent the death of the cell. In some cases the activation of multiple pathways is apparent morphologically, as in excitotoxic neuronal death in immature brains (Portera-Cailliau et al., 1997), but in other cases a new death pathway appears after protection that had been masked by the rapid death via the first pathway. For example, a predominantly apoptotic pathway in differentiated PC12 cells exposed to activated microglia is replaced by a non-apoptotic death pathway following blockage of the caspase-3 cascade (Tanabe et al., 1999). Likewise cultured cerebellar granule neurons deprived of potassium and serum undergo an apoptosis that can be inhibited by the mixed linage kinase (MLK) inhibitor CEP-1347 and apparently depends on JNK, but the protection is only temporary and 3 days later the cells die by an MLK-independent pathway (Harris et al., 2002).

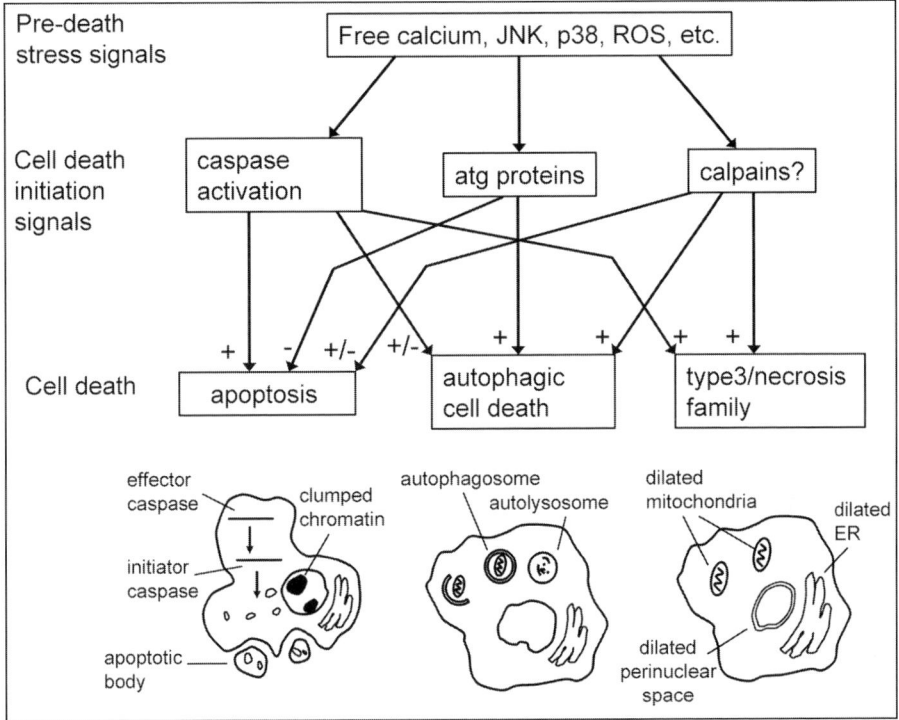

Fig. 3. Diagram showing the interactions between the three main death pathways. ER, endoplasmic reticulum; +, activation; –, inhibition.

The situation is still more complicated, however, because a given cellular signal can be involved in more than one death pathway. In some cases it may be pro-death in both pathways – for example, caspases and calpains can contribute synergistically to both apoptosis and necrosis (Yamashima, 2000; Blomgren et al., 2001; Ray, 2006) as they share many common substrates (Wang, 2000), and caspases can enhance calpain proteolysis by inhibiting calpastatin, a powerful endogenous inhibitor of calpains (Porn-Ares et al., 1998). However, mediators of one death pathway can also inhibit other death pathways. This can even be true of the interaction between caspases and calpains – for example, calpain I was shown in an excitotoxicity model to inhibit the activation of caspases-3 and -9 (Lankiewicz et al., 2000).

There are also both positive and negative interactions between the apoptotic and autophagic pathways. For example, pro-apoptotic BH3-only members of the Bcl-2 family can trigger autophagy by competitively disrupting the interaction between Beclin-1 (atg6) and Bcl-2/Bcl-X_L (Maiuri et al., 2007). However, proapoptotic caspase-8 inhibits an autophagic death pathway, so that caspase-8 inhibition can provoke cell death by the latter (Yu et al., 2004), and the removal of damaged mitochondria by autophagy protects against apoptosis (Chang & Reynolds, 2006).

There may also be interactions between the autophagic and type3/necrotic pathways, because calpains have been found to be necessary for (macro)autophagy (DeMarchi et al., 2006).

The fact that there are positive interactions between different cell death pathways is a problem for neuroprotection, because it implies that more than one pathway may need to be inhibited; however, the existence of *negative* interactions between the pathways is a far greater problem, because it implies that inhibiting one death pathway may even make matters worse, by exacerbating other death pathways.

Multiple death pathways in perinatal brain damage

The above principles were drawn from many different cell types in a variety of contexts. We here address the limited information available from animal models of perinatal brain damage. Most studies on perinatal brain damage have focused on apoptosis and necrosis in models involving hypoxia or ischaemia or both. There has been debate as to whether apoptosis contributes significantly to neuronal death in these models (Ishimaru et al., 1999) – the weight of evidence indicates that even if the cell death is not pure apoptosis, apoptotic mechanisms are at work (Portera-Cailliau et al., 1997; Northington et al., 2005). Other types of cell death have been neglected, but Zhu et al. (2005) studied the relative contributions of the three main types of cell death in cerebral hypoxia-ischaemia undertaken at various ages. They found that apoptotic mechanisms (nuclear translocation of AIF, cytochrome c release, and caspase-3 activation) were all substantially more pronounced in immature brains, whereas necrosis-related calpain activation was similar at all ages. They also state that the increase in autophagy, judged from the proportional increase in the autophagosome-related form of LC3, was more pronounced in adult brains, but this appears to reflect the fact that the control values that served as a basis for normalization were greater in the younger animals (Zhu et al., 2005).

Our own unpublished research has provided evidence for strongly enhanced autophagy in two neonatal rat models: focal cerebral ischaemia at P12 (adapted from Renolleau et al. (1998), and cerebral hypoxia-ischaemia at P7 (Vannucci-Rice model) (Vannucci et al., 1999). In both models, many neurons in the ischaemic area showed enhanced lysosomal activity, as judged from histochemical staining for acid phosphatase and β-hexosaminidase activities, and immunoreactivity for lysosomal (cathepsin D) markers from 5 to 48 hours post-ischaemia. The immunohistochemistry was confirmed with western blots or enzymatic assays, or both, and western blots showed a strong increase in the autophagic marker LC3-II (not shown). Electron microscopy revealed numerous large electron-dense membranous vacuoles or autophagosomes (Figs. 4 and 5).

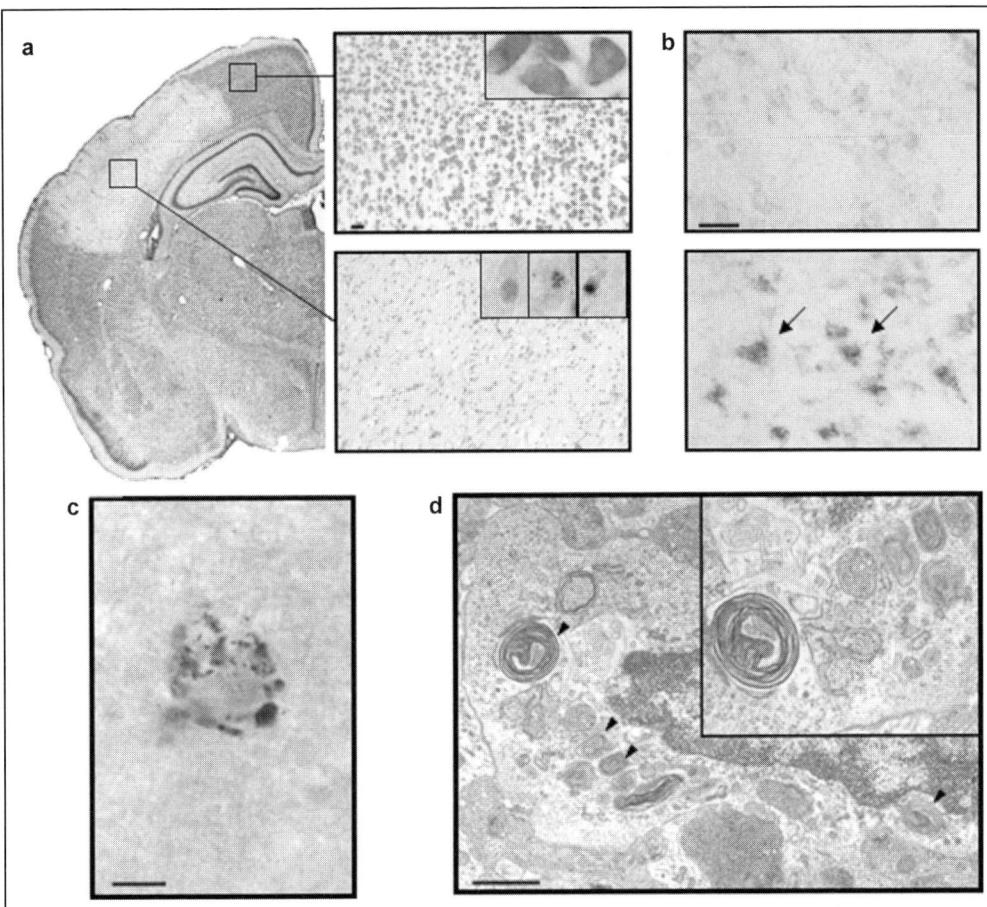

Fig. 4. Involvement of autophagy in P12-old rat following left middle cerebral artery occlusion (MCAO) in association with a 1.5 hour occlusion of the left common carotid artery (adapted from Renolleau et al., 1998). (a) Cresyl violet-stained coronal section showing an infarct in the fronto-parietal cortex and, at high magnification, the presence of numerous apoptotic-like dying neurons (chromatin fragmentation and pyknosis). (b) From 6 hours, an increase in cathepsin D labelling is detected in neurons (arrows) located in the ischaemic hemisphere (lower panel) compared with the control hemisphere (upper panel). (c) At 24 hours, numerous neurons located in the lesion were strongly positive for β-hexosaminidase histochemistry. (d) From 6 hours, neurons located in the ischaemic hemisphere displayed numerous autophagosomes (arrowheads) as observed by electron microscopy. Bars: a, b, 25 μm; c, 10 μm; d, 1 μm.

The prominence of autophagic and lysosomal activation in neonatal cerebral ischaemia and hypoxia-ischaemia raises the question of whether the autophagy is contributing to the cell death. In this context it is striking that very strong protection was found against neonatal cerebral ischaemia (Borsello et al., 2003b) using an inhibitor of the JNK pathway, D-JNKI1, that had been shown in organotypic cultures to inhibit autophagy as well as excitotoxicity (Borsello et al., 2003c). It will be important now to test directly whether inhibiting autophagy protects against the brain damage.

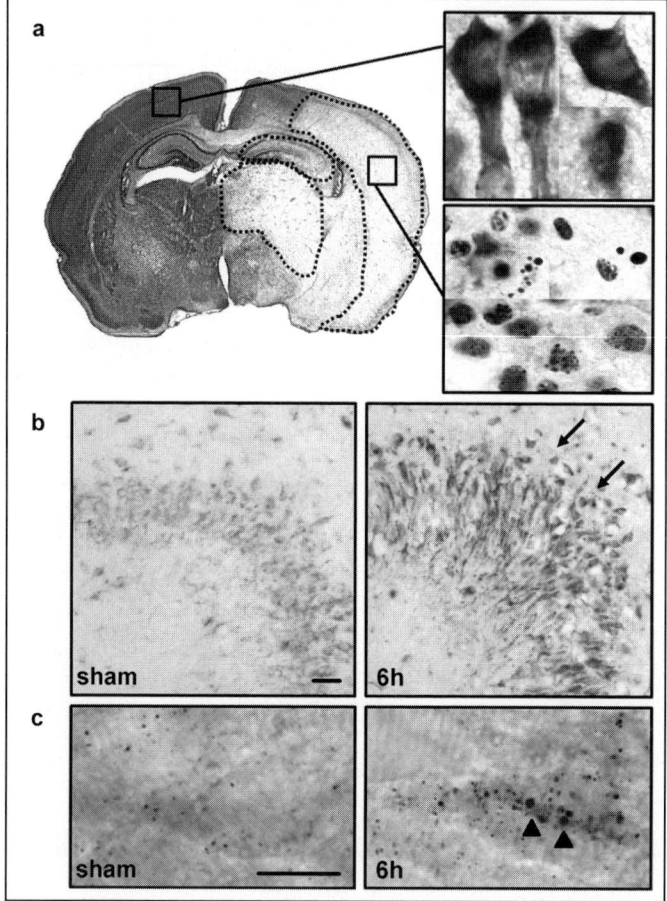

Fig. 5. Involvement of autophagy following neonatal hypoxia-ischaemia in P7-day-old rats (permanent ligation of the right common carotid artery followed by 2 hours of hypoxia at 8 per cent O_2, Rice-Vannucci model). (a) Cresyl violet-stained section 48 hours after the hypoxia, showing an extensive lesion in the hemisphere ipsilateral to the ligation involving the cerebral cortex, hippocampus, and thalamus. The striatum was also affected (not shown). At high magnification, shrunken cells can be seen in the ischaemic cortex with clumped nuclear chromatin, whereas only healthy neurons are seen in the uninjured cortex. (b) From 6 hours in the hippocampus the cathepsin-D labelling increased in CA3 neurons (arrows) compared with a control animal (sham) not exposed to hypoxia-ischaemia. (c) CA3 neurons displaying an increase in acid phosphatase activity as shown by numerous large positive vesicles (arrowheads); this is seen after 6 hours hypoxia-ischaemia but not in a control animal (sham). Bars: b, 25 µm; c, 10 µm.

Conclusions

There are at least three different morphological types of cell death, reflecting a multiplicity of different intracellular death pathways, and these can all contribute to perinatal brain damage. Our own results indicate that neuronal death following cerebral ischaemia or hypoxia-ischaemia involves enhanced autophagy, and raise the possibility that inhibition of autophagy could be a new complementary neuroprotective strategy.

Acknowledgments: The research described here was supported by grants 3100A0-101696, 3100A0-105824, and 3100A0-113925 to P.C. and A.T. from the Swiss National Science Foundation and by a grant from the Eagle Foundation to A.T.. We thank Sonia Naegele-Tollardo and Guylène Magnin for histology, and Vincent Mottier for electron microscopy.

References

Adhami, F., Liao, G.H., Morozov, Y.M., Schloemer, A., Schmithorst, V.J., Lorenz, J.N., Dunn, R.S., Vorhees, C.V., Wills-Karp, M., Degen, J.L., Davis, R.J., Mizushima, N., Rakic, P., Dardzinski, B.J., Holland, S.K., Sharp, F.R. & Kuan, C.Y. (2006): Cerebral ischemia-hypoxia induces intravascular coagulation and autophagy. *Am. J. Pathol.* **169**, 566–583.

Aggoun-Zouaoui, D., Margalli, I., Borrega, F., Represa, A., Plotkine, M., Ben-Ari, Y. & Charriaut-Marlangue, C. (1998): Ultrastructural morphology of neuronal death following reversible focal ischemia in the rat. *Apoptosis* **3**, 133–141.

Arora, A.S., de Groen, P.C., Croall, D.E., Emori, Y. & Gores, G.J. (1996): Hepatocellular carcinoma cells resist necrosis during anoxia by preventing phospholipase-mediated calpain activation. *J. Cell. Physiol.* **167**, 434–442.

Arthur, P.G., Matich, G.P., Pang, W.W., Yu, D.Y. & Bogoyevitch, M.A. (2007): Necrotic death of neurons following an excitotoxic insult is prevented by a peptide inhibitor of c-jun N-terminal kinase. *J. Neurochem.* **102**, 65–76.

Blomgren, K., Zhu, C.L., Wang, X.Y., Karlsson, J.O., Leverin, A.L., Bahr, B.A., Mallard, C. & Hagberg, H. (2001): Synergistic activation of caspase-3 by m-calpain after neonatal hypoxia-ischemia – a mechanism of 'pathological apoptosis'? *J. Biol. Chem.* **276**, 10191–10198.

Blommaart, E.F.C., Krause, U., Schellens, J.P.M., Vreeling-Sindelárová, H. & Meijer, A.J. (1997): The phosphatidylinositol 3-kinase inhibitors wortmannin and LY294002 inhibit autophagy in isolated rat hepatocytes. *Eur. J. Biochem.* **243**, 240–246.

Borsello, T., Mottier, V., Castagné, V. & Clarke, P.G.H. (2002): Ultrastructure of retinal ganglion cell death after axotomy in chick embryos. *J. Comp. Neurol.* **453**, 361–371.

Borsello, T., Bressoud, R., Mottier, V., Gonzalez, N., Gomez, G. & Clarke, P.G.H. (2003a): Kainate-induced endocytosis in retinal amacrine cells. *J. Comp. Neurol.* **465**, 286–295.

Borsello, T., Clarke, P.G.H., Hirt, L., Vercelli, A., Repici, M., Schorderet, D.F., Bogousslavsky, J. & Bonny, C. (2003b): A peptide inhibitor of c-Jun N-terminal kinase protects against excitotoxicity and cerebral ischemia. *Nat. Med.* **9**, 1180–1186.

Borsello, T., Croquelois, K., Hornung, J.P. & Clarke, P.G.H. (2003c): N-methyl-D-aspartate-triggered neuronal death in organotypic hippocampal cultures is endocytic, autophagic and mediated by the c-Jun N-terminal kinase pathway. *Eur. J. Neurosci.* **18**, 473–485.

Castagné, V. & Clarke, P.G.H. (1996): Axotomy-induced retinal ganglion cell death in development: its timecourse and its diminution by antioxidants. *Proc. R. Soc. Lond. [Biol.]* **263**, 1193–1197.

Chan, F.K., Shisler, J., Bixby, J.G., Felices, M., Zheng, L., Appel, M., Orenstein, J., Moss, B. & Lenardo, M.J. (2003): A role for tumor necrosis factor receptor-2 and receptor-interacting protein in programmed necrosis and antiviral responses. *J. Biol. Chem.* **278**, 51613–51621.

Chang, D.T. & Reynolds, I.J. (2006): Mitochondrial trafficking and morphology in healthy and injured neurons. *Prog. Neurobiol.* **80**, 241–268.

Clarke, P.G.H. (1984): Identical populations of phagocytes and dying neurons revealed by intravascularly injected horseradish peroxidase, and by endogenous glutaraldehyde-resistant acid phosphatase, in the brains of chick embryos. *Histochem. J.* **16**, 955–969.

Clarke, P.G.H. (1990): Developmental cell death: morphological diversity and multiple mechanisms. *Anat. Embryol.* **181**, 195–213.

Clarke, P.G.H. (1999): Apoptosis versus necrosis. How valid a dichotomy for neurons? In: *Cell death and diseases of the nervous system*, ed. V.E. Kaliotsos & R.R. Ratan, pp. 3–28. Totowa, NJ: Humana Press.

Clarke, P.G.H. & Martin, A.H. (1985): Effects of de-efferentation on chick spinal motoneurons: peroxidase-uptake, and activities of acid phosphatase and N-acetyl-B-glucosaminidase. *Cell Biol. Int. Rep.* **9**, 676.

Darios, F., Lambeng, N., Troadec, J.D., Michel, P.P., & Ruberg, M. (2003): Ceramide increases mitochondrial free calcium levels via caspase 8 and Bid: role in initiation of cell death. *J. Neurochem.* **84**, 643–654.

Darios, F., Muriel, M.P., Khondiker, M.E., Brice, A. & Ruberg, M. (2005): Neurotoxic calcium transfer from endoplasmic reticulum to mitochondria is regulated by cyclin-dependent kinase 5-dependent phosphorylation of tau. *J. Neurosci.* **25**, 4159–4168.

DeMarchi, F., Bertoli, C., Copetti, T., Tanida, I., Brancolini, C., Eskelinen, E.L. & Schneider, C. (2006): Calpain is required for macroautophagy in mammalian cells. *J. Cell Biol.* **175,** 595–605.

Guillon-Munos, A., van Bemmelen, M.X. & Clarke, P.G.H. (2005): Role of phosphoinositide 3-kinase in the autophagic death of serum-deprived PC12 cells. *Apoptosis* **10,** 1031–1041.

Harris, C., Maroney, A.C. & Johnson, E.M. (2002): Identification of JNK-dependent and -independent components of cerebellar granule neuron apoptosis. *J. Neurochem.* **83,** 992–1001.

Higuchi, Y., Tanii, H., Koriyama, Y., Mizukami, Y. & Yoshimoto, T. (2007): Arachidonic acid promotes glutamate-induced cell death associated with necrosis by 12-lipoxygenase activation in glioma cells. *Life Sci.* **80,** 1856–1864.

Hornung, J.P., Koppel, H. & Clarke, P.G.H. (1989): Endocytosis and autophagy in dying neurons: an ultrastructural study in chick embryos. *J. Comp. Neurol.* **283,** 425–437.

Ishimaru, M.J., Ikonomidou, C., Tenkova, T.I., Der, T.C., Dikranian, K., Sesma, M.A. & Olney, J.W. (1999): Distinguishing excitotoxic from apoptotic neurodegeneration in the developing rat brain. *J. Comp. Neurol.* **408,** 461–476.

Kawamura, M., Nakajima, W., Ishida, A., Ohmura, A., Miura, S. & Takada, G. (2005): Calpain inhibitor MDL 28170 protects hypoxic-ischemic brain injury in neonatal rats by inhibition of both apoptosis and necrosis. *Brain Res.* **1037,** 59–69.

Kerr, J.F., Wyllie, A.H. & Currie, A.R. (1972): Apoptosis: a basic biological phenomenon with wide-ranging implications in tissue kinetics. *Br. J. Cancer* **26,** 239–257.

Kuwana, T. & Newmeyer, D.D. (2003): Bcl-2-family proteins and the role of mitochondria in apoptosis. *Curr. Opin. Cell Biol.* **15,** 691–699.

Lankiewicz, S., Luetjens, C.M., Bui, N.T., Krohn, A.J., Poppe, M., Cole, G.M., Saido, T.C. & Prehn, J.H.M. (2000): Activation of calpain I converts excitotoxic neuron death into a caspase-independent cell death. *J. Biol. Chem.* **275,** 17064–17071.

Lefèvre, K., Clarke, P.G.H., Danthe, E.E. & Castagné, V. (2002): Involvement of cyclin-dependent kinases in axotomy-induced retinal ganglion cell death. *J. Comp. Neurol.* **447,** 72–81.

Maiuri, M.C., Criollo, A., Tasdemir, E., Vicencio, J.M., Tajeddine, N., Hickman, J.A., Geneste, O. & Kroemer, G. (2007): BH3-only proteins and BH3 mimetics induce autophagy by competitively disrupting the interaction between Beclin 1 and Bcl-2/Bcl-X(L). *Autophagy* **3,** 374–376.

Majno, G. & Joris, I. (1995): Apoptosis, oncosis, and necrosis: an overview of cell death. *Am. J. Pathol.* **146,** 3–15.

Muriel, M.P., Lambeng, N., Darios, F., Michel, P.P., Hirsch, E.C., Agid, Y. & Ruberg, M. (2000): Mitochondrial free calcium levels (Rhod-2 fluorescence) and ultrastructural alterations in neuronally differentiated PC12 cells during ceramide-dependent cell death. *J. Comp. Neurol.* **426,** 297–315.

Nicotera, P., Leist, M., Fava, E., Berliocchi, L. & Volbracht, C. (2000): Energy requirement for caspase activation and neuronal cell death. *Brain Pathol.* **10,** 276–282.

Niquet, J., Baldwin, R.A., Allen, S.G., Fujikawa, D.G. & Wasterlain, C.G. (2003): Hypoxic neuronal necrosis: protein synthesis-independent activation of a cell death program. *Proc. Natl. Acad. Sci. U.S.A.* **100,** 2825–2830.

Nitatori, T., Sato, N., Waguri, S., Karasawa, Y., Araki, H., Shibanai, K., Kominami, E. & Uchiyama, Y. (1995): Delayed neuronal death in the CA1 pyramidal cell layer of the gerbil hippocampus following transient ischemia is apoptosis. *J. Neurosci.* **15,** 1001–1011.

Northington, F.J., Graham, E.M. & Martin, L.J. (2005): Apoptosis in perinatal hypoxic-ischemic brain injury: how important is it and should it be inhibited? *Brain Res. Brain Res. Rev.* **50,** 244–257.

Porn-Ares, M.I., Samali, A. & Orrenius, S. (1998): Cleavage of the calpain inhibitor, calpastatin, during apoptosis. *Cell Death Differ.* **5,** 1028–1033.

Portera-Cailliau, C., Price, D.L. & Martin, L.J. (1997): Excitotoxic neuronal death in the immature brain is an apoptosis-necrosis morphological continuum. *J. Comp. Neurol.* **378,** 70–87.

Ray, S.K. (2006): Currently evaluated calpain and caspase inhibitors for neuroprotection in experimental brain ischemia. *Curr. Med. Chem.* **13,** 3425–3440.

Renolleau, S., Aggoun-Zouaoui, D., Ben-Ari, Y. & Charriaut-Marlangue, C. (1998): A model of transient unilateral focal ischemia with reperfusion in the P7 neonatal rat – morphological changes indicative of apoptosis. *Stroke* **29,** 1454–1460.

Rothman, S.M. (1994): Excitotoxic neuronal death: mechanisms and clinical relevance. *Semin. Neurosci.* **6,** 315–322.

Sandvig, K. & van Deurs, B. (1992): Toxin-induced cell lysis: protection by 3-methyladenine and cycloheximide. *Exp. Cell Res.* **200,** 253–262.

Shimizu, S., Kanaseki, T., Mizushima, N., Mizuta, T., Arakawa-Kobayashi, S., Thompson, C.B. & Tsujimoto, Y. (2004): Role of Bcl-2 family proteins in a non-apoptotic programmed cell death dependent on autophagy genes. *Nat. Cell Biol.* **6,** 1221–1228.

Sloviter, R.S., Dean, E., Sollas, A.L. & Goodman, J.H. (1996): Apoptosis and necrosis induced in different hippocampal neuron populations by repetitive perforant path stimulation in the rat. *J. Comp. Neurol.* **366**, 516–533.

Sperandio, S., De Belle, I. & Bredesen, D.E. (2000): An alternative, nonapoptotic form of programmed cell death. *Proc. Natl. Acad. Sci. U.S.A.* **97**, 14376–14381.

Sperandio, S., Poksay, K., De Belle, I., Lafuente, M.J., Liu, B., Nasir, J. & Bredesen, D.E. (2004): Paraptosis: mediation by MAP kinases and inhibition by AIP-1/Alix. *Cell Death Differ.* **11**, 1066–1075.

Tanabe, K., Nakanishi, H., Maeda, H., Nishioku, T., Hashimoto, K., Liou, S.Y., Akamine, A. & Yamamoto, K. (1999): A predominant apoptotic death pathway of neuronal PC12 cells induced by activated microglia is displaced by a non-apoptotic death pathway following blockage of caspase-3-dependent cascade. *J. Biol. Chem.* **274**, 15725–15731.

van Gurp, M., Festjens, N., Van Loo, G., Saelens, X. & Vandenabeele, P. (2003): Mitochondrial intermembrane proteins in cell death. *Biochem. Biophys. Res. Commun.* **304**, 487–497.

Vannucci, R.C., Connor, J.R., Mauger, D.T., Palmer, C., Smith, M.B., Towfighi, J. & Vannucci, S.J. (1999): Rat model of perinatal hypoxic-ischemic brain damage. *J. Neurosci. Res.* **55**, 158–163.

Walker, N.I., Harmon, B.V., Gobe, G.C. & Kerr, J.F. (1988): Patterns of cell death. *Meth. Achiev. Exp. Pathol.* **13**, 18–54.

Wang, K.K.W. (2000): Calpain and caspase: can you tell the difference? [erratum appears in *Trends Neurosci* 2000;**23**:59]. [Review; 76 references.] *Trends Neurosci.* **23**, 20–26.

Wyllie, A.H. (1987): Cell death. *Int. Rev. Cytol.* (Suppl.) **17**, 755–785.

Wyllie, A.H., Kerr, J.F. & Currie, A.R. (1980): Cell death: the significance of apoptosis [review]. *Int. Rev. Cytol.* **68**, 251–306.

Xue, L.Z., Fletcher, G.C. & Tolkovsky, A.M. (1999): Autophagy is activated by apoptotic signalling in sympathetic neurons: an alternative mechanism of death execution. *Mol. Cell. Neurosci.* **14**, 180–198.

Yamashima, T. (2000): Implication of cysteine proteases calpain, cathepsin and caspase in ischemic neuronal death of primates [review]. *Prog. Neurobiol.* **62**, 273–295.

Yu, L., Alva, A., Su, H., Dutt, P., Freundt, E., Welsh, S., Baehrecke, E.H. & Lenardo, M.J. (2004): Regulation of an ATG7-beclin 1 program of autophagic cell death by caspase-8. *Science* **304**, 1500–1502.

Yu, L., Wan, F., Dutta, S., Welsh, S., Liu, Z., Freundt, E., Baehrecke, E.H. & Lenardo, M. (2006): Autophagic programmed cell death by selective catalase degradation. *Proc. Natl. Acad. Sci. U.S.A.* **103**, 4952–4957.

Zhu, C., Wang, X., Xu, F., Bahr, B.A., Shibata, M., Uchiyama, Y., Hagberg, H. & Blomgren, K. (2005): The influence of age on apoptotic and other mechanisms of cell death after cerebral hypoxia-ischemia. *Cell Death Differ.* **12**, 162–176.

Chapter 4

Prenatal diffusion MRI characterization of fetal brain oedema

Andrea Righini, Cecilia Parazzini, Chiara Doneda, Laura Avagliano *,
Mariangela Rustico, Gaetano Bulfamante *, Alessandra Kustermann °,
Roberto Fogliani °, Umberto Nicolini and Fabio Triulzi

Children's Hospital V. Buzzi, via Castelvetro 32, 20154 Milan, Italy;
* *San Paolo Hospital, Milan, Italy;*
°*IRCCS – Fondazione Policlinico, Milan, Italy*
neurorad@icp.mi.it

Summary

We examined the possibility of investigating fetal brain lesions associated with oedema by measuring the apparent diffusion coefficient (ADC) of water molecules. In 11 cases studied, we found that determining a decrease in ADC was pivotal in the detection of acute ischaemic cytotoxic oedema. A reduction in ADC was also characteristic of the acute phase of leucomalacia, as has recently been demonstrated in premature babies. An increase in ADC helped in the characterization of chronic lesions, highlighting the presence of interstitial oedema in cases of impaired venous drainage or increased intracranial pressure, as well as identifying the presence of vasogenic oedema (for example, infection-induced focal white matter rarefaction).

Introduction

In the past 10 years, diffusion-weighted magnetic resonance imaging (DWI) has been used extensively to detect intracellular (cytotoxic) or extracellular (vasogenic and interstitial) oedema associated with brain lesions in both adult (Warach *et al.*, 1995) and paediatric patients (Barkovitch *et al.*, 2001). According to the most widely accepted model, when brownian motion of water molecules within the tissue is restricted by cell swelling (for example, in acute hypoxic-ischaemic lesions) the apparent diffusion coefficient (ADC) of water decreases in comparison with the normal values (Pierpaoli *et al.*, 1993). On the other hand, when water molecule motion is less restricted than normal, because of an increase in extracellular water volume (interstitial oedema) or blood-brain barrier failure (vasogenic oedema), the ADC increases abnormally (Ebisu *et al.*, 1993). More recently, ADC measurements have been undertaken in acute ischaemic lesions occurring during fetal life *in vivo* (Baldoli *et al.*, 2002), and normal fetal brain ADC values have been determined (Righini *et al.*, 2003; Schneider *et al.*, 2007).

In this chapter we describe how we studied the possibility of investigating fetal brain lesions associated with oedema by measuring the ADC of water molecules.

Subjects and methods

From among about 260 fetal brain DWI studies carried out at our institution between 2000 and 2007, we selected those with technically adequate DWI images and in which DWI was deemed by two senior paediatric neuroradiologists (A.R. and C. P.), with seven years' experience in fetal magnetic resonance imaging, to have provided additional information over standard conventional T2-weighted images. All studies had been done for clinical purposes, because of ultrasonic or clinical suspicion of central nervous system anomalies. No maternal or fetal sedation was given. A 1.5 Tesla scanner with a surface abdominal coil was used. Multiplanar single-shot fast spin-echo (ss-FSE) T2-weighted sequences were acquired (TR/TE 3000/180 ms, 3–4 mm thick slices, 1.16 to 1.25 mm in plane resolution). In a minority of cases only could T1-weighted FSE or gradient echo 5 mm thick sections be obtained sufficiently free from motion artefacts to be evaluated. The DWI three-axis acquisition sequence lasted about 7 to 12 seconds, with the mother holding her breath. In-plane spatial resolution was 1.9 mm^2 with a 5 mm thick slice. A maximum b-factor of 600 s/mm^2 was adopted, according to previous reports on fetal DWI (Righini *et al.*, 2003). ADC maps were calculated and regions of interest (ROIs) were placed on injured and spared brain areas by a senior paediatric neuroradiologist.

Results

We found five cases with markedly *decreased* ADC values of between 0.4 and 0.9 μm^2/ms (normal 1.7–1.9 μm^2/ms) (Righini *et al.*, 2003). These cases were as follows: acute ischaemic lesions in the survivor of monochorionic twin pregnancy, within a few days after death of the co-twin (three cases); infection-related leucomalacia in the acute/subacute phase (one case) (Fig. 1); and vein of Galen malformation associated with acute ischaemia (one case). Conventional ss-FSE T2-weighted images were less informative than DWI in most of these cases.

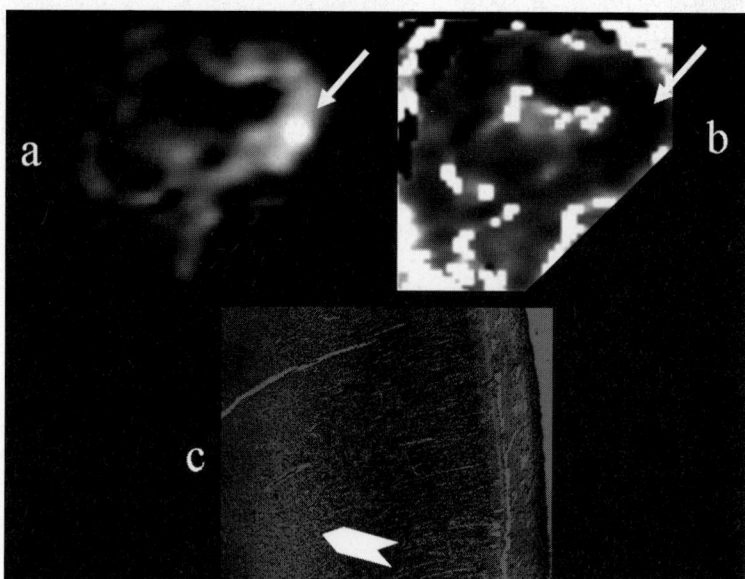

Fig. 1. 20-week gestation fetus in the acute/subacute phase of frontal-parietal leucomalacia. (a) coronal DWI section and corresponding ADC map; (b) showing large area of water diffusion restriction (ADC value = 0.7 μm^2/ms) in the left frontal subcortical parenchyma (arrows); (c) low magnification histology specimen depicting a subcortical area of tissue rarefaction, compatible with cellular swelling (arrowhead). ADC, apparent diffusion coefficient; DWI, diffusion-weighted imaging.

We found six cases with a clear *increase* in ADC value (between 2.0 and 2.6 µm²/ms). These were as follows: obstructive hydrocephalus with white matter interstitial oedema (one case); Arnold-Chiari type II malformation (one case) (Fig. 2); brain swelling and intracranial venous congestion due to probable impairment of venous drainage (one case); focal white matter rarefaction and oedema caused by cytomegalovirus infection (one case); and subacute-chronic focal ischaemia (one case). In these cases T2-weighted images generally showed blurring of the normal layering of the cerebral mantle.

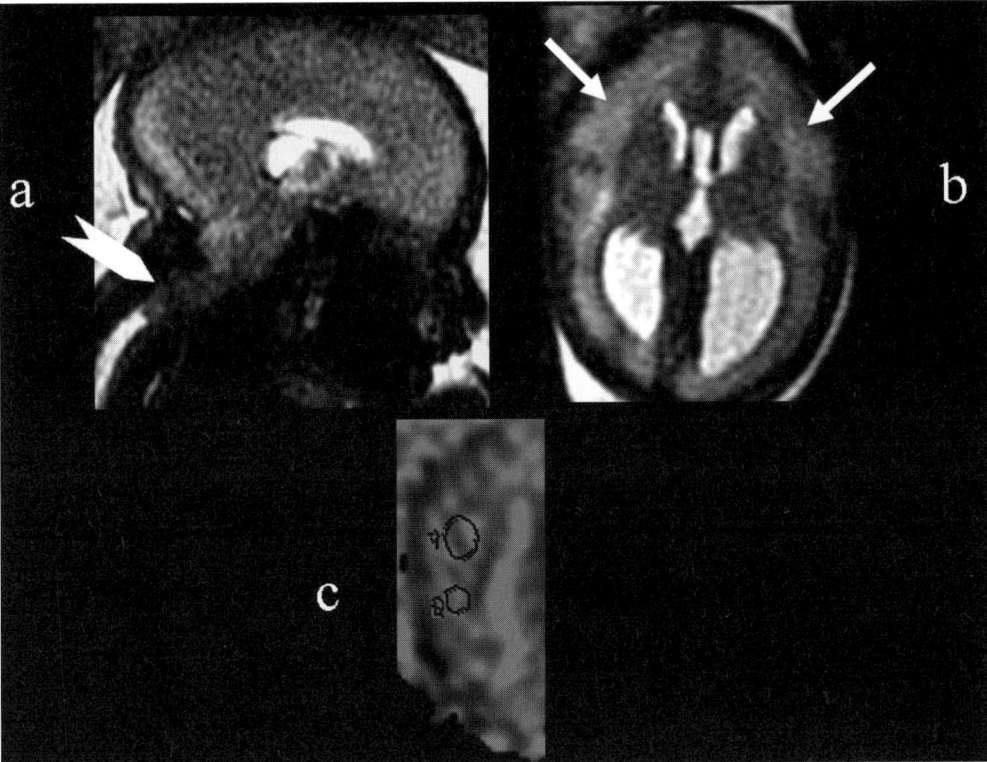

Fig. 2. 28-week gestation fetus with Arnold-Chiari II malformation. (a) Sagittal and (b) axial ss-FSE T2-weighted sections showing severe downward displacement of cerebellar tonsils (arrowhead) and general blurring of normal layering of cerebral mantle (arrows). (c) Axial ADC map showing regions of interest (ROIs), which revealed an abnormally increased ADC value of 2.5 µm²/ms. ADC, apparent diffusion coefficient.

Comment

In our limited fetal brain DWI series we found that a reduction in ADC was pivotal in the detection of acute ischaemic cytotoxic oedema, confirming previous reports (Baldoli *et al.*, 2002; Righini *et al.*, 2007). Moreover, a reduced ADC also identified the acute phase of leucomalacia, as recently demonstrated in premature babies (Inder *et al.*, 1999; Bozzao *et al.*, 2003).

On the other hand, detection of an increase in ADC may help in the characterization of chronic lesions, revealing, for example, the presence of interstitial oedema in cases of impaired venous drainage or increased intracranial pressure (hydrocephalus), which may have a long-term detrimental effect on normal brain development.

References

Baldoli, C., Righini, A., Parazzini, C., Scotti, G. & Triulzi, F. (2002): Demonstration of acute ischemic lesions in the fetal brain by diffusion magnetic resonance imaging. *Ann. Neurol.* **52,** 243–246.

Barkovich, A.J., Westmark, K.D., Bedi, H.S., Partridge, J.C., Ferriero, D.M. & Vigneron, D.B. (2001): Proton spectroscopy and diffusion imaging on the first day of life after perinatal asphyxia: preliminary report. *Am. J. Neuroradiol.* **22,** 1786–1794.

Bozzao, A., Di Paolo, A., Mazzoleni, C., Fasoli, F., Simonetti, A., Fantozzi, L.M. & Floris, R. (2003): Diffusion-weighted MR imaging in the early diagnosis of periventricular leucomalacia. *Eur. Radiol.* **13,** 1571–1576.

Ebisu, T., Naruse, S., Horikawa, Y., Ueda, S., Tanaka, C., Uto, M., Umeda, M. & Higuchi, T. (1993): Discrimination between different types of white matter edema with diffusion-weighted MR imaging. *J. Magn. Reson. Imaging* **3,** 863–868.

Inder, T., Huppi, P.S., Zientara, G.P., Maier, S.E., Jolesz, F.A., di Salvo, D., Robertson, R., Barnes, P.D. & Volpe, J.J. (1999): Early detection of periventricular leucomalacia by diffusion-weighted magnetic resonance imaging techniques. *J Pediatr.* **134,** 631–634.

Pierpaoli, C., Righini, A., Linfante, I., Tao-Cheng, J.H., Alger, J.R. & Di Chiro, G. (1993): Histopathologic correlates of abnormal water diffusion in cerebral ischemia: diffusion-weighted MR imaging and light and electron microscopic study. *Radiology* **189,** 439–448.

Righini, A., Bianchini, E., Parazzini, C., Gementi, P., Ramenghi, L., Baldoli, C., Nicolini, U., Mosca, F. & Triulzi, F. (2003): Apparent diffusion coefficient determination in normal fetal brain: a prenatal MR imaging study. *Am. J. Neuroradiol.* **24,** 799–804.

Righini, A., Kustermann, A., Parazzini, C., Fogliani, R., Ceriani, F. & Triulzi F. (2007): Diffusion-weighted magnetic resonance imaging of acute hypoxic-ischemic cerebral lesions in the survivor of a monochorionic twin pregnancy: case report. *Ultrasound Obstet. Gynecol.* **29,** 453–456.

Schneider, J.F., Confort-Gouny, S., Le Fur, Y., Viout, P., Bennathan, M., Chapon, F., Fogliarini, C., Cozzone, P. & Girard, N. (2007): Diffusion-weighted imaging in normal fetal brain maturation. *Eur. Radiol.* **17,** 2422–2429.

Warach, S., Gaa, J., Siewert, B., Wielopolski, P. & Edelmann, R.R. (1995): Acute human stroke studied by whole brain echo planar diffusion-weighted magnetic resonance imaging. *Ann. Neurol.* **37,** 231–241.

Chapter 5

Intrauterine growth restriction and neurological damage

Enrico Ferrazzi and Serena Rigano

Department of Clinical Sciences, University of Milan, via G.B. Grassi 74, 20157 Milan, Italy
enrico.ferrazzi@unimi.it

Summary

Confusion persists over the definition of growth restriction. In the year 2000 the Vermont Oxford Network reported the perinatal outcome in 19,000 growth-restricted neonates. In that study '... intrauterine growth restriction was defined as the 10th percentile for birth weight according to the 1993 US national statistics...'. However, any intention-to-treat study or follow-up study will be severely biased by the inclusion of many different abnormal conditions which comprise the small-for-gestational-age population. Possible approaches to this problem are customized reference standards derived from models of fetal growth, and the adoption of individual intrauterine growth curves. The combination of a growth-restricted fetal abdominal circumference and a raised uterine artery and umbilical artery Doppler blood flow resistance provides the most specific diagnosis of placenta-based fetal growth restriction. This stringent criterion has the advantage of focusing on a relatively homogeneous group of growth-restricted fetuses. From a perinatal perspective the definition of the severity of growth restriction and fetal condition at the time of delivery should be a sound basis for any neonatal study of growth-restricted neonates.

A series of four independent studies reported the 'natural' sequence of events which bring the growth-restricted fetus to premature delivery. Recent studies on blood flow volume measurements in fetal vessels proved that in growth-restricted fetuses, even if the umbilical blood flow per kg is severely reduced, the absolute blood flow that passes through the ductus venosus to the vital organs (brain and myocardium) is maintained within the normal range for gestational age. The cost of maintaining ductal flow is fetal hepatic perfusion. When ductal shunting is stable for more than 2 to 4 days, it is likely that the liver will be the first organ to be damaged by final attempts to compensate for worsening placental perfusion. These findings have been independently replicated by different investigators. They provide a new perspective on neonatal care: Would it be wise to give parenteral and enteral nutrients rich in amino acids to a newborn baby with abnormal liver function? How can we reverse the epigenetic effects of nutritional deprivation *in utero*? and so forth.

These findings, based on difficult blood volume flow studies, were confirmed by an international multi-centre study based on simple ductal waveform analysis which proved that between 26 and 29 weeks and above a birth weight of 600 g, abnormal ductus venosus Doppler waveform was the best predictor of neonatal mortality, and the absence or reversal of the ductus venosus a-wave predicted a significant decline in intact survival in this population of growth-restricted neonates.

How do we define intrauterine growth restriction?

Intrauterine growth restriction caused by placental insufficiency is a leading cause of neonatal mortality and morbidity and an important antecedent of poor neurodevelopment in childhood and adult life. This group accounts for most of the morbidity and mortality among small neonates.

Unfortunately for those who are trying to solve the complex issue of differentiating the various causes of growth restriction *in utero* and possibly discovering cause-related treatments, there is still much confusion over even the definition of growth restriction. In the year 2000 the Vermont Oxford Network (Bernstein *et al.*, 2000) reported the perinatal outcome of a large series of 19,000 growth-restricted neonates. They were included in the study according to the following definition: '...intrauterine growth restriction was defined as the 10th percentile for birth weight according to the 1993 US national statistics...'. This criterion has been generally adopted in both the obstetric and the neonatal literature. However, any intention-to-treat study or any follow-up study will be severely biased by the inclusion of so many different abnormal conditions which comprise the small for gestational age population, while at the same time genuinely growth-restricted fetuses may be left out on the basis of that criterion. Prenatal centile weight charts are biased by the wrong assumption that fetuses delivered prematurely before 37 weeks of gestation represent normally grown fetuses. However, it is obvious that there is no reason for a normal fetus to be delivered before term except in extraordinary circumstances, such as trauma. We know that premature delivery is mainly determined by infections or stress acting through inflammatory pathways (Gomez *et al.*, 1998). Inflammation can affect placental development and function. Figure 1 shows the odd shape of the lower centile values of the

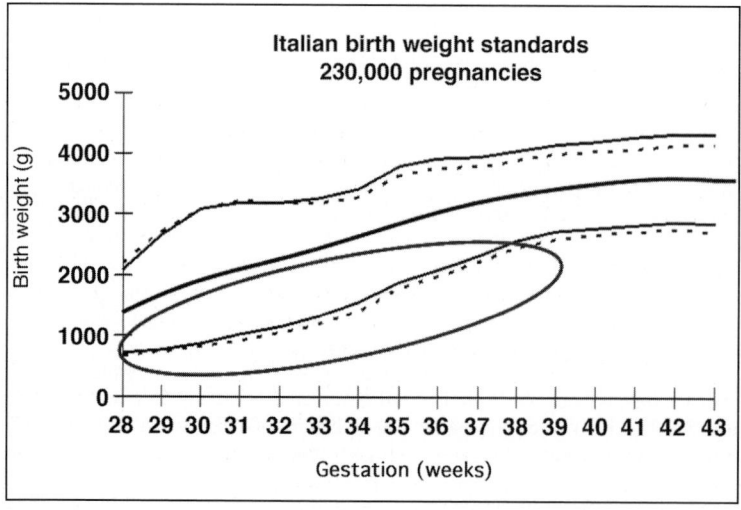

Fig. 1. Ninetieth and fifth centiles for the Italian birth weight standard. The lower centile curve has a sinusoid shape which is consistent with the inclusion of otherwise undetected growth-restricted fetuses. The weight difference from the expected growth of a non-sinusoid curve for the lower centile at 32 weeks is up to 250 g. IUGR, intrauterine growth restriction.

largest Italian study of birth weight centiles (Parazzini *et al.*, 1991). When we compare birth weight centiles after 37 weeks' gestation they are identical to any other prospective series obtained on true normal pregnancies (Todros *et al.*, 1987). When we examine birth weights before 34 weeks' gestation we can see that there is a sinusoidal shape to the lower growth curve which is consistent with the inclusion of growth-restricted fetuses. In a classical study by Bernstein *et al.* (2000), when the birth weight of fetuses delivered prematurely by 'normal' pregnant women was compared with the estimated fetal weight *in utero* of fetuses who were eventually delivered uneventfully at term, a mean weight difference of 200 grams was observed (Fig. 2).

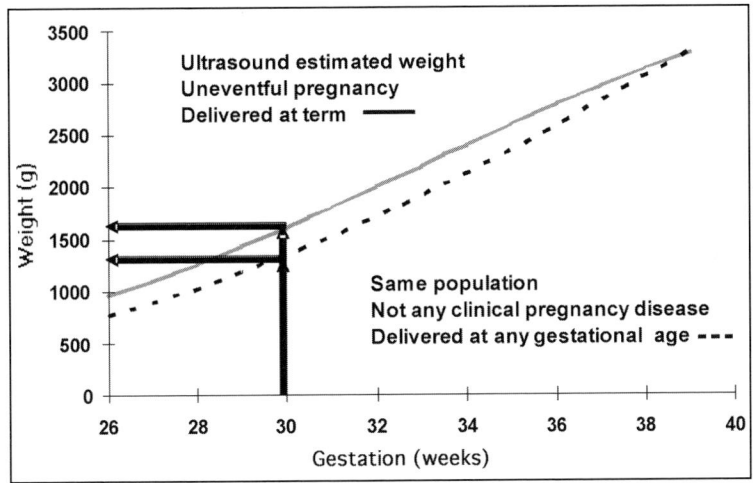

Fig. 2. Continuous line: Mean ultrasound estimated fetal weight in a cohort of pregnancies delivered uneventfully at term. Dotted line: Mean newborn weight observed at birth in a cohort of pregnancies delivered prematurely in the same years at the same referral centre. Iatrogenic premature deliveries were excluded.

A possible approach to this problem in large series is to adopt the criteria of Zeitlin *et al.* (2000), who used a customized reference standard derived from models of fetal growth (which included sex, ethnic group, body mass index, and other biological variables). That study was conducted on a sample of 4,700 preterm infants between 22 and 36 completed weeks of gestation and 6,460 control infants between 37 and 40 weeks of gestation. Using this standard, the investigators proved that the relation between growth restriction and preterm delivery was strongest for preterm births before 34 weeks' gestation, when approximately 20 per cent of neonates were below the reference standard. A more precise approach is represented by the adoption of individual intrauterine growth curves. Fetal growth restriction is defined in this case by a progressive decrease in centile rank with gestation. In our experience, up to 60 per cent of severely growth-restricted fetuses delivered before 30 weeks' gestation would have been included in the appropriate for gestational age group by traditional gestational age based newborn weight charts. An additional criterion to ensure that recruitment to intention-to-treat and follow-up studies involves only fetuses who are genuinely growth-restricted through placental insufficiency would be to include those with an abnormal umbilical pulsatility index (Pardi *et al.*, 1993) and abnormal uterine arterial Doppler velocimetry (Ferrazzi *et al.*, 1999). Figure 3 shows the correlation between abnormal uterine Doppler velocimetry and placental damage independently of maternal hypertension, as reported in that study, which was in agreement with the findings of other investigators examining fetuses with intrauterine growth retardation delivered by non-preeclamptic women (Salafia et al., 1995). The combination of a growth-restricted fetal abdominal circumference, as detected by longitudinal measurements after 12 to 14 days, and a raised uterine artery and umbilical artery Doppler blood flow resistance provides the most specific diagnosis of placenta-based fetal growth restriction. This stringent criterion has the advantage of focusing on a relatively homogeneous group of growth-restricted fetuses; a limitation is the exclusion of other causes of fetal growth restriction.

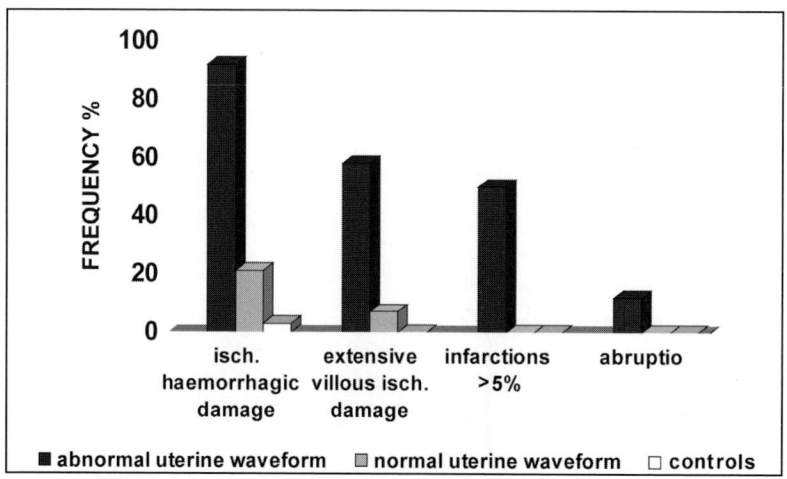

Fig. 3. Distribution of ischaemic haemorrhagic placental lesions in hypertensive patients with abnormal uterine Doppler waveform (black bars) and normal uterine Doppler waveform (white bars) versus controls (gray bars). Isch., ischaemic.

These considerations, which summarize the basic elements of a major scientific debate, should allow us to conclude once and for all that a growth-restricted fetus is not synonymous with a small for gestational age fetus. For clinical purposes this definition and its criteria should be abandoned, and clinical research should be based on homogeneous inclusion criteria relating to particular pathological conditions.

How do we define the severity of growth restriction?

From present insights and knowledge about progressive early intrauterine nutritional deprivation and worsening gas exchange, gestational-age-specific neonatal survival and complication rates in live-born growth-restricted neonates need to be considered in relation to the natural history of intrauterine growth restriction and the timing of intervention.

Doppler evaluation of fetal umbilical, cerebral, and venous circulations has increased our understanding of placental dysfunction, providing evidence that placenta-based fetal growth restriction is associated with progressive cardiovascular signs heralding fetal acidaemia and stillbirth.

Table 1 shows the perinatal outcome reported by the European Multicentre Study in 1994 (Karsdorp et al., 1994). Since then, the prognostic value of umbilical arterial Doppler velocimetry had been included in the standard diagnostic work-up of growth-restricted fetuses. Biological evidence of the correlation between umbilical Doppler velocimetry and acidaemia had been reported shortly before by our group (Pardi et al., 1993).

Table 1. Neonatal outcome according to umbilical arterial Doppler velocimetry *in utero*

	PED	AED	RED	*p* Value
Intrauterine death	6/214 (3%)	25/178 (14%)	16/67 (24%)	< 0.001
Severe RDS	4/124 (3%)	21/122 (17%)	19/46 (41%)	< 0.001
Admitted to NICU	126/208 (60%)	147/153 (96%)	50/51 (98%)	< 0.001
Cerebral haemorrhage, severe	1/124 (1%)	11/122 (9%)	16/46 (9%)	< 0.001
NEC	3/124 (3%)	6/122 (5%)	4/46 (9%)	0.2

AED, absent end-diastolic flow; NEC, necrotizing enterocolitis; NICU, neonatal intensive care unit; PED, present end-diastolic flow; RDS, respiratory distress syndrome; RED, reverse end-diastolic flow.

More recent studies have shown a significant correlation between arterial pulsatility and umbilical vein volume flow (Ferrazzi et al., 2000; Rigano et al., 2001). These studies demonstrated that when there is abnormal umbilical arterial velocimetry, a reduction in venous flow per unit weight is an early and consistent finding. Figure 4 shows the umbilical vein flow per unit fetal weight in a series of growth-restricted fetuses.

From a perinatal perspective the definition of the severity of growth restriction and fetal condition at the time of delivery should be a sound basis for any neonatal study on growth-restricted neonates. Neonatal studies on growth-restricted fetuses in which these criteria are not considered suffer major limitations owing to the wide variation in fetal condition at delivery.

How do we decide to deliver a growth-restricted fetus based on genuine fetal indication?

A series of four independent studies reported the 'natural' sequence of events which bring the growth-restricted fetus to premature delivery (Hecher et al., 2001; Baschat et al., 2001; Ferrazzi et al., 2002; Cosmi et al., 2005). These studies confirmed the prognostic value of the arterial umbilical Doppler circulation, the compensatory effect of cerebral vasodilatation as assessed by the middle cerebral artery pulsatility index, and the late changes in the fetal venous indices at the level of the ductus venosus, which dilates to increase umbilical blood shunting to the right heart (readily detectable by dramatic changes in waveform).

The ductus venosus connects the intrahepatic portion of the umbilical vein to the fetal right atrium and then, by way of the foramen ovale, to the left atrium. Bypassing the fetal liver, this provides a fraction of highly oxygenated and nutrient-rich umbilical venous blood to the myocardium and brain.

How can we prevent fetal organ damage and possibly neurological damage?

A recent paper by Bellotti (2004) proved that, in growth-restricted fetuses, even if the umbilical blood flow corrected for estimated fetal weight is severely reduced, the absolute blood flow that passes through the ductus venosus to the vital organs (brain and myocardium) is maintained within the normal range for gestational age (33.3 ± 18.1 ml/min in normal fetuses; 40.3 ± 19.4 ml/min in growth-restricted fetuses). Hence the reduction in ductal flow that is expected for the smaller fetal size is not found. These data clearly establish the role of the ductus venosus in maintaining an adequate oxygen supply to the brain and myocardium by means of constant ductal blood flow, even in the presence of placental disease which is

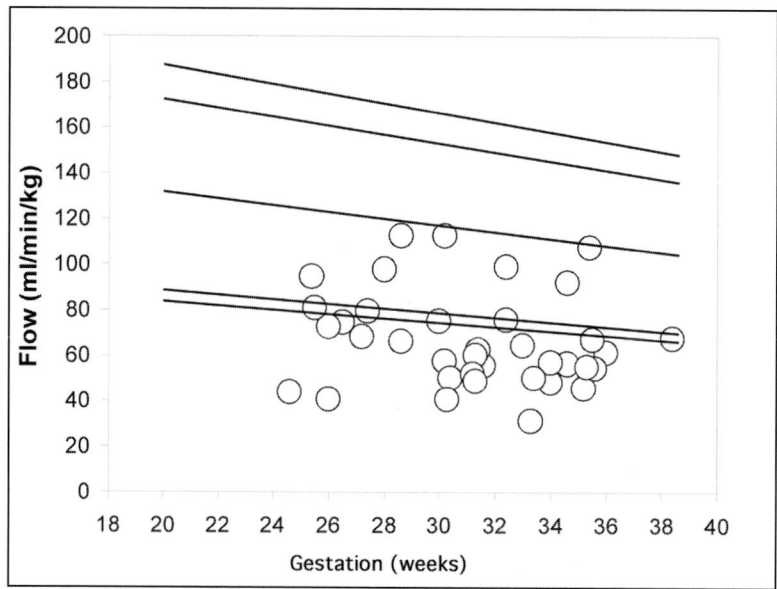

Fig. 4. Yellow dots: umbilical vein flow per unit weight in growth-restricted fetuses with abnormal umbilical velocimetry. The outcome of those within the 10th centile was uneventful.

associated with a reduced umbilical blood flow. The cost of maintaining ductal flow is fetal hepatic perfusion. When ductal shunting is stable for more than 2 to 4 days it is likely that the liver will be the first organ to be damaged by final attempts to compensate for worsening placental perfusion. These findings had been independently replicated by another group (Kiserud et al., 2006). They open a new perspective on neonatal care: Would it be wise to give parenteral and enteral nutrients rich in amino acids in a newborn baby with abnormal liver function? How can we reverse the epigenetic effects of nutritional deprivation *in utero*? and so forth.

To our knowledge the largest study on short-term neonatal outcome with a proper classification of the severity of intrauterine growth restriction was that recently reported by Baschat and co-workers (2007). The study analysed the results of a multicentre series collected in the USA and Europe, including a large dataset from our group. Major morbidity occurred in 35.9 per cent of 604 neonates, with intraventricular haemorrhage in 92 (5.2 per cent). Total mortality was 21.5 per cent (n = 130), and 58.3 per cent survived without complication (n = 352). Gestational age was the most significant determinant ($p < 0.005$) of total survival up to 26 weeks ($r^2 = 0.27$), and of intact survival up to 29 weeks ($r^2 = 0.42$). Beyond these gestational age cut-off points, and above a birth weight of 600 g, abnormal ductus venosus Doppler was the best predictor of neonatal mortality ($r^2 = 0.38$; $p < 0.001$), and the absence or reversal of the ductus venosus a-wave predicted a marked decline in intact survival in our population of growth-restricted neonates ($r^2 = 0.34$; $p < 0.001$) (Fig. 5).

This series provides for the first time neonatal outcomes that are specific for early-onset placenta-based fetal growth restriction, quantifying the impact of fetal cardiovascular parameters in addition to gestational age and birth weight. Beyond 29 weeks' gestation and 600 g birth

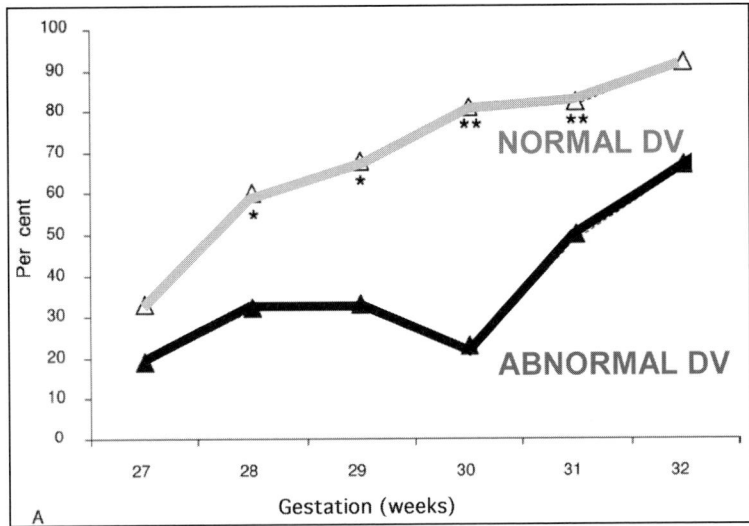

Fig. 5. Prevalence of intact neonatal survival in growth-restricted fetuses with abnormal umbilical Doppler velocimetry and normal ductus venous waveform (grey line) and abnormal ductus venosus velocimetry (black line). DV, Doppler velocimetry.

weight, ductus venosus Doppler indices emerge as the primary cardiovascular factor in predicting neonatal outcome, including early neurological damage.

Conclusions

A significant improvement in basic sciences and in diagnostic technology has resulted in major changes in the prenatal diagnosis of fetal growth restriction. It is probably now time to abandon old clinical paradigms such as postnatal criteria for growth restriction and clinical interventional and follow-up studies based on gestational age and weight at delivery, and embrace new diagnostic and prognostic criteria to classify and assess the severity of fetal growth restriction.

References

Baschat, A.A., Gembruch, U. & Harman, C.R. (2001): The sequence of changes in Doppler and biophysical parameters as severe fetal growth restriction worsens. *Ultrasound Obstet. Gynecol.* **18,** 571–577.

Baschat, A.A., Cosmi, E., Bilardo, C.M., Wolf, H., Berg, C., Rigano, S., Germer, U., Moyano, D., Turan, S., Hartung, J., Bhide, A., Müller, T., Bower, S., Nicolaides, K.H., Thilaganathan, B., Gembruch, U., Ferrazzi, E., Hecher, K., Galan, H.L. & Harman, C.R. (2007): Predictors of neonatal outcome in early-onset placental dysfunction. *Obstet. Gynecol.* **109,** 253–261.

Bellotti, M., Pennati, G., De Gasperi, C., Bozzo, M., Battaglia, F.C. & Ferrazzi, E. (2004): Simultaneous measurements of umbilical venous, fetal hepatic, and ductus venosus blood flow in growth-restricted human fetuses. *Am. J. Obstet. Gynecol.* **190,** 1347–1358.

Bernstein, I.M., Horbar, J.B., Badger, G.J., Ohlsson, A. & Golan, A., for the Vermont Oxford Network (2000): Morbidity and mortality among very-low-birth-weight neonates with intrauterine growth restriction. *Am. J. Obstet. Gynecol.* **182,** 198–206.

Cosmi, E., Ambrosini, G., D'Antona, D., Saccardi, C. & Mari, G. (2005): Doppler, cardiotocography, and biophysical profile changes in growth-restricted fetuses. *Obstet. Gynecol.* **106,** 1240–1245.

Ferrazzi, E., Bulfamante, G., Mezzopane, R., Barbera, A., Ghidini, A. & Pardi G. (1999): Uterine Doppler velocimetry and placental hypoxic-ischemic lesion in pregnancies with fetal intrauterine growth restriction. *Placenta* **20,** 389–394.

Ferrazzi, E., Rigano, S., Bozzo, M., Bellotti, M., Giovannini, N., Galan, H. & Battaglia, F.C. (2000): Umbilical vein blood flow in growth-restricted fetuses. *Ultrasound Obstet. Gynecol.* **16,** 432–438.

Ferrazzi, E., Bozzo, M., Rigano, S., Bellotti, M., Morabito, A., Pardi, G., Battaglia, F.C. & Galan, H.L. (2002): Temporal sequence of abnormal Doppler changes in the peripheral and central circulatory systems of the severely growth-restricted fetus. *Ultrasound Obstet. Gynecol.* **19,** 140–146.

Gomez, R., Romero, R., Ghezzi, F., Yoon, B.H., Mazor, M. & Berry, S.M. (1998): The fetal inflammatory response syndrome. *Am. J. Obstet. Gynecol.* **179,** 194–202.

Hecher, K., Bilardo, C.M., Stigter, R.H., Ville, Y., Hackeloer, B.J., Kok, H.J., Senat, M.V. & Visser, G.H. (2001): Monitoring of fetuses with intrauterine growth restriction: a longitudinal study. *Ultrasound Obstet. Gynecol.* **18,** 564–570.

Karsdorp, V.H., van Vugt, J.M., van Geijn, H.P., Kostense, P.J., Arduini, D., Montenegro, N. & Todros, T. (1994): Clinical significance of absent or reversed end diastolic velocity waveforms in umbilical artery. *Lancet* **244,** 1664–1668.

Kiserud, T., Kessler, J., Ebbing, C. & Rasmussen, S. (2006): Ductus venosus shunting in growth-restricted fetuses and the effect of umbilical circulatory compromise *Ultrasound Obstet. Gynecol.* **28,** 143–149.

Parazzini, F., Cortinovis, I., Bortolus, R. & Fedele, L. (1991): Standard di peso alla nascita in Italia. *Ann. Ost. Gin. Med. Perinat.* **12,** 203–246.

Pardi, G., Cetin, I., Marconi, A.M., Lanfranchi, A., Bozzetti, P., Ferrazzi, E., Buscaglia, M. & Battaglia, F.C. (1993): Diagnostic value of blood sampling in fetuses with growth retardation. *N. Engl. J. Med.* **328,** 692–696.

Rigano, S., Bozzo, M., Ferrazzi, E., Bellotti, M., Battaglia, F.C. & Galan, H.L. (2001): Early and persistent reduction in umbilical vein blood flow in the growth-restricted fetus: a longitudinal study. *Am. J. Obstet. Gynecol.* **185,** 834–848.

Salafia, C.M., Minior, V.K., Pezzullo, J.C., Popek, E.J., Rosenkrantz, T.S. & Vintzileos, A.M. (1995): Intrauterine growth restriction in infants of less than thirty-two weeks' gestation: associated placental pathologic features. *Am. J. Obstet. Gynecol.* **173,** 1049–1057.

Todros, T., Ferrazzi, E., Groli, C., Nicolini, U., Parodi, L., Pavoni, M., Zorzoli, A. & Zucca, S. (1987): Fitting growth curves to head and abdomen measurements of the fetus: a multicentric study. *J. Clin. Ultrasound* **15,** 95–105.

Vermont Oxford Network (2000): Morbidity and mortality among very-low-birth-weight neonates with intrauterine growth restriction. *Am. J. Obstet. Gynecol.* **182,** 198–206.

Zeitlin, J., Ancel, P.Y., Saurel-Cubizolles, M.J. & Papiernik, E. (2000): The relationship between intrauterine growth restriction and preterm delivery: an empirical approach using data from a European case-control study. *Br. J. Obstet. Gynaecol.* **107,** 750–758.

Chapter 6

Fetal cytomegalovirus infection: the brain as a window in the establishment of prognosis

Gustavo Malinger and Tally Lerman-Sagie *

Fetal Neurology Clinic, Prenatal Diagnosis Unit, Department of Obstetrics and Gynaecology and *Paediatric Neurology Unit, Edith Wolfson Medical Centre, P.O. Box 5, Holon, Israel
gmalinger@gmail.com

Summary

Cytomegalovirus (CMV) is the most common congenital infection in many countries. Serological or culture evidence of intrauterine infection has been reported in 0.2 to 2.2 per cent of all neonates but only 10 per cent of these are symptomatic at birth. Late sequelae may develop in another 10 to 20 per cent. A detailed study of the fetal brain by ultrasound, in some cases complemented by magnetic resonance imaging (MRI), is helpful in two different subsets: (1) Screening for fetal signs of CMV infection: the diagnosis of microcephaly, abnormal periventricular echogenicity, periventricular cysts, intraventricular adhesions, calcifications, abnormal cortical development, and callosal and/or cerebellar anomalies should raise suspicion of CMV infection. In conjunction with positive serological or polymerase chain reaction tests, these findings indicate a very poor prognosis. (2) Follow-up of fetuses with known intrauterine CMV infection and with apparently normal ultrasound examination until the end of pregnancy: sequential normal ultrasound examinations, followed by normal MRI close to term, reduce the risk of a seriously affected newborn considerably but this does not exclude the possible development of late sequelae.

Introduction

Congenital cytomegalovirus (CMV) infection is the most common intrauterine infection, affecting 0.2 to 2.2 per cent of all neonates (Stagno *et al.*, 1986; Istas *et al.*, 1995). Primary maternal infection followed by haematogenous spread to the fetus is the main source of transmission; reactivation of the disease and infection by a different CMV strain are rare but possible occurrences (Boppana *et al.*, 2001).

Affected neonates may be asymptomatic or may show a wide range of symptoms; severe cases may present with hepatosplenomegaly, haematological disturbances, microcephaly with or without intracranial findings, chorioretinitis, and sensorineural hearing loss. Intrauterine growth restriction and an increased risk of intrauterine death have also been reported.

Several studies based on imaging techniques have shown that the presence of microcephaly at birth and intracranial pathology are associated with a very high risk of neurological abnormalities and mental retardation.

The Houston Congenital CMV Longitudinal Study Group (Noyola et al., 2001) found that in a group of 41 symptomatic children evaluated serially from birth, microcephaly was the most specific predictor of mental retardation and major motor disability, while an abnormal intracranial computed tomography (CT) finding was the most sensitive predictor. Overall, children with microcephaly at birth or positive CT findings had a more than 90 per cent risk of being severely affected. Symptomatic children with a normal head circumference and without abnormal CT findings had a good cognitive outcome.

Recently, Ancora and colleagues (Ancora et al., 2007) undertook a similar study based on the use of ultrasound, with similar results. All neonates with symptoms who had abnormal ultrasound results showed at least one sequel or died, while only three of 47 with symptoms but normal ultrasound results had sensorineural hearing loss. Data on asymptomatic children were not sufficient to reach conclusions.

Studies from prenatally diagnosed fetuses are scant. Lipitz et al. (2002) found that the risk of postnatal neurological abnormalities was 19 per cent (three of 16) when there were no prenatal ultrasonographic abnormalities; two of these children had microcephaly which was not diagnosed during pregnancy. Enders et al. (2001) reported similar findings with respect to infected fetuses with ultrasonographic findings but believed that 'normal ultrasound of infected fetuses at gestational weeks 22–23 can neither completely exclude an abnormal ultrasound at a later week of gestation and the birth of a severely damaged child nor the birth of neonates which are afflicted by single manifestations at birth or later and of the kind which are not detectable by currently available ultrasonographic techniques'.

As universal scanning for CMV during pregnancy is not usually undertaken, many infected fetuses escape prenatal detection. In these cases the best chances for diagnosis are based on a high degree of suspicion for signs of fetal infection during the performance of second and third trimester ultrasound examinations.

Our aim in this chapter is to present our experience in the visualization and characterization of CNS ultrasonographic findings associated with CMV infection. We also propose a follow-up protocol in cases of known vertical CMV transmission for fetuses presenting with an apparently normal ultrasound scan.

Visualization and characterization of CNS ultrasonographic findings

Ultrasound was used to detect the presence of suspected signs of fetal infection during routine examinations in fetuses in whom the serological CMV status was unknown or in fetuses suspected of suffering from CMV disease. It was also used in pregnancies with known fetal CMV infection in order to monitor the possible development of CMV stigmata in women who were willing to continue their pregnancies if the fetus was apparently unaffected.

We retrospectively reviewed all the cases of CMV infection evaluated at our unit. We found 31 fetuses with diverse CNS ultrasonographic signs of infection; and 18 fetuses with positive polymerase chain reaction (CMV) amniocentesis but without any signs of CMV disease, where the parents were willing to continue the pregnancy. Nine fetuses with CNS ultrasound findings have been reported previously (Malinger et al., 2003).

Termination of pregnancy was offered according to the law in Israel in all cases with abnormal brain findings.

Patients with apparently subclinical CMV infections were counselled at different multidisciplinary clinics around the country regarding the disease, prognosis, and the risks of developing clinical CMV disease during pregnancy and after delivery. The possibility of terminating the pregnancy was discussed with all the families. Women who were willing to continue their pregnancies were referred to our unit for a detailed neurosonographic examination and an examination for the presence of possible non-CNS findings. The examinations were carried out at 3-to 4-week intervals until delivery and were complemented by magnetic resonance imaging (MRI) of the fetal brain between 32 and 36 weeks of pregnancy.

Fetuses with brain ultrasound signs of CMV infection

Thirty-one fetuses were identified as suspected of suffering from intrauterine CMV infection based on the presence of characteristic findings. In 28, the ultrasound examination was the first indication of the presence of an affected fetus, and the remaining three fetuses were initially referred for ultrasound examination because of positive serological findings in the mother's serum.

Gestational age at the time of the first diagnostic ultrasound ranged between 22 and 37 weeks (mean 29.1 weeks).

Abnormal hyperechogenic periventricular tissue was depicted in all fetuses; 17 also had associated periventricular cystic lesions (Fig. 1). These cysts were found in different locations, mainly close to the posterior horns but also in the parietal, frontal, and temporal lobes. In nine fetuses, associated with these cysts or probably as a result of the convergence of multiple cysts, intraventricular bands or adhesions were also observed (Fig. 2). The presence of such cysts was not always easy to identify as they could have been mistaken for normal or slightly enlarged occipital horns. Ventriculomegaly was found in only 19 fetuses, all with mild ventriculomegaly (less than 14.9 mm). Calcifications were only found in 13 fetuses. Brain parenchymal anomalies representing global brain atrophy or focal brain destruction were observed in nine fetuses (Fig. 3). In some cases the insult resulted in malformation of cortical development (seven fetuses), callosal anomalies (seven), and cerebellar anomalies (five). Seven fetuses had findings localized to the basal ganglia, comprising striatal vasculopathy or thalamic calcifications, or both (Fig. 4). Finally, the head circumference was more than 2SD below the mean at the time of the first ultrasound examination in seven fetuses.

Intrauterine CMV infection was confirmed after the performance of amniocentesis in 25 women. The remaining six women opted for termination of pregnancy without waiting for the results of laboratory confirmatory tests, and the diagnosis was based on serological studies of fetal blood or on the presence of characteristic histological findings at autopsy.

Based on the very poor prognosis associated with congenital CMV in the presence of a clear brain insult, termination of pregnancy was carried out in 25 women. Six infants were delivered, two dying during the neonatal period. Three of the remaining children suffer from severe psychomotor retardation and only one is developing normally (last developmental evaluation at 36 months of age).

Fetuses with proven intrauterine CMV infection but with normal ultrasound

From the initial group of 18 women willing to continue pregnancy in spite of an amniocentesis-proven intrauterine CMV infection, 15 had normal neurosonographic examination at the time of referral and at 3 to 4 week intervals until delivery, and a normal brain MRI examination done at 32 to 36 weeks of pregnancy. The 15 fetuses were delivered and found to be unaffected

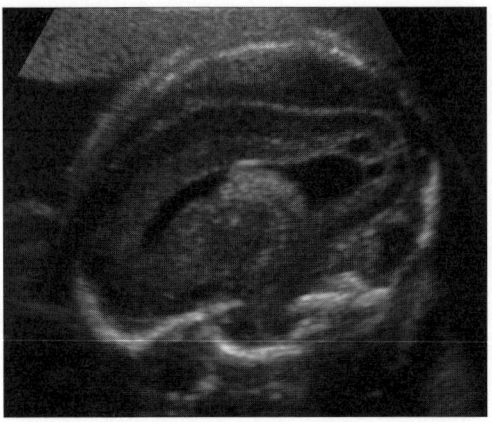

Fig. 1. Transvaginal parasagittal plane in a 24.5 week fetus with histologically proven cytomegalovirus infection. Note the sharp demarcation between the periventricular zone and the cortical plate and the cyst in the occipital lobe.

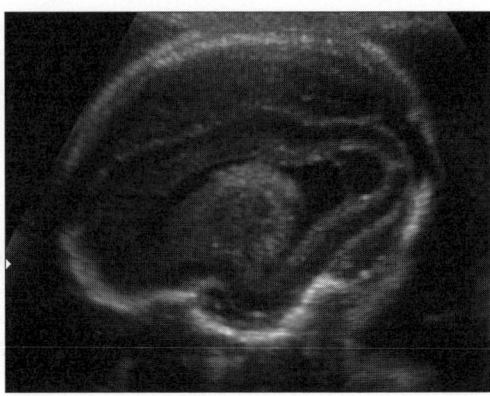

Fig. 2. The same fetus as in Fig. 1 at 26 weeks, showing the appearance of an intraventricular adhesion not present at 24.5 weeks.

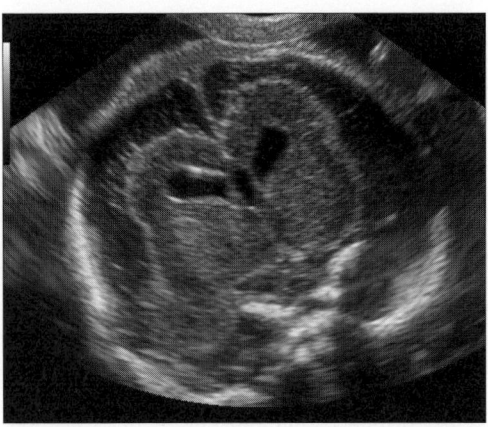

Fig. 3. Transvaginal coronal plane in a 24 week fetus, showing brain atrophy. Note the increased amount of cerebrospinal fluid around the brain and the abnormal development of the Sylvian fissures.

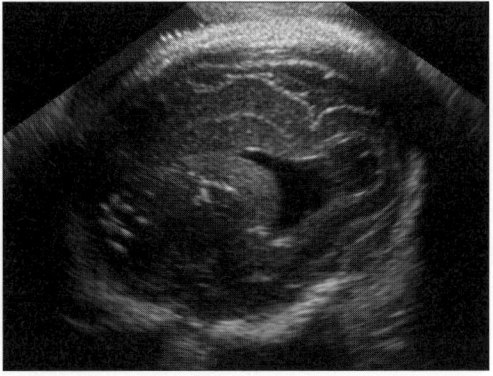

Fig. 4. Transvaginal parasagittal view of the brain at 30.5 weeks of pregnancy in a fetus with cytomegalovirus infection, showing abnormal linear echogenicity in the thalamus consistent with striatal vasculopathy. Note also the abnormal echogenicity of the periventricular zone, abnormal sulcation, and punctuate calcifications.

at the initial postnatal ultrasound examination; in all these cases the BERA test was also normal. Short-term neurodevelopmental follow-up of these children is normal.

In the remaining three fetuses, neurosonographic examinations were considered normal but MRI examinations raised the suspicion of a possible brain insult, comprising abnormal white matter or periventricular temporal cysts. All three women opted to continue pregnancy, and their neonates had normal physical and neurological examinations, brain imaging, and BERA tests. One infant received gancyclovir for 6 months.

Comments

The prenatal management of pregnant women with suspected fetal intrauterine CMV infection is complicated owing to the very broad spectrum of severity in this disease. Although most cases will be asymptomatic, the risk of neurodevelopmental damage or hearing loss remains considerable.

Based on current knowledge it is widely accepted that the presence of microcephaly or abnormal intracranial imaging findings in the newborn is associated with a bad prognosis.

We have shown that a careful neurosonographic examination carried out during the second or third trimester is a good option for the diagnosis of CMV brain involvement, especially in countries where population screening is only partially done or not done at all.

As we reported in our previous paper (Malinger et al., 2003), a hyperechogenic periventricular zone, clearly and sharply differentiated from the remaining of the brain, with or without cysts or calcifications, was present in all our patients and was highly indicative of an intrauterine infection.

Although less common, the presence of intraventricular adhesions in the occipital horn was consistently associated with CMV infection. All the fetuses with this pathology were found to be CMV positive.

Cerebral calcifications were present in only 42 per cent of the affected fetuses. A possible explanation for this relatively low prevalence is that the diagnosis in some cases was made relatively early in the course of the disease, so there was not sufficient time for them to develop.

Although data on the prognosis of symptomatic children with CMV infection seem to indicate a very good prognosis when brain ultrasound is normal, available data are still not sufficient to reach definitive conclusions (Ancona et al., 2007). Data on prenatal diagnosed cases are even more limited (Lipitz et al., 2002).

Proposed follow-up protocol

Our proposed protocol consists of performance of targeted serial ultrasound examinations at 3 to 4 week intervals, complemented by an MRI study between 34 and 36 weeks. Ultrasound examinations should include a biometric assessment with particular attention to the head circumference, a detailed neurosonographic examination, and an itemized search for characteristic non-CNS findings (intestinal echogenicity, liver size and the presence of calcifications, spleen size, presence of signs of hydrops fetalis, and heart size). Fetal brain MRI is used in order to back up the ultrasonographic examination, with particular emphasis on signs of white matter involvement and abnormal cortical formation.

Conclusions

At present our follow-up and neurological evaluation of patients secreting CMV but without fetal ultrasonographic brain findings is not complete, so we cannot yet prove that normal consecutive fetal ultrasounds are predictive of a good outcome. Therefore, the protocol for evaluation of fetuses with suspected CMV infection will remain only another option in our armamentarium until more data are obtained. Parents willing to continue pregnancy in spite of intrauterine infection may be offered this type of management after giving informed consent, following an explanation by a multidisciplinary team that includes an obstetrician or a radiologist with experience in fetal neurosonography, a specialist in paediatric infectious diseases, and a paediatric neurologist.

We believe that ultrasound has a fundamental role in the diagnosis of fetal CMV infections in the non-screened population and an even more important place in the evaluation of fetuses with known CMV infection.

References

Ancora, G., Lanari, M., Lazzarotto, T., Venturi, V., Tridapalli, E., Sandri, F., Menarini, M., Ferretti, E. & Faldella, G. (2007): Cranial ultrasound scanning and prediction of outcome in newborns with congenital cytomegalovirus infection. *J. Pediatr.* **150**, 157–161.

Boppana, S.B., Rivera, L.B., Fowler, K.B., Mach, M. & Britt, W.J. (2001): Intrauterine transmission of cytomegalovirus to infants of women with preconceptional immunity. *N. Engl. J. Med.* **344**, 1366–1371.

Enders, G., Bäder, U., Lindemann, L., Schalasta, G. & Daiminger, A. (2001): Prenatal diagnosis of congenital cytomegalovirus infection in 189 pregnancies with known outcome. *Prenat. Diagn.* **21**, 362–377.

Istas, A.S., Demmler, G.J., Dobbins, J.G. & Stewart, J.A. (1995): Surveillance for congenital cytomegalovirus disease: a report from the National Congenital Cytomegalovirus Disease Registry. *Clin. Infect. Dis.* **20**, 665–670.

Lipitz, S., Achiron, R., Zalel, Y., Mendelson, E., Tepperberg, M. & Gamzu, R. (2002): Outcome of pregnancies with vertical transmission of primary cytomegalovirus infection. *Obstet. Gynecol.* **100**, 428–433.

Malinger, G., Lev, D., Zahalka, N., Ben Aroia, Z., Watemberg, N., Kidron, D., Ben-Sira, L. & Lerman-Sagie, T. (2003): Fetal cytomegalovirus infection of the brain. The spectrum of sonographic findings. *Am. J. Neuroradiol.* **24**, 28–32.

Noyola, D.E., Demmler, G.J., Nelson, C.T., Griesser, C., Williamson, W.D., Atkins, J.T., Rozelle, J., Turcich, M., Llorente, A.M., Sellers-Vinson, S., Reynolds, A., Bale J.F.J., Gerson, P. & Yow, M.D. for the Houston Congenital CMV Longitudinal Study Group (2001): Early predictors of neurodevelopmental outcome in symptomatic congenital cytomegalovirus infection. *J. Pediatr.* **138**, 325–331.

Stagno, S., Pass, R.F., Cloud, G., Britt, W.J., Henderson, R.E., Walton, P.D., Veren, D.A., Page, F. & Alford, C.A. (1986): Primary cytomegalovirus infection in pregnancy: incidence, transmission to fetus, and clinical outcome. *JAMA* **256**, 1904–1908.

Chapter 7

Perinatal brain damage

Luca A. Ramenghi, Laura Bassi, Monica Fumagalli, Fabio Mosca

Neonatologia e Terapia Intensiva Neonatale, IRCCS Fondazione Scientifica, Policlinico, Ospedale Mangiagalli, Regina Elena, Italy
lucrameng@hotmail.com

Summary

It is difficult to clarify the temporal limits of the term 'perinatal' but its ambiguity remains appropriate since the 'prime mover' in the most frequent and important brain lesions affecting the brains of term and premature newborn babies remains unknown. In this chapter we debate how 'perinatal' are the most common brain lesions affecting neonates, such as asphyxia, arterial infarcts, intraventricular haemorrhage, and periventricular leucomalacia. The problem is further compounded by uncertainties over the functional consequences of lesions identified by diagnostic investigations. The predictive value of certain neuroradiological techniques is well recognized (for example, cavitation in the white matter on brain ultrasound is predictive of motor disability), but distinct lesions correlated with impaired cognitive outcome in preterm infants have not been identified, even with the most sophisticated applications of magnetic resonance imaging. Any attempt to improve our knowledge in this field – including a better understanding of the term 'perinatal' – should aim at minimizing the incidence of brain damage and associated disabilities.

Introduction

The terms 'perinatal' and 'brain damage' have often been linked, not only in the medical literature but also in scientific articles for the layman. The neurological integrity of the fetus during the course of pregnancy has generally been assumed, and the possibility of investigating and diagnosing neurological problems has been considered only in the most recent past, with the advent of prenatal ultrasound and neonatal magnetic resonance investigations. Therefore the consequences of a 'difficult birth' may have been too readily emphasized, as they were often the only available explanation for later neurological problems in the infant (Cowan *et al.*, 2003; Cowan & Squier, 2004; Swaiman & Wu, 2006). The concept of a difficult traumatic birth causing later neurological problems was initially described by the English orthopaedic surgeon William Little in the nineteenth century, and soon afterwards Sigmund Freud proposed that the 'difficult birth' was probably introduced by an abnormal labour, perhaps intrinsic to problems in the fetus (Little, 1861). For these reasons, insults taking place during the phase of labour and delivery have been correlated with the concept that 'perinatal trauma' is primarily related to mechanical factors, with the understanding that even under optimal conditions the process of birth is potentially traumatic. With the advent of a new form of medical practice – neonatal intensive care – the concept of 'perinatal trauma' has extended to involve the premature baby, and the vulnerability of the premature brain to the development of lesions was believed to be a result of the birth process itself – in other words the birth was 'traumatic' because it was preterm. Currently, the clinical stability of even the most premature babies, now delivered under much better conditions than a few years ago, has finally shifted interest from the process of birth to scientific research into the pathogenesis of certain prenatal disorders.

Definition

It is difficult to define the 'perinatal period', and most general dictionaries of the English language do not help to clarify the term. They state that 'perinatal' means 'relating to, or occurring in the period from about 3 months before to 1 month after birth' (Collins English Dictionary) or 'relating to the time, usually a number of weeks, immediately before and after birth' (Oxford English Dictionary). The high level of temporal ambiguity of the term 'perinatal' is not surprising, although it was originally used to express the concept of fetal and neonatal mortality. Perinatal mortality involves a period starting just before the birth until the end of the first postnatal week and includes premature birth. The earliest gestational age included in the term 'perinatal mortality' used to be 27 weeks. At present, however, because of the increased survival of very preterm babies the lower limit is uncertain; 24 weeks has been proposed, but it is probably appropriate to consider babies delivered as early as 23 weeks. The postnatal extension is 1 week, but it could be a full month if we abandon the concept of mortality originally associated with the term 'perinatal'.

The ambiguity of the term perinatal, so often used in relation to brain damage, is probably appropriate as it remains extremely difficult to identify the timing of the most frequent and important lesions affecting the brains of term and preterm neonates.

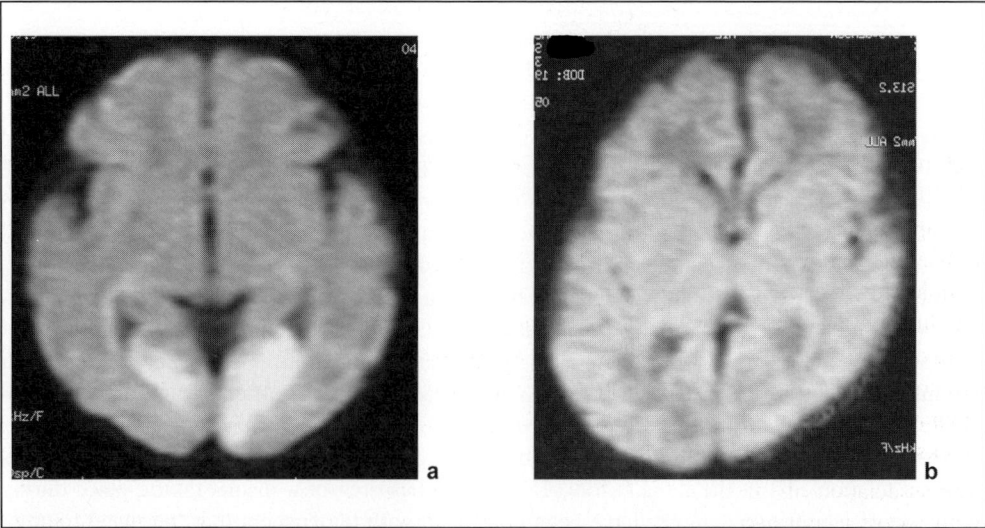

Fig. 1. Posterior bilateral 'insult'. (a) Diffusion weighted imaging at 48 hours showing the two areas of restriction. (b) Diffusion weighted imaging at 10 days showing no permanent lesion.

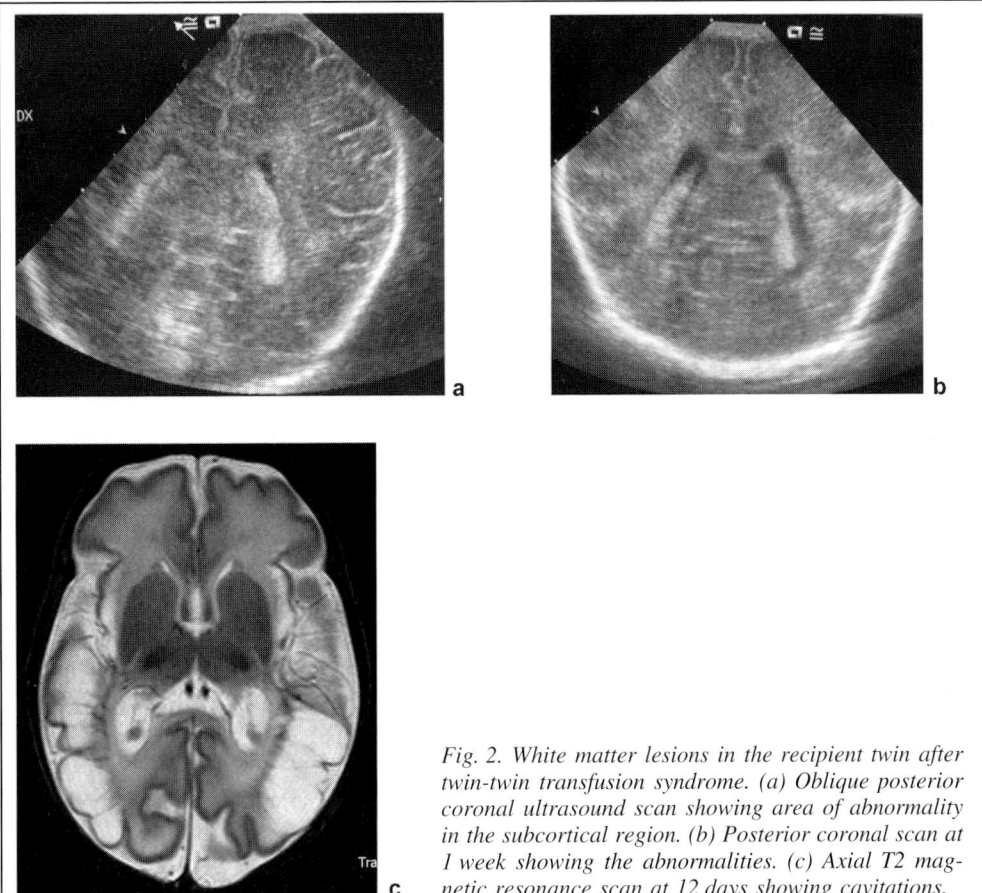

Fig. 2. White matter lesions in the recipient twin after twin-twin transfusion syndrome. (a) Oblique posterior coronal ultrasound scan showing area of abnormality in the subcortical region. (b) Posterior coronal scan at 1 week showing the abnormalities. (c) Axial T2 magnetic resonance scan at 12 days showing cavitations.

How 'perinatal' is a particular brain lesion?

Before discussing how 'perinatal' a particular brain lesion may be, it is important to understand whether a week or a month of life is a sufficient length of time for the development of brain damage. In the full-term baby this period is probably sufficient for the development of hypoxic-ischaemic lesions, arterial stroke, and venous thrombosis, because the process of damage starts with labour and current neuroimaging techniques can show evidence of acute lesions very early on. In preterm infants the most frequent lesions, such as white matter disease (WMD) and intraventricular haemorrhage (IVH), have different antenatal aetiological components which are not always correlated with labour (for example, inflammation); in addition, lesions such as cavitations in the white matter can become evident on neuroimaging carried out after the first weeks (Arthur & Ramenghi, 2001).

The association of 'perinatal' with 'asphyxia' seems to suggest a sequence of events starting with an often unknown prenatal trigger, followed by a potential intrapartum asphyxial event and resulting in hypoxic-ischaemic encephalopathy with the typical postnatal clinical signs (Cowan *et al.*, 2003; Miller *et al.*, 2005).

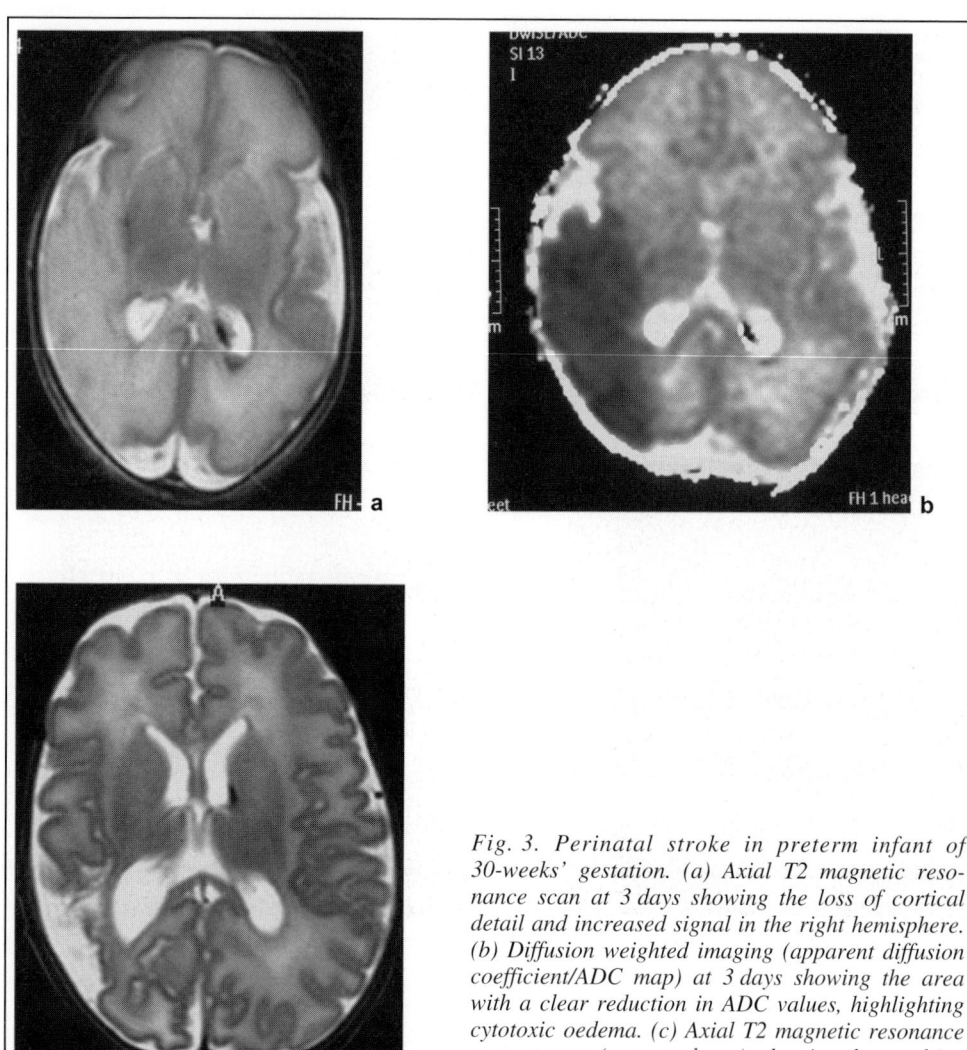

Fig. 3. Perinatal stroke in preterm infant of 30-weeks' gestation. (a) Axial T2 magnetic resonance scan at 3 days showing the loss of cortical detail and increased signal in the right hemisphere. (b) Diffusion weighted imaging (apparent diffusion coefficient/ADC map) at 3 days showing the area with a clear reduction in ADC values, highlighting cytotoxic oedema. (c) Axial T2 magnetic resonance scan at term (corrected age), showing the resulting loss of tissue, which is less than initially indicated.

The underlying causes of asphyxia in full-term infants are not clear, and controversy about the aetiology and timing of brain insult persists. Asphyxia may occur before or during labour, and rarely postnatally ('postnatal collapse syndrome'), and may be acute, subacute, or both (Cowan *et al.*, 2003; Cowan & Squier, 2004). The hypoxic-ischaemic lesions may be the final common pathway for other insults such as inflammatory-infective components and hypoxic and hypotensive neonatal insults. Postnatal hypoglycaemia, along with or in combination with other factors, also leads to apparent asphyxia.

In some cases of 'asphyxia', where infants are exposed to a defined sentinel event (for example, placental abruption, placental infarction, cord flow abnormalities, severe maternal hypotension) associated with a sudden deterioration in fetal condition (heart rate abnormalities, fetal blood acidosis, low Apgar score), there is a good evidence of hypoxia. However, for the majority of infants with asphyxia no sentinel event can be documented, although they present with fetal

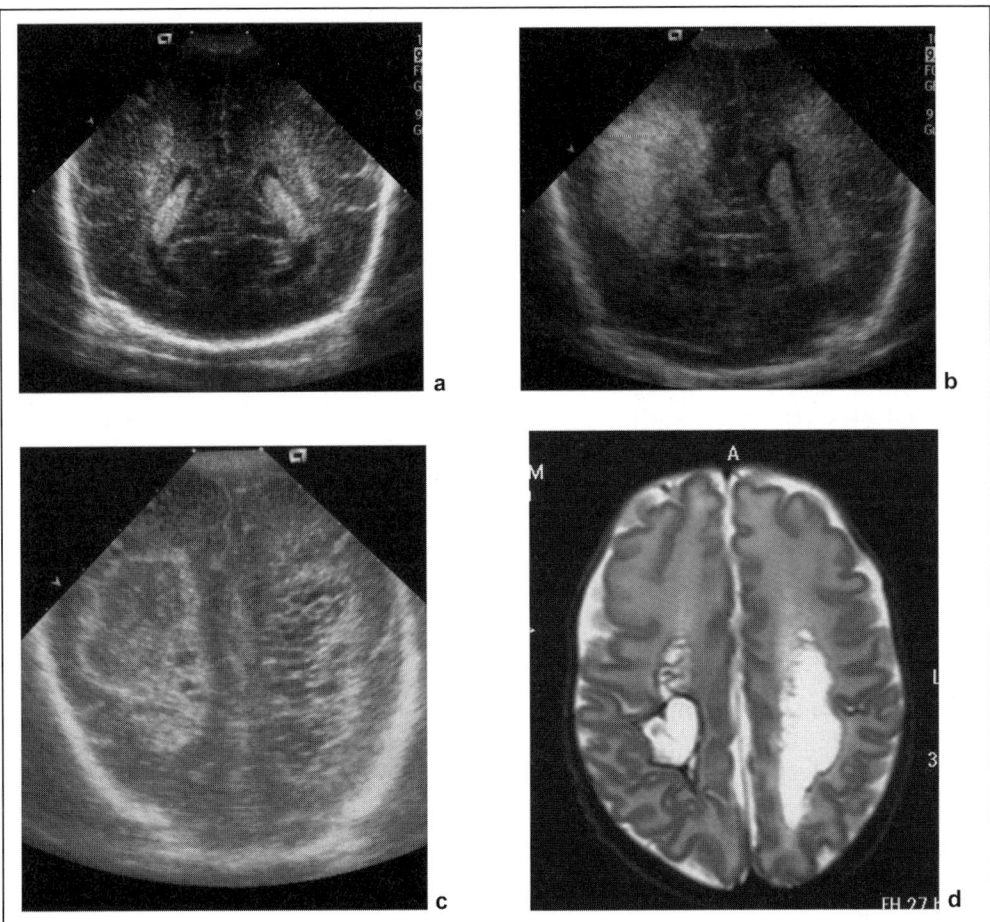

Fig. 4. A 28-week gestation baby born after severe chorioamnionitis resulting in a double lesion, periventricular leucomalacia (PVL), and intraventricular haemorrhage. (a) Posterior coronal ultrasound scan at 3 hours showing increased bilateral periventricular echogenicity. (b) Posterior coronal ultrasound scan at 96 hours showing a complicated outcome (bilateral increased echogenic areas in the right hemisphere suggesting venous infarction). (c) Posterior coronal ultrasound scan at 36 weeks of corrected age showing cavitations. (d) Axial T2 magnetic resonance scan at 40 weeks of corrected age showing bilateral cavitations (venous infarction (haemosiderin deposition) on the right; severe loss of parenchyma due to cystic PVL on the left).

distress or acidosis or both. There are also infants without evidence of fetal distress in labour who are acidotic at birth and have a clinical course suggestive of hypoxia. Risk factors may be cumulative but it remains crucial to examine the pathway that leads to asphyxia and to understand those aetiological processes associated with the final insult that dominates the outcome. The majority of infants with asphyxia and neonatal encephalopathy have more antepartum risk factors than normal controls (Little, 1861). The greater the number of risk factors the greater the chance of developing neonatal encephalopathy and of having brain damage. White matter lesions are correlated more with subacute antenatal conditions occurring days or hours before birth, while deep grey matter and cortical lesions reflect acute intrapartum events occurring in the minutes before birth.

There remain some infants with no risk factors who also develop lesions. Although almost all brain lesions are of recent onset, suggesting that the causal pathway for asphyxia may start before birth, there is a little evidence that the major component of damage occurs just before labour.

Other hypoxic-ischaemic 'perinatal' lesions include *arterial infarcts* (stroke); these lesions often lack a defined prenatal phase although they may be related to specific prenatal conditions (Lee et al., 2005; Benders et al., 2007). There is evidence that 'the process of infarction does not start until the onset of labour and delivery, suggesting that a degree of asphyxia or trauma or possibly even a "normal labour and delivery" is necessary to establish infarction in "primed" tissue' (de Vries et al., 1997; Lee et al., 2005; Benders et al., 2007) (Fig. 1).

Adverse antenatal factors, such as maternal systemic disease, intrauterine growth retardation, raised blood pressure, bleeding, infections, reduced fetal movements, trauma, maternal cocaine abuse, and maternal abdominal pain, are also more frequent than in the normal population. It is known that the haemodynamic status of the newborn infant in the first hours of life and the delivery itself make the neonate more vulnerable to thrombotic-ischaemic events, mainly in the cerebral system. There are some physiological neonatal conditions that predispose to thrombotic events, such as polycythaemia and dehydration in the first hours after delivery. There are other pathological conditions predisposing to thrombotic-embolic events such as sepsis, congenital heart disease, pulmonary hypertension, arterial catheterization, extracorporeal membrane oxygenation (ECMO), trauma, Leiden factor mutation, and congenital clotting abnormalities (Fig. 2).

In published reports, it is usual to classify strokes by the time of detection rather than the time of onset. In addition, lesions detected in the newborn period that may have occurred before the onset of labour should be kept separate from those that appear to have occurred during or just after labour (Cowan et al., 2003; Benders et al., 2007).

The time of detection can be divided into three categories, acknowledging that the moment of onset cannot always be established:

Fetal stroke: lesions detected *in utero* before the onset of labour or detected by early neonatal imaging (in the first week after birth) and with clear signs of tissue loss.

Perinatal stroke: divided by age of symptom onset into (a) those presenting with symptoms in the first week *(early neonatal)*, which are likely to be related to labour or parturition, including placental embolism, early onset infection, trauma, and diffuse hypoxic-ischaemic encephalopathy; and (b) those occurring after first week *(late neonatal)*, related to disorders of the late neonatal period, including cardiac disease, venous thrombosis with embolism, postnatal infection, and other events after birth.

In most cases, additional factors are involved in the insult but it is difficult to determine which of these are specifically associated with the presence or extent of the lesion.

The term 'perinatal' seems less appropriate for certain lesions affecting premature babies. *Intraventricular haemorrhage* (IVH) represent a typical postnatal phenomenon (onset within the first 96 hours), although it is related to the type and quality of the delivery. In published reports, opinions are divided: some data show that IVH is associated mainly with trauma and with spontaneous vaginal delivery, while others show that IVH is not associated with the mode of delivery (Ment, 2006). The major risk factor for IVH is prematurity itself and the incidence is inversely correlated with gestational age. Some antenatal conditions – such as fertility treatment, maternal illness, and thrombophilic congenital conditions – can be risk factors, but none of these is specifically associated with IVH. Other neonatal factors can also be involved in IVH, such as hypertension, haemodynamic and metabolic changes, severe hypercapnia, and clotting disorders. Hypoperfusion has often been suggested as a common denominator before the development of IVH.

More complex is the issue of how 'perinatal' is *periventricular leucomalacia* (PVL), the most representative form of white matter disease (WMD). Although PVL is traditionally considered an ischaemic lesion and many infants develop it following an evident clinical event, in others the lesions are detected incidentally by cranial ultrasound. It is clear that various different factors may play a role in the development of PVL. Perinatal infection/inflammation seems to be a major cause of both premature delivery and perinatal brain damage. Maternal intrauterine infection results in a systemic fetal inflammatory response, which can be harmful to the fetal developing brain. Immature oligodendrocytes are vulnerable to proinflammatory cytokines, an important factor in white matter damage. Inflammation may play a major role at any time before delivery. On the other hand inadvertent postnatal hypocapnia, which is not always caused by hyperventilation, is associated with WMD as well as with cerebral palsy. Neonates, and particularly preterm infants, are at high risk of oxidative stress because they are susceptible to free radicals. These free radicals are mainly generated by hyperoxia and hypoxia, ischaemia-reperfusion, and neutrophil activation. In the preterm infant there is an imbalance between antioxidant and oxidant systems which causes the cellular damage. These components can all be present in the very low birthweight infant and it is difficult to determine which plays the principal part in the damage. Neuroimaging abnormalities can appear early but in some cases not until 2 to 3 weeks after the insult, which makes it difficult to time the lesions accurately (Arthur & Ramenghi, 2001; de Vries & Levene, 2001).

Definition of injury

Neonatal brain injury encompasses a wide spectrum of conditions that result in damage to the nervous system, ultimately causing impaired function. As any abnormal appearance on imaging can be defined as an injury, further evaluation of the shape, size, structure, and signal intensity of the lesion is important. An abnormality can be identified as a lesion if it can be seen in more than one sequence and in more than one plane. In addition it should be possible to determine whether the lesion is evolving and in what way (Fig. 3). One should then evaluate whether the baby has an appropriate clinical presentation and specific signs on subsequent follow-up, as an important further step is to correlate the cerebral damage with the clinical outcome (Rutherford *et al.*, 1995; Triulzi *et al.*, 2001; Righini *et al.*, 2003; Rutherford *et al.*, 2004; Righini *et al.*, 2005; Swaiman & Wu, 2006). Very subtle injuries, barely visible on magnetic resonance imaging (MRI), may cause severe clinical problems (for example, brain stem lesions) while other more obvious abnormalities, such as intraventricular haemorrhage, may have no specific clinical outcome.

The appearance of the lesion is influenced by several different factors, for example the timing of the scan (ultrasound or MRI) from the onset of the insult, the gestation of the infant, and the imaging sequences used (especially for MRI). In the neonate these appearances will be modified by continuing growth and development. Repeated scans can show whether or not an injury is permanent, and the effects on the developing brain (Fig. 4).

What is the correlation between injury and functional consequence?

Lesions detected by MRI in the white matter may be associated with cognitive problems in term infants, while lesions to the basal ganglia or abnormal signals in the posterior limbs of internal capsule are associated with motor problems (Rutherford et al., 1995; Rutherford et al., 2004; Swaiman & Wu, 2006).

No distinct lesion correlated with impaired cognitive outcome in preterm infants has been identified by neuroradiological techniques, even with MRI. Advances in MRI seem to show that premature babies have microstructural differences in cerebral white matter compared with term-born control infants in the absence of focal abnormalities (overt pathology) and there is evidence that cognitive impairment may be associated with more subtle abnormalities of cerebral white matter. These can appear as a diffuse excessive high signal intensity (DEHSI) on T2-weighted images or increases in the apparent diffusion coefficient on diffusion-weighted imaging (Childs et al., 1998; Childs et al., 2001a; Childs et al., 2001b; Counsell et al., 2003; Counsell et al., 2006).

'Major disability' is usually defined as 'cerebral palsy and/or mental retardation' and it is not easy to diagnose before 1 to 2 years of age. In younger babies it remains very difficult to differentiate delay from disability. The incidence of disability increases with age (Swaiman & Wu, 2006). The most important issue remains how to minimize the incidence of disabilities.

Neuroprotective strategies focusing on term newborn infants involve prompt and effective resuscitation of asphyxiated babies and vigilant surveillance for conditions such as hypoglycaemia, excessive hyperbilirubinaemia, and dehydration in all low-risk term infants.

Despite the fact that 'perinatal brain injury' seems a more appropriate expression for preterm than full-term infants, a simple neuroprotective strategy is less obvious in preterm infants. Many aspects of intensive care medicine of very premature babies – such as ventilation, infection, and nutrition – are likely to play an important role in influencing the neurological outcome. The reduction in the incidence of brain lesions in these babies is far from being fully understood.

References

Arthur, R. & Ramenghi, L.A. (2001): Imaging of the neonatal brain. In: *Fetal and neonatal neurology and neurosurgery*. Edinburgh: Churchill Livingstone.

Benders, M.J., Groenendaal, F., Uiterwaal, C.S., Nikkels, P.G., Bruinse, H.W., Nievelstein, R.A. & de Vries, L.S. (2007): Maternal and infant characteristics associated with perinatal arterial stroke in the preterm infant. *Stroke* **38,** 1759–1765.

Childs, A.M., Ramenghi, L.A., Evans, D.J., Ridgeway, J., Saysell, M., Martinez, D., Arthur, R., Tanner, S. & Levene, M.I. (1998): MR features of developing periventricular white matter in preterm infants: evidence of glial cell migration. *Am. J. Neuroradiol.* **19,** 971–976.

Childs, A.M., Cornette, L., Ramenghi, L.A., Tanner, S.F., Arthur, R.J., Martinez, D. & Levene, M.I. (2001a): Magnetic resonance and cranial ultrasound characteristics of periventricular white matter abnormalities in newborn infants. *Clin. Radiol.* **56,** 647–655.

Childs, A.M., Ramenghi, L.A., Cornette, L., Tanner, S.F., Arthur, R.J., Martinez, D. & Levene, M.I. (2001b): Cerebral maturation in premature infants: quantitative assessment using MR imaging. *Am. J. Neuroradiol.* **22,** 1577–1582.

Counsell, S.J., Allsop, J.M., Harrison, M.C., Larkman, D.J., Kennea, N.L., Kapellou, O., Cowan, F.M., Hajnal, J.V., Edwards, A.D. & Rutherford, M.A. (2003): Diffusion-weighted imaging of the brain in preterm infants with focal and diffuse white matter abnromality. *Pediatrics* **112,** 1–7.

Counsell, S.J., Shen, Y., Boardman, J.P., Larkman, D.J., Kapellou, O., Ward, P., Allsop, J.M., Cowan, F.M., Hajnal, J.V., Edwards, A.D. & Rutherford, M.A. (2006): Axial and radial diffusivity in preterm infants who have diffuse white matter changes on magnetic resonance imaging at term-equivalent age. *Pediatrics* **117,** 376–386.

Cowan, F. & Squir, W. (2004): The value of autopsy in determining the cause of failure to respond to resuscitation at birth. *Semin. Neonatol.* **9,** 331–345.

Cowan, F., Rutherford, M., Groenendaal, F., Eken, P., Mercuri, E., Bydder, G.M., Meiners, L.C., Dubowitz, L.M. & de Vries, L.S. (2003): Origin and timing of brain lesions in term infants with neonatal encephalopathy. *Lancet* **361,** 736–742.

de Vries, L.S. & Levene, M.I. (2001): Cerebral ischemic lesions. In: *Fetal and neonatal neurology and neurosurgery.* Edinburgh: Churchill Livingstone.

de Vries, L.S., Groenendaal, F., Eken, P., van Haastert, I.C., Rademaker, K.J. & Meiners, L.C. (1997): Infarcts in the vascular distribution of the middle cerebral artery in preterm and full-term infants. *Neuropediatrics* **28,** 88–96.

Lee, J., Croen, L.A., Backstrand, K.H., Yoshida, C.K., Henning, L.H., Lindan, C., Ferriero, D.M., Fullerton, H.J., Barkovich, A.J. & Wu, Y.W. (2005): Maternal and infant characteristics associated with perinatal arterial stroke in the infant. *JAMA* **293,** 723–729.

Little, W.J. (1861): On the influence of abnormal parturition, difficult labours, premature birth, and asphyxia neonatorum on the mental and physical condition of the child, especially in relation to deformities. *Trans. Obstet. Soc. Lond.* **3,** 293.

Ment, L.R. (2006): Intraventricular hemorrhage of the preterm neonate. In: *Pediatric neurology*, eds. K.F. Swaiman, S. Ashwal & D.M. Ferriero. Philadelphia: Mosby Elsevier.

Righini, A., Ramenghi, L.A., Parini, R., Triulzi, F. & Mosca, F. (2003): Water apparent diffusion coefficient and T2 changes in the acute stage of maple syrup urine disease: evidence of intramyelinic and vasogenic interstitial edema. *J. Neuroimaging* **13,** 162–165.

Righini, A., Ramenghi, L., Zirpoli, S., Mosca, F. & Triulzi, F. (2005): Brain apparent diffusion coefficient decrease during correction of severe hypernatremic dehydration. *Am. J. Neuroradiol.* **26,** 1690–1694.

Rutherford, M.A., Pennock, JM, Schwieso, JE, Cowan, FM, Dubowitz, LM. (1995): Hypoxic ischaemic encephalopathy: early magnetic resonance imaging findings and their evolution. *Neuropediatrics* **26,** 83–191.

Rutherford, M.A., Counsell, S., Allsop, J., Boardman, J., Kapellou, O., Larkman, D., Hajnal, J., Edwards, D. & Cowan, F. (2004): Diffusion weighted magnetic resonance imaging in term perinatal brain injury: a comparison with site of lesion and time from birth. *Pediatrics* **114,** 1004–1014.

Swaiman, K.F. & Wu, Y. (2006): Cerebral palsy. In: *Pediatric neurology*, ed. K.F. Swaiman, S. Ashwal & D.M. Ferriero. Philadelphia: Mosby Elsevier.

Triulzi, F., Baldoli, C. & Parazzini, C. (2001): Neonatal MR imaging. *Magn. Reson. Imaging Clin. North Am.* **9,** 57–82.

Chapter 8

Is intensive care for all very immature babies justified?

Malcolm Levene

Academic Department of Paediatrics, Leeds General Infirmary, Belmont Grove, LS2 9NS Leeds, UK
m.i.levene@leeds.ac.uk

Summary

The survival of extremely preterm infants has never been higher, and increasing numbers of very immature babies are being born. In recent years some concern has been expressed about whether the outcome in terms of a high prevalence of neurodevelopmental disability justifies the introduction of intensive care in the most immature infants of 22 to 24 weeks' gestation. In this chapter I review the variabilities that may influence published outcome in these groups and explore confounding variables.

Introduction

The development of neonatal intensive care over the past 50 years has been one of the great success stories of modern medicine. Very immature babies are now surviving intact more than ever before and as a result of this success, neonatologists need to be more critical of the quality of life in survivors rather than just the number of babies who survive to go home. The lower limit of viability is currently 22 to 23 weeks of gestation, and it is exceptional for babies of 22 weeks or below to survive. Evidence is accumulating that the neurodevelopmental outcome in survivors at the edge of viability is poor. A British study (Marlow *et al.*, 2005) reported the outcome of 308 surviving infants at 6 years who had been born at 25 weeks' gestation or less in 1995. Of these, 44 per cent had moderate to severe disability and 34 per cent had mild disability; only 20 per cent were considered normal.

In the light of the reportedly poor outcome, this chapter examines the question of whether neonatologists are justified in providing neonatal intensive care for infants of 22 to 24 weeks' gestation.

To make sense of outcome data in very immature babies and to ensure that the researcher is comparing like with like, it is necessary to critically review the studies that have reported both survival rates and rates of disability in survivors. Table 1 lists some variables that may affect the comparability of outcome data between different studies. Some of these variables will be considered here in more detail.

Table 1. Variables that may affect the comparability of outcome data between different studies

- Survival and outcome data in the modern era
- Reporting gestational age rather than birth weight
- Denominator data and age at death
- Reports on regional outcome *vs.* hospital specific data
- Follow-up compliance
- Proportion of babies with growth restriction
- Sex
- Numbers of multiple births
- Racial characteristics
- 'Lethal' congenital malformations

Survival in the modern era

The two most important interventions in neonatal medicine that have been shown to improve survival rates are the widespread administration of antenatal steroids by obstetricians and the introduction of early surfactant instillation in premature babies. Although antenatal steroids were first shown to be effective in reducing mortality in the 1970s, it was not until the early to mid-1990s that they became widely used. Surfactant trials were still recruiting babies in the early 1990s and it was not until the mid-1990s that the use of surfactant became widespread in developed countries. Therefore although the 'modern era' of neonatal intensive care has been taken from 1990, it is probably more appropriate for the year 1995 to be the cusp for the widespread introduction of modern neonatal care with the application of these treatments. Consequently, studies before 1995, and certainly before 1990, cannot be considered to offer the same quality of care as from 1995 onwards. Studies before this time reporting outcome should not be included for the purposes of determining outcome today.

Unfortunately it takes a long time to collect outcome data on surviving infants. The most severe forms of neurodevelopmental disability can usually be recognized by the time the baby is 18 to 24 months old, but more subtle though still important disabilities may take up to 5 years or longer to become manifest. Consequently very premature babies born in 1995 require follow-up in 2000 to assess their 5-year outcome, and it may take a further 2 years for the data to be published in full. Some readers of those data will then consider that neonatal care has moved on and that data from 1995 are no longer relevant in 2002. This circular argument is discussed later in the chapter.

Several reports have described follow-up in adolescence or adult life of cohorts of prematurely-born babies (Hack *et al.*, 2002). To obtain this type of data will take decades to achieve, and those young adults whose outcome is now reported were born in 1977 to 1979. In the intervening years there have been many changes in clinical management.

Gestational age *vs.* birth weight

Birth weight was generally more reliable than gestational age and is the reason that historically many studies have reported outcome by birth weight rather than by gestational age. In developed countries most women now have an ultrasound dating scan early in pregnancy which allows the investigator to be much more confident about reporting the outcome of pregnancy by gestational age.

There are various methodological problems with using birth weight categories. These include the skewing of data in centres with a high proportion of growth-restricted fetuses or where there are increased numbers of multiple births, as these sibships are likely to comprise babies whose growth might have been restricted *in utero*. A second problem is the classification of birth weight groups. Studies also report birth weight categories differently. For example, one study may describe outcome of babies weighing less than 1,000 g (that is, 999 g and less) while another may report categories of babies weighing 1,000 g or less (that is, < 1,001 g). Although this difference in weight may not seem significant, most obstetric units record birth weight to the nearest 5 or 10 g, thereby tending to bias these categories.

Gestational age as assessed by an early ultrasound scan must be the gold standard for measuring outcome. This is particularly important when an obstetrician or neonatologist counsels parents in preterm labour about the likely outcome as the birth weight will not be known at that time, though there should be an accurate assessment of gestation.

Denominators and time of death

A major variable in determining mortality and morbidity data is the use of different denominators. In a systematic review (Evans & Levene, 2000), we determined three different denominators that had been reported in papers describing outcome in peer-reviewed journals. We divided them into three categories: grade A, studies reporting on the outcome of all babies who were alive in labour (this included babies who died in labour before birth) and represented the highest standard of reporting outcome; grade B included the outcome of babies who were born alive but did not include stillbirths; grade C included only babies admitted alive to the neonatal intensive care unit.

Fig. 1 shows the results of data reported by these three grades. For babies born at less than 26 weeks' gestation there was a significant trend towards increased survival into more selective groups (grade C > grade B > grade A; $p < 0.001$). In addition, for infants of 25 weeks' gestation there was an 18 per cent improvement in outcome when grade C was compared with grade A; for babies born at 24 weeks and 23 weeks this difference between these two grades was 56 per cent and 100 per cent, respectively. Hence these very large differences at the extremes of prematurity are likely to skew outcome data significantly.

Another variable which may have a significant effect on reported survival rates is the cut-off time when the baby died. Some data may report perinatal survival rates (that is, only those babies who are still alive at 7 days of age, irrespective of later death). Others may report neonatal survival rates (deaths only up to 28 days), and others may report deaths before discharge home. Rarely, reports may include babies who died at any age before the assessment of outcome. Clearly, censoring the data in these different ways may also have a major effect on reported outcome.

Regional data *vs.* centre data

Many published reports on outcome describe the results of one centre or a small number of selected neonatal intensive care units. For many reasons these may not be representative of the region within which they work. Reports on outcome are often from centres of excellence where the results may not be representative of other similar sized hospitals which are perhaps not as well staffed or equipped. Some centres may have selective admission policies, such as not taking babies with surgical abnormalities, and others may be heavily oversubscribed with referrals and are selective in whom they admit. Some major centres which publish outcome data

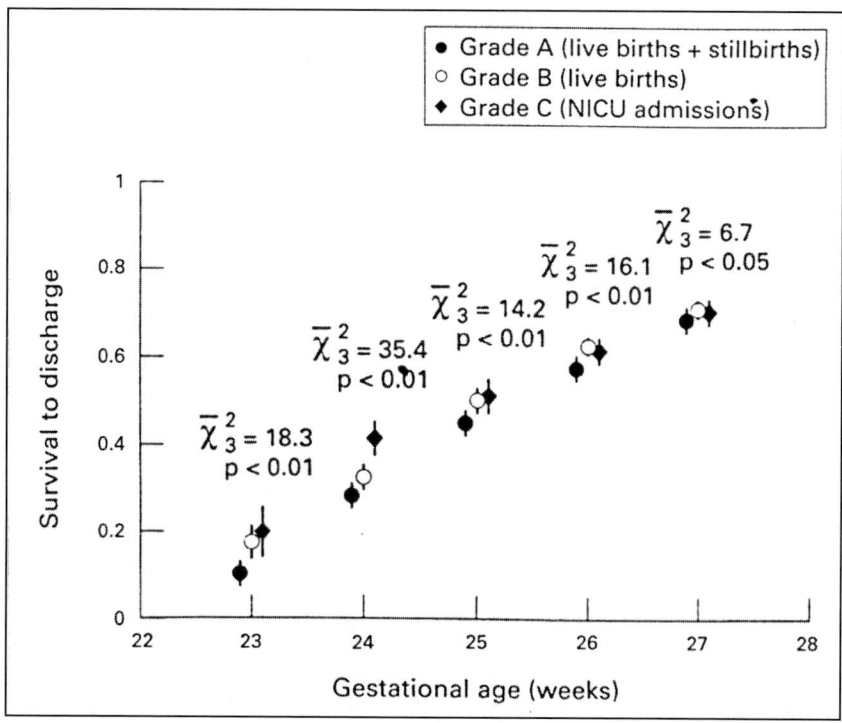

Fig. 1. Survival of preterm infants by gestational age and classification of cohort study. Bars indicate 95 per cent confidence intervals. NICU, neonatal intensive care unit. Reproduced with permission of Archives of Disease in Childhood (Evans & Levene, 2000).

have no obstetric unit on-site so all referrals will come from other hospitals. Clearly only babies who are alive at the time of referral will be transferred and this will cause data skewing similar to that described above for selective admission (Evans & Levene, 2001). In a study comparing outcome variables at 18 to 22 months in a group of babies born weighing less than 1 kg in 12 centres of excellence in the USA, there were major differences in most measures of outcome. The best centre reported that 4.5 per cent of survivors had cerebral palsy, compared with the worst centre where the rate was 23.1 per cent (Vohr et al., 2004).

The alternative strategy is to report outcome in all babies of a similar gestational age group born in a geographically-based region. The larger the region, the more representative the data will be for any particular baby. This also acts as a benchmark by which to audit individual centres. Geographically-based data have been published from regional health authorities in the United Kingdom (Bohin et al., 1996; Tin et al., 1997), states in Australia (Sutton et al., 1999; Doyle et al., 2001), and whole countries such as the United Kingdom (Wood et al., 2000), Finland (Tommiska et al., 2007), and Belgium (Vanhaesbrouck et al., 2004).

Levene (2004) published a review of survival in geographically-based studies describing deaths within the first year of life with a birth cohort during or after 1990, expressed by gestational age and where all liveborn infants were reported, including those who were not offered intensive care. Only seven studies fulfilled these five criteria. The survival rate by week of gestational age is shown in Table 2. There is clearly a very close relation between reducing gestational age and increased mortality. A similar study of centre-based outcome was carried out using the criteria described above. Only five studies fulfilled all these criteria (Lefebre et al., 1996;

Bottoms et al., 1997; Hack et al., 1999; El-Metawally et al., 2000; Jacobs et al., 2000) and all were from North America (USA, three centres; Canada, two centres). Fig. 2 shows a comparison of survival between geographically-based studies and centre-based studies. For each week of gestational age from 22 to 27 weeks there is a lower mortality in centre-based studies than in geographically-based studies. The survival rate for centre-based studies is about one week better than for geographically-based studies for each individual week of gestational age.

Table 2. Overall mortality and major morbidity rates by gestational ages from selected published studies (see text)

	Weeks of gestational age						
	21	22	23	24	25	26	27
Per cent survival	0	2	8	26	46	63	74
Per cent severe morbidity	–	–	24	30	22.5	12	12

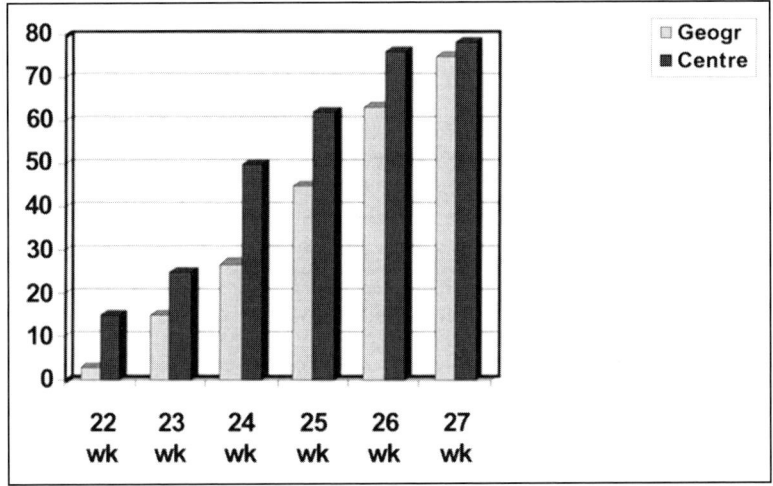

Fig. 2. Centre-based outcome data (dark columns) against geographically based survival data (lighter columns).

The same protocol was also applied to studies that reported neurodevelopmental outcome by gestational age. The criteria for those studies were cohorts born largely during or after 1990 and where there was a follow-up compliance of at least 85 per cent of all surviving infants. Only five studies were found that fulfilled these requirements. Each study used a slightly different threshold for major disability, but Table 2 shows the data where major disability was defined as including severe cerebral palsy rendering the child unable to walk independently, a DQ/IQ below 70, or registered blind or deaf (requiring hearing aids). There appears to be a much less close relation between gestational age and adverse outcome than between gestational age and mortality. Approximately 20 to 30 per cent of babies born at 23 to 25 weeks had a major disability compared with 12 per cent in those born at 26 to 27 weeks.

It is possible to interpolate the outcome data from these two analyses to produce a histogram showing the chances of babies surviving without major disability (Fig. 3). According to these data, for babies born at 25 weeks only 37 per cent survived without major disability, compared with 54 per cent at 26 weeks.

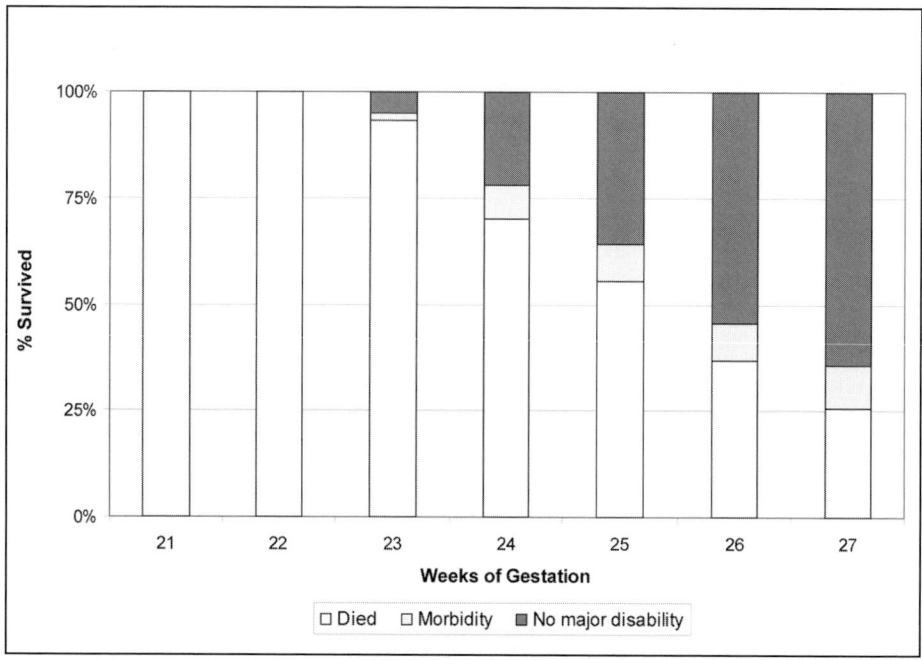

Fig. 3. Combined mortality and morbidity data. Reproduced with permission of Acta Paediatrica (Levene, 2004).

Hard-to-find babies

A well recognized weakness of follow-up studies reporting neurodevelopmental outcome is the fact that compliance figures are often poor for ascertaining all surviving babies. Some follow-up studies report outcome in cohorts where barely 50 per cent of babies have been seen at the census date. There is evidence that the babies who are hardest to find at follow-up are those with a higher incidence of disability, so the compliance rate is an important factor in the introduction of bias. Tin et al. (1998) reported outcome in a group of very preterm babies who had reached the age of 2 years. They followed up all 566 surviving infants and found that 61 (11 per cent) were hard to trace. When these children were eventually contacted and examined they found that there was a fivefold increase in disability in the hard-to-find group compared with the standard follow-up group ($p < 0.001$). An Australian study reported that the 25 per cent of children most difficult to find for follow-up at 5 years had a 41 per cent disability rate compared with 19 per cent in the group that was easy to find (Callanan et al., 2001).

What is the most up-to-date evidence?

Since my original publication in 2004 and as described above, there have been several further papers on the long-term outcome in babies born in the latter half of the 1990s and early 2000s which are reviewed here.

Hintz et al. (2005) compared two cohorts of infants of 24 weeks' gestation and below, the first born between 1993 and 1996 and the second born between 1996 and 1999. They showed no difference in outcome (cerebral palsy, developmental index < 70, and neurodevelopmental impairment) between the two cohorts, but there was a higher incidence of bronchopulmonary dysplasia and retinopathy of prematurity in the more recent cohort, while the incidence of severe intraventricular haemorrhage was reduced.

In a national study from Finland (Tommiska et al., 2007), a comparison was made between two cohorts of babies with birth weight < 1,000 g and < 27 weeks of gestation born in 1996 to 1997 and those born in 1999 to 2000. The rate of cerebral palsy and severe visual impairment showed no difference between the two periods.

Wilson-Costello et al. (2007) compared three birth epochs – 1982–1989, 1990–1999, and 2000–2002 – in groups of babies weighing 500 to 999 g born in a single American centre. They showed a statistically significant reduction in cerebral palsy, neurodevelopmental impairment, blindness, and deafness when the three cohorts were compared. The major improvement had occurred in the most recent two epochs, and the incidence of most disabilities had increased in the middle epoch compared with the earliest one.

In summary, there is no consensus view as to whether there has been an improvement in recent years in the survival of extremely tiny infants without severe neurodevelopmental disability. Two of the three most recent studies do not suggest any improvement, but the single centre study from the USA did report a reduction in a variety of disabilities in a 2000–2002 cohort, although that study has many of the methodological pitfalls discussed above.

Other factors

Intrauterine growth restriction appears to have an effect on mortality. A national survey of all babies born in Israel (Regev et al., 2003) showed that for every week of gestational age the mortality was higher in small-for-gestational-age infants than in those who were appropriately grown. In addition, the mortality for extremely low birth weight twins (< 1000 g) was higher than for singletons of the same birth weight, although this trend was reversed for larger twins compared to singletons (Glinianaia et al., 2000).

Sex is also important and there is a greater risk of adverse outcome in boys than in girls. The British Epicure study of the outcome of babies born at a gestational age of 25 weeks and assessed at 6 years showed that boys had on average a 10 point reduction in cognitive skills compared with similarly prematurely born girls, as well as a significant increase in the risk of overall disability (Marlow et al., 2005). In another American study of babies born at less than 28 weeks of gestation the risk of cerebral palsy, mental or physical developmental index (MDI, PDI) < 70, deafness, or blindness was significantly increased for boys compared with girls (Hintz et al., 2006).

References

Bohin, S., Draper, E.S. & Field, D.J. (1996): Impact of extremely immature infants on neonatal services. *Arch. Dis. Child. Fetal Neonat. Ed.* **74**, F110–F113.

Bottoms, S.F., Paul, R.H., Iams, J.D., Mercer, B.M., Thom, E.A. & Roberts, J.M. (1997): Obstetrical determinants of neonatal survival: influence of willingness to perform cesarean section delivery on survival of extremely-low-birth-weight infants. National Institute of Child Health and Human Development Network of Maternal-Fetal Medicine Units. *Am. J. Obstet. Gynecol.* **176**, 960–966.

Callanan, C., Doyle, L.W., Rickards, A.L., Kelly, E.A., Ford, G.W. & Davis, N.M. (2001): Children followed with difficulty: how do they differ? *J. Paediatr. Child Health* **37**, 152–156.

Doyle, L.W. (2001): Outcome at 5 years of age of children 23 to 27 weeks' gestation: refining the prognosis. *Pediatrics* **108,** 134–141.

El-Metwally, D., Vohr, B. & Tucker, R. (2000): Survival and neonatal morbidity at the limits of viability in the mid 1990s: 22 to 25 weeks. *J. Pediatr.* **137,** 616–622.

Evans, D.J. & Levene, M.I. (2001): Evidence of selection bias in preterm survival studies: a systematic review. *Arch. Dis. Child. Fetal Neonat. Ed.* **84,** F79–F84.

Hack, M. & Fanaroff, A.A. (1999): Outcomes of children of extremely low birthweight and gestational age in the 1990s. *Early Hum. Dev.* **53,** 193–218.

Hack, M., Flannery, D.J., Schluchter, M., Cartar, L., Borawski, E. & Klein, N. (2002): Outcomes in young adulthood for very-low-birth-weight infants. *N. Engl. J. Med.* **346,** 149–157.

Glinianaia, S.V., Pharoah, P. & Sturgiss, S.N. (2000): Comparative trends in cause-specific fetal and neonatal mortality in twin and singleton births in the North of England, 1982–1994. *Br. J. Obstet. Gynaecol.* **107,** 452–460.

Hintz, S.R., Kendrick, D.E., Vohr, B.R., Poole, W.K. & Higgins, R.D. for National Institute of Child Health and Human Development Neonatal Research Network (2005): Changes in neurodevelopmental outcomes at 18 to 22 months' corrected age among infants of less than 25 weeks' gestational age born in 1993–1999. *Pediatrics* **115,** 1645–1651.

Hintz, S.R., Kendrick, D.E. & Vohr, B.R. (2006): Gender differences in neurodevelopmental outcomes among extremely preterm, extremely-low-birthweight infants. *Acta Paediatr.* **95,** 1239–1248.

Jacobs, S.E., O'Brien, K., Inwood, S., Kelly, E.N. & Whyte, H.E. (2000): Outcome of infants 23–26 weeks' gestation pre- and post-surfactant. *Acta Paediatr.* **89,** 959–965.

Lefebvre, F., Glorieux, J. & St-Laurent-Gagnon, T. (1996): Neonatal survival and disability rate at age 18 months for infants born between 23 and 28 weeks of gestation. *Am. J. Obstet. Gynecol.* **174,** 833–838.

Levene, M. (2004): Is intensive care for very immature babies justified? *Acta Paediatr.* **93,** 149–152.

Marlow, N., Wolke, D., Bracewell, M.A. & Samara, M., for the EPICure Study Group (2005): Neurologic and developmental disability at six years of age after extremely preterm birth. *N. Engl. J. Med.* **352,** 9–19.

Regev, R.H., Lusky, A., Dolfin, T., Litmanovitz, I., Arnon, S. & Reichman, B. for the Israel Neonatal Network (2003): Excess mortality and morbidity among small-for-gestational-age premature infants: a population-based study. *J. Pediatr.* **143,** 186–191.

Sutton, L., Bajuk, B. & The NSW Neonatal Intensive Care Unit Study Group (1999): Population-based study of infants born at less than 28 weeks' gestation in New South Wales, Australia, in 1992–3. *Pediatr. Perinat. Epidemiol.* **13,** 288–301.

Tin, W., Fritz, S., Wariyar, U. & Hey, E. (1998): Outcome of very preterm birth: children reviewed with ease at 2 years differ from those followed up with difficulty. *Arch. Dis. Child. Fetal Neonat. Ed.* **79,** F83–F87.

Tin, W., Wariyar, U. & Hey, E. for the Northern Neonatal Network (1997): Changing prognosis for babies of less than 28 weeks' gestation in the north of England between 1983 and 1994. *BMJ* **314,** 107–111.

Tommiska, V., Heinonen, K., Lehtonen, L., Renlund, M., Saarela, T., Tammela, O., Virtanen, M. & Fellman, V. (2007): No improvement in outcome of nationwide extremely low birth weight infant populations between 1996–1997 and 1999–2000. *Pediatrics* **119,** 29–36.

Vanhaesebrouck, P., Allegaert, K., Bottu, J., Debauche, C., Devlieger, H., Docx, M., François, A., Haumont, D., Lombet, J., Rigo, J., Smets, K., Vanherreweghe, I., Van Overmeire, B., Van Reempts, P. for the Extremely Preterm Infants in Belgium Study Group (2004): The EPIBEL study: outcomes to discharge from hospital for extremely preterm infants in Belgium. *Pediatrics* **114,** 663–675.

Vohr, B.R., Wright, L.L., Dusick, A.M., Perritt, R., Poole, W.K., Tyson, J.E., Steichen, J.J., Bauer, C.R., Wilson-Costello, D.E. & Mayes, L.C. for the Neonatal Research Network (2004): Center differences and outcomes of extremely low birth weight infants. *Pediatrics* **113,** 781–789.

Wilson-Costello, D., Friedman, H., Minich, N., Siner, B., Taylor, G., Schluchter, M. & Hack, M. (2007): Improved neurodevelopmental outcomes for extremely low birth weight infants in 2000–2002. *Pediatrics* **119,** 37–45.

Wood, N.S., Marlow, N., Costeloe, K., Gibson, A.T. & Wilkinson, A.R. (2000): Neurologic and developmental disability after extremely preterm birth. *N. Engl. J. Med.* **343,** 378–384.

Chapter 9

Twins and triplets: relative effect of plurality and prematurity on neurological outcome

Olivier Baud *°, Romain H. Fontaine °, Gauthier Loron ° and Paul Olivier °

Service de Réanimation et de Pédiatrie Néonatales;
° *Équipe Avenir R05230HS, INSERM U676, Université Paris 7, Hôpital Robert-Debré, 48 Bd Sérurier,*
75019 Paris, France
olivier.baud@rdb.aphp.fr

Summary

Spontaneously conceived and iatrogenic multiple pregnancies following assisted reproductive techniques remain a public health issue. An increased incidence of neonatal mortality and neurological morbidity in twins is mainly a reflection of the rate of very preterm birth, monochorionicity, and the occurrence of twin-twin transfusion syndrome. Dramatic improvements in the prognosis of twin-twin transfusion syndrome following laser coagulation surgery involved reduction in prematurity and severe brain lesions. Triplets and higher order multiples seem to have a significant increase in neurological morbidity before 32 weeks' gestation but very few reliable studies have addressed the long-term follow-up of these multiple pregnancies. Prevention of prematurity associated with multiple pregnancies, together with the early diagnosis and laser treatment of a twin-twin transfusion syndrome, appear to be the most valuable goals in preventing neurological impairment in multiple gestations.

Introduction

The increasing number of multiple gestations is having an important impact because of higher complication rates. The incidence of very low birth weight infants has increased markedly, leading to a greater risk of major neonatal morbidity and mortality. In the 1990s, preterm births occurred in 9.7 per cent of singleton gestations, compared with 48 per cent of twins and 88 per cent of triplets or higher order births (Luke, 1994). Gestational age-adjusted comparisons of outcome between singletons and multiples have shown conflicting results owing to several confounding variables. The purpose of this comprehensive review is to provide evidence-based data and conclusions to answer to this crucial question: are multiple gestations at increased risk of neurological impairment?

Plurality and chorionicity

There are two types of twins – monozygotic and dizygotic. Monozygotic twins develop from a single fertilized ovum which splits into two fetuses with the same genetic material. Dizygotic twins arise from more than one fertilized ovum and are as genetically similar as any full siblings. While the rate of dizygotic twins varies by population, the incidence of monozygotic twins is constant throughout the world at 3.5 per 1,000 and is not influenced by race, maternal age, nutrition, or other factors (Benirschke & Kim, 1973). Dizygotic twins always have a dichorionic diamniotic placenta. They can have completely separate placentas or fused placentas and, with extremely rare exceptions, there should not be vascular connections across the placenta. In contrast, monozygotic twins can have any form of placentation depending on when the splitting of the zygote occurred. If the separation occurs early after fertilization (2 to 3 days before the inner cell mass forms), the placenta will be dizygotic diamniotic, with the same four layers and appearance as with dizygotic twins. If the splitting occurs between the third and the eighth day, the placenta will be monochorionic diamniotic. Almost all monochorionic twins have interfetal blood vessel connections in their placenta. If the division occurs beyond the eighth day, the twins will be monochorionic monoamniotic, without dividing membranes (Endres & Wilkins, 2005).

Triplets and higher order multiples are most likely to be multizygotic from superovulation. They can also be monozygotic or have a combination of zygosity owing to splitting of one or more zygotes when multiple oocytes were fertilized.

Multiple pregnancies, prematurity, and mortality

Twins, triplets, and higher order multiples carry a greater risk of prematurity and subsequent higher morbidity and mortality. In 2002, the average gestational age at delivery of twins, triplets, and quadruplets was reported to be 35.3, 32.2, and 29.9 weeks, respectively (Martin et al., 2003).

Infants from multiple pregnancies are at increased risk of cerebral palsy, learning disabilities, slow language development, and behavioural difficulties (ESHRE Capri workshop group, 2000), as well as of chronic lung disease, neuromuscular developmental delay, and death. This excess neonatal and long-term morbidity and mortality in multiples has been attributed to the higher incidence of prematurity but also to other aetiological factors (Grether et al., 1993; Leonard et al., 1994; Pharoah & Cookie, 1996).

Current data are conflicting regarding the mortality associated with multiple gestations (Buekens & Wilcox, 1993; Donovan et al., 1998). When adjusted for gestational age, mortality was significantly higher in extremely low birth weight twins but was found to be quite similar after 28 weeks' gestation. The differences in mortality were limited to the susceptible high risk premature subsets rather than being applied to all premature infants. When considering each week of gestational age, perinatal mortality is more strongly dependent on the use of antenatal steroid therapy than on plurality (Garite et al., 2004). In the same cohort, twin mortality did not appear to be dependent on the route of delivery or the birth order.

The birth order of multiples has been studied as a prognostic factor because of the increased incidence of operative delivery and hypoxia-ischaemia in second twins (Young et al., 1985). With contemporary obstetric practice, most complications specific to second twins in terms of perinatal morbidity and mortality have disappeared (Chen et al., 1993; Lee et al., 2003).

Neurological outcomes of twins

Long-term outcomes including neurological outcome are a critical part of preconceptional and early pregnancy counselling for parents faced with a multiple gestation or considering assisted reproductive technology (ART). However, several limitations have impaired the conclusions from most of the published studies. Few of these studies were population-based and most of them lacked long-term follow-up of both children. The presence of intrauterine growth retardation (IUGR), which is independently associated with an excess of neurodevelopmental abnormalities (Luke et al., 1993; Kilpatrick et al., 1996) and the use of ART, influencing the rate of monochorionicity, is frequently not accounted for. Neurological handicaps, often not diagnosed until years after birth, occur within a spectrum that is wide and variable, from minor learning and behavioural disability to major cerebral palsy. It is sometimes challenging to attribute accurately the true causal factor in a minor or subtle neurological impairment, whether from singleton or multiple pregnancies. Finally, other confounding adverse long-term outcomes in multiple pregnancies are the socioeconomic and cultural issues. Thus it is easy to understand why data examining these outcomes should be interpreted with caution.

An increased rate of cerebral palsy?

Neurological impairment is the most significant long-term outcome variable in surviving twins. Impairments may include cerebral palsy, learning disability, and cognitive disability, with a broad spectrum that is relatively undefined in published reports.

In 1992, a meta-analysis by Laplaza et al. (1992) reviewed 12 relevant studies and concluded that the incidence of cerebral palsy in twin pregnancies was greater than in singletons. More recently, population-based cerebral palsy registers have been established to compare the prevalence rates of cerebral palsy in twins and singletons according to birth weight and gestational age (Pharoah & Cookie, 1996; Williams et al., 1996).

In three of these population-based studies (Petterson et al., 1993; Pharoah & Cookie, 1996; Williams et al., 1996), from the Mersey region of the United Kingdom, Western Australia, and the North East Thames region of the United Kingdom, twins had an approximately fivefold increased risk of cerebral palsy when compared with singletons, while triplets had a 17-fold increased risk compared with singletons. When the cerebral palsy prevalence was stratified by birth weight, no significant difference in the prevalence was seen between twins and singletons among lower birth weight groups (< 1,500 g or between 1,500 and 2,499 g).

Neurological outcome in surviving twin after a co-twin death

The surviving twin after a co-twin death is at a significantly high risk for cerebral palsy, with the majority of these twins being monozygotic/monochorionic. Population-based studies have confirmed this high risk despite the lack of zygosity status in these studies (Grether et al., 1993; Pharoah & Cookie, 1996). It is unlikely that cerebral palsy in the surviving co-twin after an infant death is secondary to the effects of prematurity. It seems more likely to be a result of an early antenatal aetiology, attributable potentially to monochorionicity. Although some reports have denied any adverse effect on the surviving twin when the co-twin dies in early gestation (Prompeler et al., 1994), there have been numerous reports of cerebral palsy in the surviving twin following second trimester and first trimester loss of a co-twin (Rand et al., 2005).

In contrast to Pharoah's findings (2002), Monset-Couchard et al. (2004) found only a minimally increased rate of cerebral palsy in twin sets in a study evaluating the long-term outcome of intrauterine growth retarded *versus* appropriate for gestational age co-twins in the study set. In many cases, subsequent cerebral palsy appeared to be related to the death of a co-twin *in utero*, especially in a monochorionic pregnancy or one affected by twin-twin transfusion syndrome.

The twin survivor with cerebral palsy has been shown to display a wide variety of anatomical abnormalities, particularly if the co-twin's death has occurred *in utero*. These defects include white matter infarction, hydrocephalus, multicystic encephalomalacia, cortical atrophy, ventriculomegaly, holoprosencephaly, polymicrogyria, and periventricular heterotropia (Larroche *et al.*, 1994). The type of anatomical abnormality correlates with the timing of the damaging event according to the brain's developmental stage. White matter infarction and multicystic encephalomalacia correlated with third trimester events and were particularly emphasized as affecting monochorionic twins.

Chorionicity and neurological outcome

Zygosity seems to have a significant and prominent role in the long-term outcome of multiple gestations. One third of monozygotic twins and all dizygotic twins will become dichorionic. Two thirds of monozygotic twins are monochorionic. This differentiation is crucial because much of the long term morbidity and mortality occurs with monochorionic placentation. Monochorionic twinning is associated with the effects of placental anastomoses with or without the risk of twin-twin transfusion syndrome. Thus monochorionic twins are at increased risk of poor short-term and long-term outcomes when compared with dizygotic twins. In a recent report comparing neurological morbidity, preterm monochorionic infants had a sevenfold greater risk of cerebral palsy than dichorionic infants because of chronic twin-twin transfusion syndrome, discordant birth weight, and the co-twin's death *in utero* (Adegbite *et al.*, 2004).

In 1961, Benirschke published a case report of a twin with cerebral and renal cortical necrosis and splenic infarcts associated with the co-twin's death and maceration. It was postulated that this was caused by thrombotic material passing from the dead to the living twin through placental anastomoses and ultimately causing disseminated intravascular coagulopathy. Since then, this pathological theory has been implicated in findings such as multicystic brain lesions, splenic and renal infarcts, and renal cortical necrosis (Bejar *et al.*, 1990).

Fusi & Gordon (1990) proposed an alternative theory based on acute haemodynamic changes. A dramatic decrease in the blood pressure of the dead twin leads to an immediate (and unavoidable) relative exsanguination of the surviving twin, with the development of severe hypotension and ischaemic damage to the heart, brain, kidneys, and gastrointestinal tract. These consequences of vascular anastomoses may be also observed in dichorionic placentas early in gestation, with subsequent resolution (Blickstein, 1990).

In the twin-twin transfusion syndrome, poor perinatal outcome is determined largely by prematurity and by haemodynamic instability. Serial amnioreduction and fetoscopic laser surgery with selective coagulation of placental inter-twin anastomoses are the most widely used therapeutic options (Robyr *et al.*, 2005). The incidence of perinatal mortality and morbidity (with a twofold reduction in the occurrence of severe brain lesions) has been shown to be lower after laser treatment, both in observational studies and in randomized controlled trials (Senat *et al.*, 2004; Lenclen *et al.*, 2007). However, the incidence of long-term neurodevelopmental impairment remains high (17 per cent at 2 years of age) (Lopriore *et al.*, 2007). Improvement in the prognosis of the twin-twin transfusion syndrome after laser coagulation reflects a reduction in both the specific complications of this condition and in severe prematurity. After 30 weeks of gestation, the neonatal prognosis is similar to that of dichorionic preterm neonates (Lenclen et al., 2007).

Neurological outcome of triplets and higher order multiples

With current ART use, the incidence of higher-order multiples has become an increasing issue, and knowledge of the long-term outcome is relevant in considering the option of fetal reduction. Most reports on the outcomes of higher-order multiples are based on small single centre populations.

Yokoyama et al. (1995) investigated the risk of handicap in twins, triplets, quadruplets, and quintuplets in Japan. In that study, the risk of developing at least one impaired infant was approximately 7.4 per cent in twins, 20 per cent in triplets, and 50 per cent in quadruplets. Four significant risk factors were reported for such handicaps, demonstrated by logistic regression: gestation number, low gestational age, premature rupture of the membranes, and pre-eclampsia.

In their analysis of twins and triplets in the cerebral palsy registry of Western Australian births between 1980 and 1990, Petterson et al. (1993) found that cerebral palsy occurred 17 times more often in triplet pregnancies than in singletons. A confounding factor for these numbers is the incidence of intrauterine growth retardation, which, as mentioned previously, occurs in half or more of all triplet and quadruplet pregnancies (Skrablin et al., 2000).

Based on American birth statistics between 1983 and 1988, fetal mortality was compared by categories of birth weight and gestational age for twins and triplets *versus* singletons (Luke, 1996). After correcting for gestational age, triplets had a higher mortality (ranging from five- to 20-fold depending on birth weight). Similar results were reported in a Swedish registry of infants born between 1973 and 1988 (Ericson et al., 1992).

In contrast, two recent single centre studies found no difference in mortality for premature singletons, twins, and higher order multiples when corrected for gestational age (Nielsen et al., 1997; Kaufman et al., 1998). In these studies, triplets did have a higher incidence of short-term morbidity such as respiratory distress syndrome, patent ductus arteriosus, intraventricular haemorrhage, or retinopathy of prematurity. Unfortunately, these studies examined neonatal outcome alone and did not include long-term follow-up. Thus it seems that higher-order multiples may be at increased risk for short-term and long-term adverse outcomes, but further controlled, population-based studies are needed to quantify their risks adequately.

In spontaneously conceived triplets, dichorionicity is very common (Adegbite et al., 2005). Dichorionic triamniotic triplets have a fivefold increased risk of adverse perinatal outcomes, predominantly because of twin-twin transfusion syndrome and premature rupture of the membranes. In triplets conceived by assisted reproductive techniques, this increase in perinatal mortality reached eightfold (Bajoria et al., 2006).

Conclusions

In addition to an increased risk of mortality, neonates born from multiple pregnancies appear to have higher rates of morbidity and mental retardation when compared with singleton controls. The two main reasons for these findings are the increased incidence of preterm birth observed in multiple gestations and the occurrence of monochorionicity associated with the risk of twin-twin transfusion syndrome, with its associated high rate of perinatal neurological morbidity and mortality. Multiple pregnancies remain a major problem associate with assisted reproductive techniques, and very few reliable studies have addressed the issue of the long term follow-up of iatrogenic multiples. Finally, chorionicity is essential for counselling families accurately on the neonatal and long term prognosis.

References

Adegbite, A., Castille, S., Ward, S. & Bajoria, R. (2004): Neuromorbidity in preterm twins in relation to chorionicity and discordant birth weight. *Am. J. Obstet. Gynecol.* **190,** 156–163.

Adegbite, A.L., Ward, S.B. & Bajoria, R. (2005): Perinatal outcome of spontaneously conceived triplet pregnancies in relation to chorionicity. *Am. J. Obstet. Gynecol.* **193,** 1463–1471.

Bajoria, R., Ward, S.B. & Adegbite, A.L. (2006): Comparative study of perinatal outcome of dichorionic and trichorionic iatrogenic triplets. *Am. J. Obstet. Gynecol.* **194,** 415–424.

Bejar, R., Vigliocco, G., Gramajo, H., Solana, C., Benirschke, K., Berry, C., Coen, R. & Resnik, R. (1990): Antenatal origin of neurologic damage in newborn infants. II. Multiple gestations. *Am. J. Obstet. Gynecol.* **162,** 1230–1236.

Benirschke, K. (1961): Twin placenta in perinatal mortality. *N. Y. State J. Med.* **61,** 1499–1507.

Benirschke, K. & Kim, C.K. (1973): Multiple pregnancy. *N. Engl. J. Med.* **288,** 1276–1284.

Blickstein, I. (1990): The twin-twin transfusion syndrome. *Obstet. Gynecol.* **76,** 714–722.

Buekens, P. & Wilcox, A. (1993): Why do small twins have a lower mortality rate than small singletons? *Am. J. Obstet. Gynecol.* **168,** 937–941.

Chen, S.J., Vohr, B.R. & Oh, W. (1993): Effects of birth order, gender, and intrauterine growth retardation on the outcome of very low birth weight in twins. *J. Pediatr.* **123,** 132–136.

Donovan, E.F., Ehrenkranz, R.A., Shankaran, S., Stevenson, D.K., Wright, L.L., Younes, N., Fanaroff, A.A., Korones, S.B., Stoll, B.J., Tyson, J.E., Bauer, C.R., Lemons, J.A., Oh, W. & Papile, L.A. (1998): Outcomes of very low birth weight twins cared for in the National Institute of Child Health and Human Development Neonatal Research Network's intensive care units. *Am. J. Obstet. Gynecol.* **179,** 742–749.

Endres, L. & Wilkins, I. (2005): Epidemiology and biology of multiple gestations. *Clin. Perinatol.* **32,** 301–314.

Ericson, A., Gunnarskog, J., Källén, B. & Olausson, P.O. (1992): A registry study of very low birthweight live born infants in Sweden, 1973-1988. *Acta Obstet. Gynecol. Scand.* **71,** 342–348.

ESHRE Capri workshop group (2000): Multiple gestation pregnancy. *Hum. Reprod.* **15,** 1856–1864.

Fusi, L. & Gordon, H. (1990): Twin pregnancy complicated by single intrauterine death. Problems and outcome with conservative management. *Br. J. Obstet. Gynaecol.* **97,** 511–516.

Garite, T.J., Clark, R.H., Elliott, J.P. & Thorp, J.A. (2004): Twins and triplets: the effect of plurality and growth on neonatal outcome compared with singleton infants. *Am. J. Obstet. Gynecol.* **191,** 700–707.

Grether, J.K., Nelson, K.B. & Cummins, S.K. (1993): Twinning and cerebral palsy: experience in four northern California counties, births 1983 through 1985. *Pediatrics* **92,** 854–858.

Kaufman, G.E., Malone, F.D., Harvey-Wilkes, K.B., Chelmow, D., Penzias, A.S. & D'Alton, M.E. (1998): Neonatal morbidity and mortality associated with triplet pregnancy. *Obstet. Gynecol.* **91,** 342–348.

Kilpatrick, S.J., Jackson, R. & Cougham-Minihane, M.S. (1996): Perinatal mortality in twins and singletons matched for gestational age at delivery at > or = 30 weeks. *Am. J. Obstet. Gynecol.* **174,** 66–71.

Laplaza, F.J., Root, L., Tassanawipas, A. & Cervera, P. (1992): Cerebral palsy in twins. *Dev. Med. Child Neurol.* **34,** 779–782.

Larroche, J.C., Girard, N., Narcy, F. & Fallet, C. (1994): Abnormal cortical plate (polymicrogyria), heterotopias and brain damage in monozygous twins. *Biol. Neonate* **65,** 343–352.

Lee, K.H., Hwang, S.J., Kim, S.H., Lee, S.H., Yu, D.K., Hwang, J.H., Choi, C.W., Shim, J.W., Chang, Y.S. & Park, W.S. (2003): Comparison of mortality and morbidity in multiple versus singleton very low birth weight infants in a neonatal intensive care unit. *J. Korean Med. Sci.* **18,** 779–782.

Lenclen, R., Paupe, A., Ciarlo, G., Couderc, S., Castela, F., Ortqvist, L. & Ville, Y. (2007): Neonatal outcome in preterm monochorionic twins with twin-to-twin transfusion syndrome after intrauterine treatment with amnioreduction or fetoscopic laser surgery: comparison with dichorionic twins. *Am. J. Obstet. Gynecol.* **196,** 450.e1–7.

Leonard, C., Piecuch, R., Ballard, R. & Cooper, B.A. (1994): Outcome of very low birth weight infants: multiple gestation versus singletons. *Pediatrics* **93,** 611–615.

Lopriore, E., Middeldorp, J. & Sueters, M. (2007): Long-term neurodevelopmental outcome in twin-to-twin transfusion syndrome treated with fetoscopic laser surgery. *Am. J. Obstet. Gynecol.* **196**, 231.e1–4.

Luke, B., Minogue, J. & Witter, F.R. (1993): The role of fetal growth restriction in gestational age on length of hospital stay in twin infants. *Obstet. Gynecol.* **81**, 949–953.

Luke, B. (1994): The changing pattern of multiple births in the United States: maternal and infant characteristics, 1973 and 1990. *Obstet. Gynecol.* **84**, 101–106.

Luke, B. (1996): Reducing fetal deaths in multiple births: optimal birthweights and gestational ages for infants of twin and triplet births. *Acta Genet. Med. Gemellol.* **45**, 333–348.

Martin, J.A., Hamilton, B.E., Sutton, P.D., Ventura, S.J., Menacker, F. & Munson, M.L. (2003): Births: final data for 2002. *Natl. Vital Stat. Rep.* **52**, 1–113.

Monset-Couchard, M., de Bethmann, O. & Relier, J.P. (2004): Long term outcome of small versus appropriate size for gestational age co-twins/triplets. *Arch. Dis. Child. Fetal Neonat. Ed.* **89**, F310–F314.

Nielsen, H.C., Harvey-Wilkes, K., MacKinnon, B. & Hung, S. (1997): Neonatal outcome of very premature infants from multiple and singleton gestations. *Am. J. Obstet. Gynecol.* **177**, 653–659.

Petterson, B., Nelson, K.B., Watson, L. & Stanley, F. (1993): Twins, triplets, and cerebral palsy in births in Western Australia in the 1980s. *BMJ* **307**, 1239–1242.

Pharoah, P.O. & Cookie, T. (1996): Cerebral palsy and multiple births. *Arch. Dis. Child. Fetal Neonat. Ed.* **75**, F174–F177.

Pharoah, P.O. (2002): Neurological outcome in twins. *Semin. Neonatol.* **7**, 223–230.

Prompeler, H.J., Madjar, H., Klosa, W., du Bois, A., Zahradnik, H.P., Schillinger, H. & Breckwoldt, M. (1994): Twin pregnancies with single fetal death. *Acta Obstet. Gynecol. Scand.* **73**, 205–208.

Rand, L., Eddleman, K.A. & Stone, J. (2005): Long-term outcomes in multiple gestations. *Clin. Perinatol.* **32**, 495–513.

Robyr, R., Quarello, E. & Ville, Y. (2005): Management of fetofetal transfusion syndrome. *Prenat. Diagn.* **25**, 786–795.

Senat, M.V., Deprest, J., Boulvain, M., Paupe, A., Winer, N. & Ville, Y. (2004): Endoscopic laser surgery versus serial amnioreduction for severe twin-to-twin transfusion syndrome. *N. Engl. J. Med.* **351**, 136–144.

Skrablin, S., Kuvacic, I., Pavicic, D., Kalafatic, D. & Goluza, T. (2000): Maternal neonatal outcome in quadruplets and quintuplet versus triplet gestations. *Eur. J. Obstet. Gynecol. Reprod. Biol.* **88**, 147–152.

Williams, K., Hennessy, E. & Alberman, E. (1996): Cerebral palsy: effect of twinning, birthweight and gestational age. *Arch. Dis. Child. Fetal Neonat. Ed.* **75**, F178–F182.

Yokoyama, Y., Shimizu, T. & Hayakawa, K. (1995): Prevalence of cerebral palsy in twins, triplets and quadruplets. *Int. J. Epidemiol.* **24**, 943–948.

Young, B.K., Suidan, J., Antoine, C., Silverman, F., Lustig, I. & Wasserman, J. (1985): Differences in twins: the importance of birth order. *Am. J. Obstet. Gynecol.* **151**, 915–921.

Chapter 10

Cerebral ischaemia: still a plausible pathway to white matter injury in the preterm infant?

Gorm Greisen

Department of Neonatology, Righospitalet, Blegdamsvej 9, 2100 Copenhagen, Denmark
greisen@rh.dk

Summary

Ischaemia means a blood flow that is too low to allow normal tissue function. The association of low cerebral blood flow (CBF) with electrical dysfunction, white matter damage, and cerebral palsy is weak, and the association with damage does not necessarily signify causation. The associations with low blood pressure or low cardiac output are also weak, and appear mostly related to periventricular haemorrhage, and thus less directly to white matter damage. Hypocapnia caused by inadvertent hyperventilation of preterm infants, on the other hand, is robustly associated with damage to white matter as well as with cerebral palsy. Are these associations causal? The CBF-CO_2 response is developed even in the most immature infants and usually preserved in infants under intensive care. Simple hyperventilation causes damage to DNA in newborn piglets. In the Levene model of hypoxic-ischaemic brain injury, the addition of CO_2 to the hypoxic gas mixture ameliorates the injury, whereas treatment with doxapram to decrease PCO_2 aggravates the injury. Is the mechanism ischaemia? CO_2 and pH both have metabolic effects as such and have effects on neural excitability. These effects could be part of the pathogenesis. Furthermore, hyperventilation is likely to be associated with increased intrathoracic pressure and decreased cardiac output, and hypocapnia and alkalosis cause a left shift of the haemoglobin-oxygen dissociation curve and reduce tissue PO_2 at a given level of oxygen delivery. In summary, it is likely, but not proven, that cerebral ischaemia is a significant contributor to the burden of white matter damage in preterm infants.

Introduction

It has traditionally been assumed that hypoxia-ischaemia is the principal pathway to white matter injury. During the past 15 years, the specific vulnerability of the immature cells in white matter, particularly the oligodendrocyte, as well as the potent effects of inflammation in the nervous system have received more attention. Furthermore, it is now clear that birth asphyxia, or postnatal episodes of cardiovascular collapse – prototypic situations of cerebral hypoxia-ischaemia – are not important as risk factors for white matter injury in the preterm infant. It is therefore proper to re-examine the hypoxic-ischaemic pathway.

Three arguments are relevant: first, the nature of the lesion – cystic or gliotic degeneration with no or little evidence of haemorrhage; second, the end-zone character of the anatomy and physiology of arterial vascular supply to the periventricular white matter; and third, the associations between circulatory compromise and hyperventilation/hypocapnia on the one hand and white matter injury/neurodevelopmental deficit in children born preterm on the other. The focus of this review is on the last two points and on the clinical data. The purpose of the review is to add to the rational basis for the care of preterm infants in the neonatal period.

Cerebral blood flow, oxygen uptake, and ischaemic thresholds

Global cerebral blood flow (CBF) is about 15 ml/100 g/min in healthy preterm infants during the first days after birth. Mechanical ventilation may be associated with slightly lower values, about 10 ml/100 g/min (Greisen, 1986). This is one-fifth to one-third of the normal values in human adults (about 45 ml/100 g/min). Why CBF is lower during mechanical ventilation is not obvious. Several factors may play a role: reduced levels of PCO_2, sedation and immobilisation, and circulatory aspects of the respiratory distress syndrome, which is a common reason for mechanical ventilation.

Cerebral oxygen uptake has been studied by near-infrared spectroscopy. Head-down tilting or compression of the jugular veins gives rise to pooling of venous blood in the brain. The oxygenation of the pooling blood can be estimated by near infrared spectroscopy (NIRS). It is not certain that white matter and deep grey matter structures are equally well represented in the results. The mean cerebral venous oxygen saturation was 55 per cent in a small group of preterm infants. The normal adult cerebro-venous oxygen saturation is about 65 per cent, and a similar value was found in healthy, term newborn infants (Buchvald et al., 1999). A cerebro-venous oxygen saturation of less than this indicates a global CBF that is lower than normal at a given level of oxygen delivery – that is, relative ischaemia.

The normal rate of global oxygen consumption ($CMRO_2$) in preterm infants is about 1 ml O_2/100 g/min (40 µmol O_2/100 g/min) (Skov et al., 1992). In ill preterm infants during the first days of life $CMRO_2$ as low as 20 µmol O_2/100 g/min has been measured, suggesting delivery limitation in the human preterm brain – that is, a reduction in oxygen consumption due to ischaemia (Kissack et al., 2005).

One way the brain may reduce metabolic needs when the supply is failing is to reduce or completely switch off electrical function. Brain electrical function fails when CBF falls under the 'electrical threshold'. EEG is often unduly discontinuous in sick preterm infants and, whereas some EEG activity was seen in infants with global CBF as low as 5 ml/100 g/min, a continuous EEG is unusual at a CBF below 10 ml/100 g/min (Greisen & Pryds, 1990). Continuous EEG background activity is likely to reflect thalamo-cortical coordination and it is possible that the discontinuity reflects marginal ischaemia and dysfunction of the white matter. In contrast, visual evoked responses were unaffected at global flow levels well below 10 ml/100 g/min (Pryds & Greisen, 1990). One possible explanation for this difference is that the visual tracts project through less vulnerable white matter, as indicated by the fact that the neurodevelopmental consequences of white matter injury only include blindness if very severe.

The few data that are available in the human preterm infant indicate that blood flow to the white matter is much below global average, as would be expected from studies in human adults and perinatal animals (Børch & Greisen 1998; Miranda et al., 2006), and it may even be relatively lower. In the former study, carefully attending to the problems of quantitation, the rate of blood flow to white matter flow was only 17 per cent [95 per cent confidence interval (CI), 12 to 22] of that to grey matter. This is significantly lower than in any of the commonly used experimental animal models – dog pup, 0.33; piglet, 0.44; lamb, 0.77 – and underlines the need for caution when data from these animals are put into a clinical perspective.

Decreased blood flow, cerebral ischaemia, and brain injury when blood pressure is low

No relation of global CBF to mean arterial blood pressure has been found in stable very preterm infants, even at pressures well below 30 mmHg (Pryds et al., 1989; Tyszczuk et al., 1998). In contrast, in ill preterm infants receiving dopamine for hypotension a significant positive pressure-flow relation was found at 1.9 per cent/mmHg (CI, 0.8 to 3.0) (Jayasinghe et al., 2003) and at a surprising 6 per cent/mmHg (Munroe et al., 2004). It is unclear if the discrepancy between these results and those cited above reflects an interaction between hypotension and dopamine action, the statistical uncertainty of small studies, or methodological or clinical differences.

Arterial blood pressure thus is not closely linked to cerebral blood flow, and blood pressure is not closely associated with systemic cardiac output, as measured by blood flow in the superior vena cava (Kluckow & Evans, 2000). Brain electrical activity, however, was reduced when arterial blood pressure was below 23 mmHg in very preterm infants (Victor et al., 2006), and blood pressure below 30 mmHg on two occasions or more was associated with a 10-fold increased risk of periventricular leucomalacia and a twofold increased risk of suboptimal neurological status at term age (Martens et al., 2003).

The 'common sense' lower limit of mean arterial blood pressure of 30 mmHg for very preterm infants may be reasonable in view of the possibility that the arterial end-territory of the periventricular white matter is more sensitive to a low perfusion pressure than the brain as a whole. This question has been studied by imaging of cerebral blood flow during hypotension with single photon emission computed tomography (SPECT) to detect a selective disadvantage of the white matter in 24 infants, gestational age 25 to 32 weeks (Greisen & Børch, 2001). Seven of the infants had blood pressures below 30 mmHg and in the group as a whole the fractional flow to white matter was indeed directly proportional to mean arterial blood pressure. No association between flow distribution and blood pressure was found in infants with higher blood pressures.

Blood flow, brain damage, and neurodevelopmental deficit associated with hypocapnia

Arteries and arterioles constrict with hypocapnia and dilate with hypercapnia. In normocapnic adults, small changes in arterial carbon dioxide tension ($PaCO_2$) result in a change in CBF by 30 per cent/kPa (4 per cent/mmHg). Similar reactivity has been demonstrated in the normal human neonate by venous occlusion plethysmography (Leahy et al., 1980; Rahilly, 1980) and in stable preterm ventilated infants without major germinal layer haemorrhage by ^{133}Xe after intravenous injection (Greisen & Trojaborg, 1987). Reactivity was less than 30 per cent/kPa during the first 24 hours (Pryds et al., 1989) and CO_2 reactivity is reduced in states of hypoxia or hypotension.

CBF adapts over time – on the one hand such an adaptation will tend to reduce an ischaemic insult; on the other, once an infant has adapted to an abnormally high PCO_2 – for example, due to chronic lung disease – and then is intubated and mechanically ventilated, as for a surgical procedure, a rapid normalisation of PCO_2 may possibly cause cerebral ischaemia.

Carbon dioxide acts mainly through pH – that is, the H^+ concentration. Perivascular pH has a direct effect on the membrane potential of arterial smooth muscle cells as the extracellular H^+ concentration is a principal determinant of the potassium conductance of the plasma membrane of arterial smooth muscle cells and hence of the outward K^+ current (Pearce & Harder, 1996). Because of the endothelial blood-brain barrier, the buffer mechanisms of blood do not work on the extracellular environment of the cerebrovascular smooth muscle cells; therefore the effects of CO_2 are more marked in the brain than in other organs.

In contrast to the weak relation of arterial hypotension to cerebral blood flow and poor outcomes, hypocapnia is likely to be a most important risk factor in the preterm infant (Greisen & Vannucci, 2001). Hypocapnia is associated with periventricular leucomalacia in preterm infants (Calvert et al., 1987; Hashimoto et al., 1991; Graziani et al., 1992) and cerebral palsy (Greisen et al., 1987; Collins et al., 2001). Is it a question of whether hypocapnia alone can cause ischaemia, or whether it works in combination with other factors, such as hypoxaemia, hypoglycaemia, sympathetic activation, or seizures.

The Rice-Vannucci model of focal hypoxia-ischaemia in the 7-day-old rat uses a combination of unilateral carotid artery ligation followed by several hours of exposure to a hypoxic gas mixture. The hypoxic gas mixture induces hyperventilation. Adding CO_2 to the gas mixture decreases the degree of hypocapnia and the extent of the brain damage (Vannucci et al., 1995). Furthermore, in a similar hypoxic-ischaemic brain damage model in the 4-day-old rat aiming at producing selective damage to the white matter, a large dose of doxapram induced hypocapnia and did aggravate the damage (Uehara et al., 2000).

A quasi-experiment has given further weight to the suspicion that inappropriate hyperventilation of preterm infants may be a quantitatively significant contributor to the burden of cerebral palsy. At Rigshospitalet in Copenhagen, mild hyperventilation of preterm infants was instituted during the early 1980s. The aim was to prevent intraventricular haemorrhage by extending the autoregulatory interval (Lou et al., 1982). In 1985–1986 the treatment policy was changed from almost routine intubation and mechanical ventilation of very preterm babies to primary nasal CPAP (Jacobsen et al., 1993) following the experience from Odense (Kamper & Ringsted, 1990) (Fig. 1). Fifteen years later, data from the routine registration of cerebral palsy showed a fall in the incidence of cerebral palsy in children born at 31 weeks of gestation or less, from 123 to 83 per 1,000 between the periods 1983–1986 and 1987–1990 for the region of Eastern Denmark (Topp et al., 2001) (Fig. 2). This fall was exclusively due to a decrease in the number of children with cerebral palsy who had been cared for at Rigshospitalet in the neonatal period. The decrease was from 87 to 47.

Other potential mechanisms linking hypocapnia, ischaemia, and brain damage

The traditional concept is that ischaemia leads to a sequence of events starting with anaerobic glycolysis and lactic acidosis, proceeding to electrical failure, membrane pump failure, efflux of potassium, and influx of sodium and calcium. The influx of sodium may lead to osmotic swelling and necrosis. Influx of calcium may lead to microstructural damage and cell death. If this does not occur the cell recovers.

After cerebral hypoxia-ischaemia in term infants, however, much of the brain damage occurs after primary cellular recovery when secondary energy failure is followed by cell death by apoptosis. As apoptosis is a normal cellular reaction it is possible that even relatively mild insults may push cells on that path and it is likely that their ultimate fate will depend on added adverse factors such as nutritional insufficiency, inflammation, and inhibition of normal synaptic transmission by drugs, pain, or stress. Such more subtle mechanisms may be induced by hyperventilation and hypocapnia in newborn piglets – that is, increased expression of bax (a pro-apoptotic protein) without a simultaneous increase in the anti-apoptotic bcl-2 protein, an

Chapter 10 Cerebral ischaemia: still a plausible pathway to white matter injury in the preterm infant?

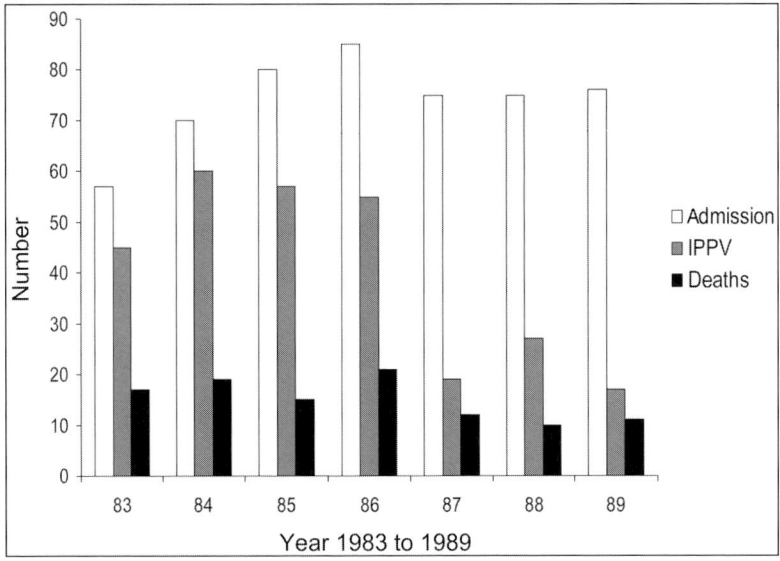

Fig. 1. The number of children with gestational age below 30 weeks born in Rigshospitalet in Copenhagen and admitted to the department of neonatology in the period 1983 to 1989, when a change of policy regarding the early management of very preterm infants was implemented. As a result the fraction of infants who were mechanically ventilated decreased from three quarters to one quarter. Mortality gradually declined over the period.

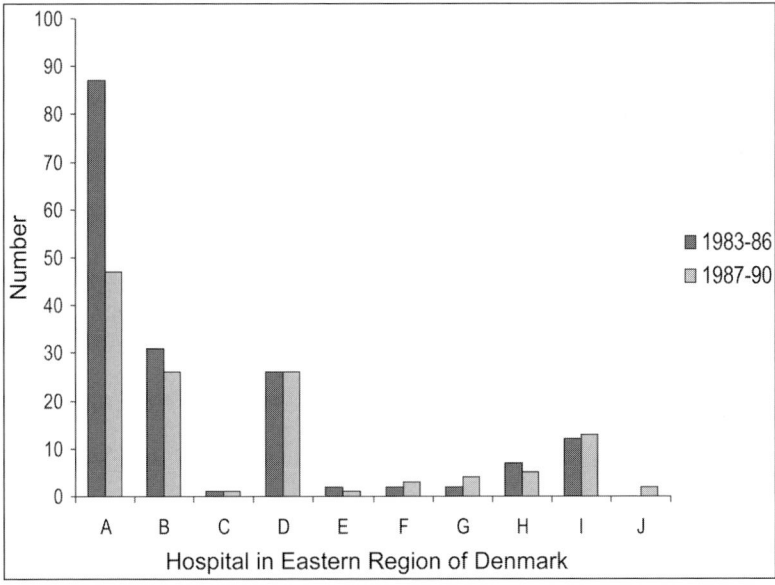

Fig. 2. The number of preterm children (gestational age < 37 weeks) with cerebral palsy in the Eastern Region of Denmark, according to year and hospital of birth. Hospitals differed much in size. Hospital A is Righospitalet in Copenhagen. This hospital received antenatal referrals for threatened very preterm birth, complications of pregnancy, and fetal malformations from most other hospitals in the region. Total numbers of preterm births in the two 4-year periods were 5,893 and 6,580, respectively. The rate of cerebral palsy in term infants remained the same over the two periods, at 1.5 per 1,000 live births (modified from Topp et al., 2001).

85

increase in conjugated dienes as evidence of plasma membrane peroxidation, and increased DNA fragmentation, all induced by severe hypocapnia (Fritz et al., 2001; Pirot et al., 2007).

Finally, hypocapnic alkalosis inhibits O_2 unloading at the capillary level, thereby aggravating the effects of marginal ischaemia, and hypocapnia sensitizes the NMDA receptor complex of cortical neurones in newborn piglets (Graham et al., 1996), possibly preventing the necessary decrease in metabolic needs during ischaemia.

Implications for clinical practice

It seems prudent to be careful to avoid hyperventilation and hypocapnia in preterm infants. All the evidence in the human relates to mechanically ventilated infants and therefore it is uncertain whether hypocapnia in the spontaneously breathing infant is a problem. It also appears prudent to pay attention to the systemic circulation – and to arterial blood pressure, as its most readily measurable parameter. Personally, I would not attempt to keep the blood pressure in the smallest infants above 30 mmHg; rather I would use the empirical limit of 'gestational age in weeks', and even leave untreated blood pressures below this level in infants without other signs of circulatory insufficiency. Clearly, the evidence basis of the latter is much weaker than that of the former.

References

Buchvald, F.F., Keshe, K. & Greisen, G. (1999): Measurement of cerebral oxyhaemoglobin saturation and jugular blood flow in term healthy newborn infants by near-infrared spectroscopy and jugular venous occlusion. *Biol. Neonate* **75**, 97–103.

Børch, K. & Greisen, G. (1998): Blood flow distribution in the normal human preterm brain. *Pediatr. Res.* **43**, 28–33.

Calvert, S.A., Hoskins, E.M., Fong, K.W. & Forsyth, S.C. (1987): Etiological factors associated with the development of periventricular leucomalacia. *Acta Paediatr. Scand.* **76**, 254–259.

Collins, M.P., Lorent, J.M., Jetton, J.R. & Paneth, N. (2001): Hypocapnia and other ventilation-related risk factors for cerebral palsy in low birth weight infants. *Pediatr. Res.* 50, 712–719.

Fritz, K.I., Ashraf, Q.M., Mishra, O.M.P. & Delivoria-Papadopoulos, M. (2001): Effect of moderate hypocapnic ventilation on nuclear DNA fragmentation and energy metabolism in the cerebral cortex of newborn piglets. *Pediatr. Res.* **50**, 586–589.

Graham, E.M., Apostolon, M., Mishra, O.P. & Delivoria-Papadopoulos, M. (1996): Modification of the N-methyl-D-aspartate (NMDA) receptor in the brain of newborn piglets following hyperventilation induced ischemia. *Neurosci. Lett.* **218**, 29–32.

Graziani, L.J., Spitzer, A.R., Michell, D.G., Merton, D.A., Stanley, C., Robinson, N. & McKee, L. (1992): Mechanical ventilation in preterm infants: neurosonographic and developmental studies. *Pediatrics* **90**, 515–522.

Greisen, G. (1986): Cerebral blood flow in preterm infants during the first week of life. *Acta Paediatr. Scand.* **75**, 43–51.

Greisen, G. & Børch, K. (2001): White matter injury in the preterm neonate: the role of perfusion. *Dev. Neurosci.* **23**, 209–212.

Greisen, G., Munck, H. & Lou, H. (1987): Severe hypocarbia in preterm infants and neurodevelopmental deficit. *Acta Paediatr. Scand.* **76**, 401–404.

Greisen, G. & Pryds, O. (1990): Low CBF, discontinuous EEG activity, and periventricular brain injury in preterm neonates. *Brain Dev.* **11**, 164–168.

Greisen, G. & Trojaborg, W. (1987): Cerebral blood flow, $PaCO_2$ changes, and visual evoked potentials in mechanically ventilated, preterm infants. *Acta Paediatr. Scand.* **76**, 394–400.

Greisen, G. & Vannucci, R.C. (2001): Is periventricular leucomalacia a result of hypoxic ischaemic injury? Hypocapnia and the preterm brain. *Biol. Neonat.* **79**, 194–200.

Chapter 10 Cerebral ischaemia: still a plausible pathway to white matter injury in the preterm infant?

Hashimoto, K., Takeuchi, Y. & Takashima, S. (1991): Hypocarbia as a pathogenic factor in pontosubicular necrosis. *Brain Dev.* **13,** 155–157.

Jacobsen, T., Grønvall, J., Petersen, S. & Andersen, G.E. (1993): 'Minitouch' treatment of very low birth weight infants. *Acta Paediatr.* **82,** 934–938.

Jayasinghe, D., Gill, A.B. & Levene, M.I. (2003): CBF reactivity in hypotensive and normotensive preterm infants. *Pediatr. Res.* **54,** 848–853.

Kamper, J. & Ringsted, C. (1990): Early treatment of idiopathic respiratory distress syndrome using binasal continuous positive airway pressure. *Acta Paediatr. Scand.* **79,** 581–586.

Kissack, C.M., Garr, R., Wardle, S.P. & Weindling, A.M. (2005): Cerebral factional oxygen extraction is inversely correlated with cerebral oxygen delivery in the sick, newborn, preterm infant. *J. Cereb. Blood Flow Metab.* **25,** 545–553.

Kluckow, M. & Evans, N. (2000): Low superior vena cava flow and intraventricular haemorrhage in preterm infants. *Arch. Dis. Child. Fetal Neonat. Ed.* **82,** 188–194.

Leahy, F.A.N., Cates, D., MacCallum, M. & Rigatto, H. (1980): Effect of CO_2 and 100 per cent O_2 on cerebral blood flow in preterm infants. *J. Appl. Physiol.* **48,** 468–472

Lou, H.C., Phibbs, R.H., Wilson, S.L. & Gregory, G.A. (1982): Hyperventilation at birth may prevent early periventricular haemorrhage. *Lancet* i, 1407.

Martens, S.E., Rijken, M., Stoelhorst, G.M.S.J., van Zwieten, P.T.H., Swinderman, A.H., Wit, J.M., Hadders-Algra, M. & Veen, S. (2003): Is hypotension a major risk factor for neurological morbidity at term age in very preterm infants? *Early Hum. Dev.* **75,** 79–89.

Miranda, M.J., Olofsson, K. & Sidaros, K. (2006): Non invasive measurements of regional cerebral perfusion in preterm and term neonates by magnetic resonance arterial spin labeling. *Pediatr. Res.* **60,** 359–363.

Munro, M.J., Walker, A.M. & Barfield, C.P. (2004): Hypotensive extremely low birth weight infants have reduced cerebral blood flow. *Pediatrics* **114,** 1591–1596.

Pearce, W.J. & Harder, D.R. (1996): Cerebrovascular smooth muscle and endothelium. In: *Neurophysiological basis of cerebral blood flow control: an introduction*, ed. S. Mraovitch & R. Sercombe, pp. 153–158. London: John Libbey.

Pirot, A.L., Fritz, K.I., Mishra, O.P. & Delivoria-Papadopoulos, M. (2007): Effects of severe hypocapnia on expression of bax and bcl-2 proteins, DNA-fragmentation, and membrane peroxidation products in cerebral cortical mitochondria of newborn piglets. *Neonatology* **91,** 20–27.

Pryds, O. & Greisen, G. (1990): Preservation of single flash visual evoked potentials at very low cerebral oxygen delivery in sick, newborn, preterm infants. *Pediatr. Neurol.* **6,** 151–158.

Pryds, O., Greisen, G., Lou, H. & Friis-Hansen, B. (1989): Heterogeneity of cerebral vasoreactivity in preterm infants supported by mechanical ventilation. *J. Pediatr.* **115,** 638–645.

Rahilly, P.M. (1980): Effects of 2 per cent carbon dioxide, 0.5 per cent carbon dioxide and 100 per cent oxygen on cranial blood flow of the human neonate. *Pediatrics* **66,** 685–689.

Skov, L., Pryds, O., Greisen, G. & Lou, H. (1992): Estimation of cerebral venous oxygen saturation in newborn infants by near infrared spectroscopy. *Pediatr. Res.* **32,** 52–55.

Topp, M., Uldall, P. & Greisen, G. (2001): Cerebral palsy births in eastern Denmark, 1987–90: implications for neonatal care. *Paediatr. Perinat. Epidemiol.* **15,** 271–277.

Tyszczuk, L., Meek, J., Elwell, C. & Wyatt, J. (1998): Cerebral blood flow is independent of mean arterial blood pressure in preterm infants undergoing intensive care. *Pediatrics* **102,** 337–341.

Uehara, H., Yosioka, H., Najai, H., Ochiari, R., Naito, T., Hasegowa, K. & Sadawa, T. (2000): Doxapram accentuates white matter injury in neonatal rats following bilateral carotid artery occlusion. *Neurosci. Lett.* **281,** 191–194.

Vannucci, R.C., Towfighi, J., Heitjan, D.F. & Brucklacher, R.M. (1995): Carbon dioxide protects the perinatal brain from hypoxic-ischaemic damage: an experimental study in the immature rat. *Pediatrics* **95,** 868–874.

Victor, S., Marson, A.G., Appleton, R.E., Beirne, M. & Weindling, A.M. (2006): Relationship between blood pressure, cerebral electrical activity, cerebral fractional oxygen extraction and peripheral blood flow in very low birth weight newborn infants. *Pediatr. Res.* **59,** 314–319.

Chapter 11

Oxidative stress in the developing brain

Giuseppe Buonocore, Serafina Perrone and Maria Carmela Muraca

Department of Paediatrics, Obstetrics, and Reproductive Medicine, University of Siena, viale Bracci 36, 53100 Siena, Italy
buonocore@unisi.it

Summary

Oxidative stress presents numerous opportunities for tissue injury through the formation of reactive oxygen or nitrogen species. It is becoming evident that oxidative stress is the final common pathway for a complex convergence of events, some genetically determined and some triggered by stressors acting *in utero*. Oxidative stress affects a complex array of genes involved in inflammation, coagulation, fibrinolysis, the cell cycle, signal transduction, and programmed cell death. It is now clear that a single pathway may be insufficient to explain the actions of oxidative stress in the pathogenesis of the so-called free radical diseases of the newborn.
The developing brain is prone to produce free radicals from various pathways. Free radicals operate intramitochondrial protein nitrosylation, triggering cell death or apoptosis or both. It is also plausible that the intramitochondrial scavenging system in the developing brain fails to detoxify nitrogen and oxygen free radicals.
The mitochondria play a crucial role in the activation of apoptotic mechanisms; they are both the initiators and the targets of oxidative stress. The immature brain is more susceptible than the mature brain to oxidative stress and more prone to the activation of an apoptotic cascade. The different ways in which the immature brain suffers from perinatal stress are related to anatomical and biochemical substrates.

Introduction

Oxidative stress *in vivo* is a degenerative process caused by overproduction of free radicals and the propagation of their reactions (Halliwell, 1994). Free radicals are highly reactive chemical molecules containing one or more unpaired electrons. They donate or accept electrons from other molecules to create electron pairs for a more stable species. Oxygen-derived free radicals – such as superoxide anions ($°O_2^-$), hydroxyl radicals ($°OH$), hydrochlorous acid (HOCL), and metabolites of hydrogen peroxide (H_2O_2), collectively termed reactive oxygen species (ROS) – are produced in healthy living organisms. When overproduced, they are major mediators of cell and tissue injury. Free radical reactions lead to the oxidation of lipids, proteins, and polysaccharides and to DNA damage (fragmentation, apoptosis, base modifications, and strand breakage) (Saugstad, 1996). Free radicals may be generated by mechanisms such as hyperoxia, ischaemia-reperfusion, hypoxia, neutrophil and macrophage activation, Fenton chemistry, endothelial cell xanthine oxidase, and free fatty acid and prostaglandin metabolism.

Newborns, and particularly preterm infants, are at high risk of oxidative stress and are very susceptible to free radical oxidative damage. In these individuals there is evidence of an imbalance between antioxidant- and oxidant-generating systems which causes oxidative damage. At birth the neonate encounters a world much higher in oxygen than in the intrauterine environment. The changes from the *in utero* milieu (PO_2 20–25 torr) to the *ex utero* milieu (PO_2 100 torr) is accompanied by a four- to fivefold increase in environmental oxygen. This hyperoxic challenge is exacerbated by the low efficiency of natural antioxidant systems in the newborn, especially the preterm neonate (Frank & Sosenko, 1991). Other important factors contribute to augmenting oxidative stress and to vulnerability in the early phase of life, including increased susceptibility to infection and inflammation, which increases oxidative stress, and the presence of free iron in the plasma and tissue of premature infants to a greater extent than in term infants (Speer & Silverman, 1998; Ciccoli *et al.*, 2003).

In many animals, especially humans, the brain undergoes substantial quantitative and qualitative changes that occur primarily, or solely, during development. These include cell division, differentiation and migration, axonal and dendritic proliferation, synaptogenesis, myelination, programmed cell death, and the formation of neuronal networks. These processes need a complex network of signalling molecules, ion channels, cerebral expression, receptor maturation, and growth factor synthesis (Erecinska *et al.*, 2004).

Because of its growth the mammalian brain can be considered a steady state system in which ATP production matches ATP utilization. Energy metabolism is central to life because cells cannot exist without an adequate supply of ATP. The brain is particularly sensitive to any disturbances of energy generation, and even a short term interruption can lead to long lasting, irreversible damage. Whenever there is energy failure, brain damage can occur.

Antepartum and intrapartum asphyxia is generally recognized as the most common cause of brain damage, though not the only one (Ferriero, 2004; Nelson & Lynch, 2004; Hagberg *et al.*, 2006). An increasing body of experimental and epidemiological evidence suggests that antenatal factors predispose to brain injury events in the immediate perinatal period. According to current views, the pathophysiology of brain injury almost always involves multiple factors: genetic, haemodynamic, metabolic, nutritional, endocrinological, toxic, and infectious mechanisms, acting in the antenatal or postnatal periods. In most cases the conjunction of these factors ultimately triggers neuronal death processes (Saliba & Marret 2001; Terzidou & Bennett, 2001; Bracci & Buonocore, 2003; Sullivan *et al.*, 2004).

Mechanisms of injury

There are considerable differences between the adult brain and the developing brain. The cerebral metabolic rate for glucose, the metabolic rate for oxygen, energy utilization, and cerebral blood flow increase dramatically during perinatal brain development. The metabolic rate in the developing brain has been shown to be higher than in mature brain. These biochemical changes are accompanied by modifications to mitochondrial structure and functional activity, including the number of mitochondria per cell, mitochondrial protein and respiratory enzyme content, mitochondrial matrix density, and the height of the crysts (Pysh & Khan, 1972; Erecinska *et al.*, 2004). Energy failure during the development period has more dramatic consequences in the fetal or neonatal brain than in the adult brain.

The vulnerability of the developing brain to hypoxic-ischaemic injury may be related to intrinsic regional metabolic factors (Blumberg, 1997). First, the telencephalic white matter – particularly in the depths of the sulci – represents a border zone of blood supply between the major cerebral arteries. The relative sparing of cerebral grey matter is explained on the basis of the presence of numerous leptomeningeal anastomoses between the major cerebral arteries, a characteristic feature in fetal brain (Volpe, 1995).

Hypoxia may also result in an increase in anaerobic metabolism, leading to a rapid rise in the levels of lactic acid and oxygen free radicals (Mishra & Delivoria-Papadopoulos, 1999; Buonocore & Perrone 2004). The neonatal brain has high concentrations of unsaturated fatty acids, so it is prone to generating and propagating free radicals. Polyunsaturated fatty acid constituents of membrane lipids in white matter are highly susceptible to free radical damage. Free radical attacks on immature myelin sheaths would lead to lipid peroxidation, and lipid peroxides are themselves free radicals (Halliwell, 1992). Antioxidant defences during a hyperoxic challenge are impaired in neonatal life. Specifically, the antioxidant enzyme systems superoxide dismutase, catalase, and glutathione peroxidase display lower concentration and reduced activity in the immature brain than in the mature brain (Fullerton et al., 1998; Baud et al., 2004).

It has been suggested that a transient increase in the density and distribution of glutamate receptors in developing brains contributes to the vulnerability of such regions to hypoxic damage (Ikonomidou et al., 1999).

Free iron release under hypoxic conditions from neonatal erythrocytes and from other storage sites can increase cerebral oxidative stress and oligodendrocyte damage (Buonocore & Perrone, 2002; Blomgren & Hagberg, 2006).

There are several defence systems against free radicals and several pathways for their inactivation. α-Tocopherol (vitamin E) prevents lipid peroxidation, acting as a radical scavenger in human tissue. Iron chelation is another endogenous system for neutralizing free radical formation. We showed that treatment with deferoxamine, an iron chelator, improved cerebral recovery after hypoxia-ischaemia in immature brain but not in adult brain, consistent with the view that the immature brain is more prone to suffer from oxidative stress than the adult brain (Buonocore & Groenendaal, 2007). The superoxide anion is dismutated *in vivo* by superoxide dismutase with the participation of catalase and glutathione peroxidase. There are three major forms of superoxide dismutase (SOD): Cu,Zn-SOD (or SOD1), Mn-SOD (or SOD2), and EC-SOD (SOD3). SOD1 and SOD2 are located into the intracellular space, SOD2 in the mitochondrial matrix, and SOD3 into the extracellular space. In the immature brain, especially under stress conditions (such as hypoxia), SOD is overexpressed (Okado-Matsumoto & Fridovich, 2001). Immature oligodendroglial cells are glutathione peroxidase and catalase deficient, so overexpression of SOD can be dangerous instead of protective. Accumulating evidence has also implicated free radical production and subsequent oxidative damage as major contributing factors in brain aging and declining cognitive function (Hyman et al., 1992; Lipton et al., 1993; Kraus et al., 2005). Individuals suffering from Down syndrome are at high risk of dementia and Alzheimer's disease. Down syndrome is caused by the presence of excess chromosome 21 in the cellular karyotype, and SOD gene is localized on chromosome 21. We have detected an increase in 8-iso-PGF2a isoprostane, a reliable biomarker of oxidative stress, in amniotic fluid from pregnancies with a Down syndrome fetus (Perrone et al., 2007). It is likely that overexpression of SOD, derived from the excess chromosome 21, is implicated in the early occurrence of oxidative stress in pregnancy, and in subsequent oxidative damage as a major contributing factor to brain aging and decline in cognitive function.

Mature oligodendrocytes are highly resistant to oxidative stress, owing in part to differences in the levels of expression of antioxidant enzymes and proteins involved in programmed cell death. These characteristics of oligodendrocytes may explain why white matter often is injured selectively in the brains of premature neonates.

One aspect of cell damage in the developing brain is related to the pivotal role of the mitochondria in cell metabolism under normal conditions and after hypoxia-ischaemia. After hypoxia the mitochondria develop a degree of swelling related to calcium deposition (Puka-Sundvall et al., 2000), and cells containing swollen calcium-containing mitochondria show cromatin condensation, a feature of apoptosis. Cerebral apoptosis starts with cytochrome c translocation from the mitochondria, followed by caspase 9 activation and then caspase 3 activation (Zhu et al., 2005). Many apoptosis-related factors, such caspase-3, Apaf-1, Bcl-2, and Bax, are upregulated in the immature brain (Ota et al., 2002). In the developing brain, NMDA receptor activation depresses mitochondrial respiration and induces apoptosis, a phenomenon not seen in adult brain (the so-called NMDA paradox) (Ikonomidou et al., 1999). For antiapoptotic signalling, the integrity of amino acid receptors of the NMDA subtype is essential.

The developing brain is prone to produce free radicals from oxygen and NO; these cause intramitochondrial protein nitrosylation, triggering cell death or apoptosis. It is thus plausible that intramitochondrial scavenging systems in the developing brain fail to detoxify nitrogen and oxygen free radicals (Peeters-Scholte et al., 2002).

It is clear that mitochondria play crucial roles in the activation of the apoptotic mechanism – they are both initiators and targets of oxidative stress. The immature brain is more susceptible to oxidative stress and more prone to activate the apoptotic cascade.

The different ways in which the immature brain suffers from perinatal stress have both anatomical and biochemical substrates.

Biomarkers of oxidative stress in the early phases of life

During the intrapartum period, the relative inaccessibility of the fetus and the complexity of the pathophysiology of fetal oxygenation makes it difficult to obtain and interpret information on the fetal response to stress. Recent data suggest that a delicate redox balance must exist to allow for proper growth and development (Dennery, 2004). When oxidative stress occurs, overproduction of free radicals becomes dangerous. The damaging effect of free radicals in the perinatal period may be demonstrated by measuring biochemical markers of oxidative stress in amniotic fluid and cord blood.

We have reported increased plasma total hydroperoxide, advanced oxidative protein products, and carbonyl groups as indices of lipid and protein oxidation in cord blood of hypoxic fetuses (Buonocore et al., 2000). We also found that total hydroperoxides and advanced oxidative protein products increased from birth to 7 days of life in both preterm and term babies, indicating that oxidative stress occurs early in life and that neonates are particularly susceptible to oxidative damage (Buonocore et al., 2002).

Intrauterine hypoxia may induce free radical generation and fetal oxidative stress. We demonstrated oxidative stress in pregnancies with fetal growth restriction. Fetal growth restriction is often complicated by intrauterine hypoxia and impaired blood flow to the fetus (Thaete et al., 2004). Chronic restriction of uterine blood flow elicits placental and fetal responses in the form of growth adaptation to hypoxia. Intrauterine hypoxia may induce free radical generation and fetal oxidative stress. We found that isoprostane concentrations in amniotic fluid have a significant predictive value in fetuses suffering from growth restriction because of oxidative stress (Longini et al., 2005).

Isoprostanes are a family of prostaglandin isomers derived from polyunsaturated fatty acids through free radical catalysed peroxidation of arachidonic acid (Morrow & Roberts, 1996). They can be measured in biofluids such as circulating plasma, and later in urine. In particular, 8-iso-PGF2, a major isoprostane that is relatively stable chemically and measurable in biofluids, is a reliable biomarker of oxidative stress. We measured levels of F(2)-isoprostanes (F2-IP) in neonatal plasma by gas chromatography/mass spectrometry and found they were significantly increased in preterm and term neonates compared with healthy adults (Comporti et al., 2004). A significant inverse correlation was found between the plasma levels of isoprostanes and gestational age. Because no increase in F2-IP levels was found in plasma from mothers at delivery or during pregnancy, and no correlation was found between plasma F2-IP in mothers and newborns, the results suggested that some form of lipid peroxidation is active in the fetus.

Another aspect of the importance of ROS-induced damage to amniotic epithelium and chorioamniotic collagen was clarified by our recent data showing that F2-IP concentrations were significantly higher in pregnancies with premature rupture of the membranes than in normal pregnancies (Longini et al., 2007). ROS may disrupt amino acid binding in proteins and polyunsaturated fatty acids of the membrane lipid bilayers, causing cell dysfunction and modification of chorioamniotic biology, and predisposing to premature rupture of the membranes.

Considering the close relations between free radical release and phagocyte function and the relation between phagocyte activation and infection, additional markers of infection could be exploited to determine the occurrence of oxidative stress. Activated phagocytes release large quantities of oxygen radicals and proteases (Buonocore et al., 1994). Superoxide anion – the most abundant radical species – is also the first stage of the bacterial killing reaction, which is followed by production of other free radicals, such as hydrogen peroxide (H_2O_2) by superoxide dismutase, hydroxyl radicals catalysed by transition metals, and $HOCl^-$ catalysed by myeloperoxidase. These substances contribute to bacterial killing but also favour tissue damage. Moreover, they produce increased capillary permeability which facilitates the passage of cytokines. The precise mechanisms of interaction between inflammation and oxidative stress are not known. Preceding infection with cytokine production amplifies the effect of hypoxic-ischaemic insults. It has also been suggested that the effect of infection may be mediated through hypoxia-ischaemia. Finally, it should be noted that, while pro-inflammatory cytokines are liberated in response to infection, several other conditions including ischaemia and non-specific inflammation are also known to cause cytokine production. These cytokines could therefore enter a 'final common pathway' in the cascade of molecular interaction leading to tissue damage, whether triggered by infection or ischaemia (Dietrich et al., 2004). It is known that FiO_2 activates lung phagocytes and enhances ROS release in the lung and brain tissues (Kelly & Lubec, 1995). In an interesting multicentre study of the problem of inflammatory mediators and cerebral palsy, Kaukola et al. (2004) found that B-lymphocyte chemoattractants, ciliary neutrophil factor, epidermal growth factor, interleukin (IL)-5, IL-12, IL-13, and IL-15, macrophage migration inhibitory factor, monocyte chemoattractant protein-3, monokine induced by interferon-γ, and tumour necrosis factor-related, apoptosis-inducing ligands were significantly raised in subjects with cerebral palsy.

The roles of inflammatory responses by the fetal system and multiorgan failure seem to be critically important for understanding the genesis of oxidative stress related diseases of the newborn. It is not known whether the inflammatory response is causal or modulatory in the cascade of events that occurs during an intrauterine or perinatal oxidative insult to the newborn.

Free iron

In the absence of efficient protection by antioxidant factors, oxidative stress is responsible for a release of the reactive form of iron, predisposing neonates to the risk of severe oxidative damage caused by the production and propagation of free radical reactions. Iron is normally sequestered in transport proteins such as transferrin and lactoferrin and is stored in proteins such as ferritin and haemosiderin that maintain it in a non-toxic form, unable to engage in the Fenton reaction (Papanikolaou & Pantopoulos, 2005). During situations of iron overload and low plasma pH, as occurs during ischaemia, transferrin releases its iron, and chelatable forms of Fe (non-protein-bound iron, NPBI) escape sequestration in biological systems, producing free radicals (Papanikolaou & Pantopoulos, 2005). These free radicals release even more iron by mobilizing it from ferritin (Buonocore *et al.*, 1998a; Buonocore *et al.*, 1998b). This may lead to a cascade of iron release and free radical production, causing extensive cell damage.

Erythrocytes were the first cells from newborns to reveal the susceptibility of the neonate to oxidative stress (Bracci *et al.*, 2001). Oxidative stress leads to oxidation of haemoglobin and damage to the erythrocyte membrane. Extensive investigations by our research group showed the key role of oxidative stress and iron release in a reactive form, causing membrane protein damage mediated by the Fenton reaction and hydroxyl radical production (Buonocore *et al.*, 1998a; Buonocore *et al.*, 1998b). Intraerythrocytic NPBI has been found to be particularly elevated in cord blood of hypoxic newborns. Release of NPBI was associated with increased lipoperoxide products in plasma (Buonocore *et al.*, 1998a; Buonocore *et al.*, 1998b; Comporti *et al.*, 2002). When experiments were carried out by incubating neonatal red cells under hypoxic conditions, we found a much greater release of iron than in an equal period of normoxia. It is interesting that membrane protein damage was related to the appearance of the senescence antigen (Rossi *et al.*, 2006). In neonates, the release of NPBI in erythrocytes is correlated with plasma NPBI: the released iron has a tendency to diffuse from erythrocytes into the surrounding medium, suggesting the appearance of plasma NPBI (Comporti *et al.*, 2002).

After asphyxia in newborn infants there is an increase in intraerythrocyte and plasma NPBI, significantly correlated with neurodevelopmental outcome (Buonocore *et al.*, 2003). Leakage of plasma NPBI into the brain through a compromised blood-brain barrier may occur and is particularly damaging, as it is taken up directly by cells in a manner that is independent of transferrin. Oxidative stress may also result from iron delocalization induced by the superoxide anion, acidosis, and anoxia (Oubidar *et al.*, 1994). Enhanced proteolytic activity occurring in injured tissue also releases iron from storage proteins (Rothman *et al.*, 1992). When non-protein-bound iron gains access to the extracellular space, its uptake by cells is enhanced by intracellular calcium and paradoxically also by increased levels of intracellular iron (Cozzi *et al.*, 1990). The toxicity of iron is inversely proportional to the availability of ferritin for sequestering and detoxifying ferrous ion, and directly proportional to the quantity of hydrogen peroxide producing hydroxyl radicals by the Fenton reaction. After hypoxia, the expression of transferrin receptors on brain macrophages increases (Kaur & Ling, 1999). This is a protective mechanism to facilitate the active uptake of excess iron that may be released by iron-rich oligodendrocytes, or may accumulate because of disruption of its normal transport after a hypoxic insult.

Conclusions

The developing brain is prone to produce free radicals from various pathways. Free radicals cause intramitochondrial protein nitrosylation, triggering cell death or apoptosis, or both. It is also plausible that the intramitochondrial scavenging system in the developing brain fails to detoxify nitrogen and oxygen free radicals.

Mitochondria play a crucial role in the activation of the apoptotic mechanism, being both initiators and targets of oxidative stress. The immature brain is more susceptible to oxidative stress and more prone to activation of the apoptotic cascade than the mature brain. The different ways in which the immature brain suffers from perinatal stress are related to anatomical and biochemical substrates.

Acknowledgments: We acknowledge the receipt of grants from the University of Siena (PAR 2005): 'Early markers of perinatal hypoxic-ischaemic brain damage'.

References

Baud, O., Greene, A.E., Li, J., Wang, H., Volpe, J.J. & Rosenberg, P.A. (2004): Glutathione peroxidase-catalase cooperativity is required for resistance to hydrogen peroxide by mature rat oligodendrocytes. *J. Neurosci.* **24**, 1531–540.

Blomgren, K. & Hagberg, H. (2006): Free radicals, mitochondria, and hypoxia-ischemia in the developing brain. *Free Radic. Biol. Med.* **40**, 388–397.

Blumberg, R.M. (1997): Relation between delayed impairment of cerebral energy metabolism and infarction following transient focal hypoxia-ischaemia in the developing brain. *Exp. Brain Res.* **113**, 130–137.

Bracci, R., Perrone, S. & Buonocore, G. (2001): Red blood cell involvement in fetal/neonatal hypoxia. *Biol. Neonate* **79**, 210–212.

Bracci, R. & Buonocore, G. (2003): Chorioamnionitis: a risk factor for fetal and neonatal morbidity. *Biol. Neonate* **83**, 85–86.

Buonocore, G. & Perrone, S. (2002): Iron: a potent prooxidant. In: *Infant formula: closer to the reference*, ed. N.C.R. Raiha & F.F. Rubaltelli, vol. 47S, pp. 85–96. Philadelphia: Lippincott Williams and Wilkins.

Buonocore, G. & Perrone, S. (2004): Biomarkers of hypoxic brain injury in the neonate. *Clin. Perinatol.* **31**, 107–116.

Buonocore, G. & Groenendaal, F. (2007): Anti-oxidant strategies. *Semin. Fetal Neonat. Med.* **12**, 287–295.

Buonocore, G., Gioia, D., De Filippo, M., Picciolini, E. & Bracci R. (1994): Superoxide anion release by polymorphonuclear leukocytes in whole blood of newborns and mothers during the peripartal period. *Pediatr. Res.* **36**, 619–622.

Buonocore, G., Zani, S., Perrone, S., Caciotti, B. & Bracci, R. (1998a): Intraerythrocyte nonprotein-bound iron and plasma malondialdehyde in the hypoxic newborn. *Free Radic. Biol. Med.* **25**, 766–770.

Buonocore, G., Zani, S., Sargentini, I., Gioia, D., Signorini, C. & Bracci, R. (1998b): Hypoxia-induced free iron release in the red cells of newborn infants. *Acta Paediatr.* **87**, 77–81.

Buonocore, G., Perrone, S., Longini, M., Terzuoli, L. & Bracci, R. (2000): Total hydroperoxide and advanced oxidation protein products in preterm hypoxic babies. *Pediatr. Res.* **47**, 221–224.

Buonocore, G., Perrone, S., Longini, M., Vezzosi, P., Marzocchi, B., Paffetti, P. & Bracci, R. (2002): Oxidative stress in preterm neonates at birth and on the seventh day of life. *Pediatr. Res.* **52**, 46–49.

Buonocore, G., Perrone, S., Longini, M., Paffetti, P., Vezzosi, P., Gatti, M.G., & Bracci, R. (2003): Non protein bound iron as early predictive marker of neonatal brain damage. *Brain* **126**, 1224–1230.

Ciccoli, L., Rossi, V., Leoncini, S., Signorini, C., Paffetti, P., Bracci, R. & Comporti, M. (2003): Iron release in erythrocytes and plasma non protein-bound iron in hypoxic and non hypoxic newborns. *Free Radic. Res.* **37**, 51–58.

Comporti, M., Signorini, C., Buonocore, G. & Ciccoli, L. (2002). Iron release, oxidative stress and erythrocyte ageing. *Free Rad. Biol. Med.* **32**, 568–576.

Comporti, M., Signorini, C., Leoncini, S., Buonocore, G., Rossi, V. & Ciccoli L. (2004): Plasma F(2)-isoprostanes are elevated in newborns and inversely correlated to gestational age. *Free Radic. Biol. Med.* **37**, 724–732.

Cozzi, A., Santambrogio, P., Levi, S. & Arosio, P. (1990): Iron detoxifying activity of ferritin. Effects of H and L human apoferritins on lipid peroxidation in vitro. *FEBS Lett.* **277**, 119–122.

Dennery, P.A. (2004): Role of redox in fetal development and neonatal diseases. *Antioxid. Redox Signal* **6,** 147–153.

Dietrich, N., Thastrup, J., Holmberg, C., Gyrd-Hansen, M., Fehrenbacher, N., Lademann, U., Lerdrup, M., Herdegen, T., Jäättelä, M. & Kallunki, T. (2004): JNK2 mediates TNF-induced cell death in mouse embryonic fibroblasts via regulation of both caspase and cathepsin protease pathways. *Cell Death Differ.* **11,** 301–313.

Erecinska, M., Cherian, S. & Silver, I. A. (2004): Energy metabolism in mammalian brain during development. *Prog. Neurobiol.* **73,** 397–345.

Ferriero, D.M. (2004): Neonatal brain injury. *N. Engl. J. Med.* **351,** 1985–1995.

Frank, L. & Sosenko, I.R. (1991): Failure of premature rabbits to increase antioxidant enzymes during hyperoxic exposure, increased susceptibility to pulmonary oxygen toxicity compared with term rabbits. *Pediatr. Res.* **29,** 292–296.

Fullerton, H.J., Ditelberg, J.S., Chen, S.F., Sarco, D.P., Chan, P.H., Epstein, C.J. & Ferriero, D.M. (1998):Copper/zinc superoxide dismutase transgenic brain accumulates hydrogen peroxide after perinatal hypoxia ischemia. *Ann. Neurol.* **44,** 357–364.

Hagberg, H., Rousset, C.I., Wang, X. & Mallard, C. (2006): Mechanisms of perinatal brain damage and protective possibilities. Drug discovery today: disease mechanisms. *Perinat. Disord.* **3,** 397–407.

Halliwell, B. (1992): Reactive oxygen species and the central nervous system. *J. Neurochem.* **59,** 1609–1623.

Halliwell, B. (1994): Free radicals, antioxidants and human disease: curiosity, cause, or consequence? *Lancet* **344,** 721–724.

Hyman, B.T., Marzloff, K., Wenniger, J.J., Dawson, T.M., Bredt, S.D. & Snyder, S.H. (1992): Relative sparing of nitric oxide synthetase-containing neurons in the hippocampal formation in Alzheimer's disease. *Ann. Neurol.* **32,** 818–820.

Ikonomidou, C., Bosch, F., Miksa, M., Bittigau, P., Vockler, J., Dikranian, K., Tenkova, T.I., Stefovska, V., Turski, L. & Olney, J.W. (1999): Blockade of NMDA receptors and apoptotic neurodegeneration in the developing brain. *Science* **283,** 70–74.

Kaukola, T., Satyaraj, E., Patel, D.D., Tchernev, V.T., Grimwade, B.G., Kingsmore, S.F., Koskela, P., Tammela, O., Vainionpaa, L., Pihko, H., Aarimaa, T. & Hallman M. (2004): Cerebral palsy is characterized by protein mediators in cord serum. *Ann. Neurol.* **55,** 186–194.

Kaur, C. & Ling, E.A. (1999). Increased expression of transferrin receptors and iron in amoeboid microglial cells in postnatal rats following an exposure to hypoxia. *Neurosci. Lett.* **262,** 183–186.

Kelly, F.J. & Lubec, G. (1995): Hyperoxic injury of immature guinea pig lung is mediated via hydroxyl radicals. *Pediatr. Res.* **38,** 286–291.

Kraus, L.R., Pasieczny, R., Lariosa-Willingham, K., Turner, M.S., Jiang, A. & Trauger, J.W. (2005): Antioxidant properties of minocycline: neuroprotection in an oxidative stress assay and direct radical-scavenging activity. *J. Neurochem.* **94,** 819–827.

Lipton, S.A., Choi, Y.B., Pan, Z.-H, Lei, S.Z., Chen, H.S., Sucher, N.J., Loscalzo, J., Singel, D.J. & Stamler, J.S. (1993): A redox-based mechanism for the neuroprotective and neurodestructive effects of nitric oxide and related compounds. *Nature* **364,** 626–632.

Longini, M., Perrone, S., Kenanidis, A., Vezzosi, P., Marzocchi, B., Petraglia, F. & Buonocore, G. (2005): Isoprostanes in amniotic fluid, a predictive marker for fetal growth restriction in pregnancy. *Free Radic. Biol. Med.* **38,** 1537–1541.

Longini, M., Perrone, S., Vezzosi, P., Marzocchi, B., Kenanidis, A., Centini, G., Petraglia, F. & Buonocore, G. (2007): Oxidative stress in amniotic fluid and premature rupture of membranes in preterm and term pregnancies. *Clin. Biochem.* **40,** 793–797.

Mishra, O.P. & Delivoria-Papadopoulos, M. (1999): Cellular mechanisms of hypoxic injury in the developing brain. *Brain Res. Bull.* **48,** 233–238.

Morrow, J. & Roberts, L. (1996): The isoprostanes. Current knowledge and directions for future research. *Biochem. Pharmacol.* **12,** 1–9.

Nelson, K.B. & Lynch, J.K. (2004): Stroke in newborn infants. *Lancet Neurol.* **3,** 150–158.

Okado-Matsumoto, A. & Fridovich, I. (2001): Subcellular distribution of superoxide dismutases (SOD) in rat liver: Cu,Zn-SOD in mitochondria. *J. Biol. Chem.* **276,** 38388–38393.

Ota, K., Yakovlev, A.G., Itaya, A., Kameoka, M., Tanaka, Y. & Yoshihara, K. (2002): Alteration of apoptotic protease-activating factor-1 (APAF-1)-dependent apoptotic pathway during development of rat brain and liver. *J. Biochem.* **131,** 131–135.

Oubidar, M., Boquillon, M., Marie, C., Schreiber, L. & Bralet, J (1994): Ischemia-induced brain iron delocalization, effect of iron chelators. *Free Radic. Biol. Med.* **16,** 861–867.

Papanikolaou, G. & Pantopoulos, K. (2005): Iron metabolism and toxicity. *Toxicol. Appl. Pharmacol.* **202,** 199–211.

Peeters-Scholte, C., Koster, J., Veldhuis, W., van den Tweel, E., Zhu, C., Kops, N., Blomgren, K., Bar, D., van Buul-Offers, S., Hagberg, H., Nicolay, K., van Bel, F. & Groenendaal, F. (2002): Neuroprotection by selective nitric oxide synthase inhibition at 24 hours after perinatal hypoxia-ischemia. *Stroke* **33**, 2304–2310.

Perrone, S., Longini, M., Bellieni, C.V., Centini, G., Kenanidis, A., De Marco, L., Petraglia, F. & Buonocore, G. (2007): Early oxidative stress in amniotic fluid of pregnancies with Down syndrome. *Clin. Biochem.* **40**, 177–180.

Puka-Sundvall, M., Gajkowska, B., Cholewinski, M., Blomgren, K., Lazarewicz, J.W. & Hagberg, H. (2000): Subcellular distribution of calcium and ultrastructural changes after cerebral hypoxia-ischemia in immature rats. *Brain Res. Dev. Brain Res.* **125**, 31–41.

Pysh, J.J. & Khan, T. (1972): Variations in mitochondrial structure and content of neurons and neuroglia in rat brain: an electron microscopic study. *Brain Res.* **36**, 1–8.

Rossi, V., Leoncini, S., Signorini, C., Buonocore, G., Paffetti, P., Tanganelli, D., Ciccoli, L. & Comporti, M. (2006): Oxidative stress and autologous immunoglobulin G binding to band 3 dimers in newborn erythrocytes. *Free Radic. Biol. Med.* **40**, 907–915.

Rothman, R.J., Serroni, A. & Farber, J.L. (1992): Cellular pool of transient ferric iron, chelatable by deferoxamine and distinct from ferritin, that is involved in oxidative cell injury. *Mol. Pharmacol.* **42**, 703–710.

Saliba, E. & Marret, S. (2001): Cerebral white matter damage in the preterm infant: pathophysiology and risk factors. *Semin. Neonatol.* **6**, 121–133.

Saugstad, O.D. (1996): Mechanisms of tissue injury by oxygen radicals, implications for neonatal disease. *Acta Paediatr.* **85**, 1–4.

Speer, C.P. & Silverman, M. (1998): Issues relating to children born prematurely. *Eur. Respir. J. Suppl.* **27**, 13s–16s.

Sullivan, M.H., Steel, J., Kennea, N., Feldman, R.G. & Edwards, A.D. (2004): The role of intrauterine bacteria in brain injury. *Acta Paediatr. Suppl.* **93**, 4–5.

Terzidou, V. & Bennett, P. (2001): Maternal risk factors for fetal and neonatal brain damage. *Biol. Neonate.* **79**, 157–162.

Thaete, L.G., Dewey, E.R. & Neerhof, M.G. (2004): Endothelin and the regulation of uterine and placental perfusion in hypoxia-induced fetal growth restriction. *J. Soc. Gynecol. Investig.* **11**, 16–21.

Volpe, J.J., ed. (1995): Hypoxic-ischemic encephalopathy neuropathology and pathogenesis. In: *Neurology of the newborn*, 2nd edition, pp. 168–202. Philadelphia: WB Saunders.

Zhu, C., Wang, X., Xu, F., Bahr, B.A., Shibata, M., Uchiyama, Y., Hagberg, H. & Blomgren, K. (2005): The influence of age on apoptotic and other mechanisms of cell death after cerebral hypoxia-ischemia. *Cell Death Differ.* **12**, 162–176.

Chapter 12

Infection/inflammation – a complex hot topic in perinatal brain white matter damage aetiology

Olaf Dammann

Tufts Floating Hospital for Children at Medical Center, BOX 854, 800 Washington St, Boston, MA 02111, USA, and Hannover Medical School, Hannover, Germany
ODammann@tuftsmedicalcenter.org; dammann.olaf@mh-hannover.de

Summary

Over the past decades, a theory has been developed that helps to clarify the observed association between prematurity and brain white matter damage (WMD) among infants born preterm. In essence, this theory suggests that antenatal maternal intrauterine infection induces a fetal inflammatory response, which contributes to both preterm delivery and brain injury. In this chapter, I summarize the ongoing story of how this theory developed, illustrating important concepts by epidemiological and experimental data.

Introduction

In 1962, Banker and Larroche coined the term 'periventricular leucomalacia' (PVL) in a paper that described the observation of frank necrosis in the white matter of babies who would nowadays be considered near term. The inference derived from the observation that most of these children had 'trouble breathing' was that anoxia was a major causal contributor. Only a few years later, Gilles and Murphy (Gilles & Murphy, 1969) described a similar neuropathological condition in newborn infants, which they called 'perinatal telencephalic leukoencephalopathy' (PTL), an arguably difficult term which might have contributed to its failure to survive intact to the present day. Beyond the observation of frank necrosis which Banker and Larroche had described, Gilles and Murphy also listed histological factors apart from necrosis, including hypertrophic astrocytes and areas of acutely damaged glia. In a subsequent epidemiological investigation into the origins of PTL, Leviton and co-workers found that infants who died with PTL were five times more likely than their peers without PTL to have bacteria cultured from postmortem blood cultures (Leviton & Gilles, 1973). The hypothesis that circulating correlates of infection (for example, endotoxin) might be involved in PTL pathogenesis was explored in a subsequent experimental study in which Gilles and colleagues provided proof of the principle that intraperitoneal application of endotoxin to newborn kittens results in cerebral astrogliosis and focal necroses, both of which are characteristics of PTL (Gilles *et al.*, 1976).

The cytokine hypothesis

Despite this initial convincing epidemiological and experimental evidence, the concept of endotoxin-induced PTL went into hibernation for two decades, until new developments in immunology led to a new twist to the story by introducing the concept of cytokine-induced damage to the developing brain.

In 1993, two annotations published back-to-back provided the basis for a new concept of neonatal/childhood brain damage as a consequence of intrauterine infection. Adinolfi suggested that intrauterine infection could induce a cytokine response in the maternal-fetal compartment, which contributes to brain injury (Adinolfi, 1993). At the same time, Leviton suggested that the major culprit among such cytokines might be tumour necrosis factor (TNF)α (Leviton, 1993), which received its name from research into mouse tumours that underwent necrotic cell death after exposure to TNF.

Based on this suggestion, we developed an integrative model looking at the complex relationship between infection, inflammation, prematurity, and brain damage by considering the uterine environment, the fetal systemic circulation, and the fetal brain as three compartments separated by the boundaries of the placenta and the blood-brain barrier (Dammann & Leviton, 1997). The literature at that time suggested that pro-inflammatory cytokines are present in all three compartments, and can cross the boundaries of interest, thereby providing an explanatory framework for the scenario in question. Only a few years later, Cai and colleagues provided experimental evidence in support of this concept by showing that exposure of pregnant rats to intraperitoneal endotoxin led to an upregulation of pro-inflammatory cytokines in the fetal brain, an upregulation of glial fibrillary acidic protein (an astrocyte marker, probably supporting the observation of astrocytosis described above), and a downregulation of myelin basic protein (an oligodendrocyte marker) (Cai *et al.*, 2000), probably supporting the notion of hypomyelination postulated as one characteristic of WMD (Leviton & Gilles, 1996).

The fetal inflammatory response

One of the most interesting phenomena in the context of preterm WMD is that, in contrast to conventional infections in pregnancy (for example, rubella, toxoplasma, or cytomegalovirus), we have no evidence for the presence of infectious organisms in the fetal brain. This has led to the suggestion that it is not brain infection but infection remote from the brain that leads to WMD (Dammann & Leviton, 1998). Thus, we assume that it might not be infection itself but an inflammatory response that contributes to WMD causation.

In the past years, we have come to use the term 'fetal inflammatory response' (Leviton *et al.*, 1999) to encompass fetal vasculitis, cytokinaemia, white cell activation, and neuroinflammation (for an overview see Dammann & Leviton, 2004). In essence, we have evidence now that fetal vasculitis, an invasion of the fetal vessel walls in the chorionic plate and umbilical cord, is associated with WMD (Leviton *et al.*, 1999). Multiple studies suggest that raised levels of circulating cytokines are associated with WMD (for an overview see Dammann & Leviton, 2004). Fetal white cell activation (Dammann *et al.*, 2001) appears to occur before birth to a greater extent in children who later develop MRI-defined WMD than in controls (Duggan *et al.*, 2001). Finally, a neuroinflammatory component characterized by increased blood-brain barrier leakage and white cell invasion (Yan *et al.*, 2004), as well as the presence of microglia in white matter lesions of animals exposed to a systemic endotoxin challenge (Mallard *et al.*, 2003), appears to be part of the fetal inflammatory response to remote infection. Both the latter and another study in fetal sheep (Peebles *et al.*, 2003) suggest that the damage induced by endotoxin exposure in the fetus is *not* due to haemodynamic suppression which might lead to hypoxia-ischaemia.

Complexity

In the light of the wide variety of theories and data in WMD aetiology research, it seems rather unlikely that only one of these alone can explain the entire phenomenology of WMD. In deep appreciation of such complexities, we have recently suggested that the infection-associated inflammation can intersect with other cascades.

First, one way to integrate the above concepts with the suggested causal pathway leading to WMD via hypoxia-ischaemia (see Greisen in this volume, chapter 10) is by employing the concept of sensitization/preconditioning (Hagberg *et al.*, 2004). This paradigm states that a sub-threshold first hit does not do harm, but paves the way for damage after a second hit, which might be much increased compared with individuals who sustain the initial hit only. Indeed, exactly this was observed in 7-day-old rats pretreated with endotoxin which were subsequently exposed to 20 minutes of hypoxia-ischaemia and developed much more prominent brain injury than controls exposed to hypoxia-ischaemia only (Eklind *et al.*, 2001).

Second, it is most likely that inflammatory mechanisms interact with the coagulation cascade. Indeed, inflammation and coagulation are mutually stimulatory phenomena, thereby potentially prolonging pro-inflammatory processes (see below) and increasing the likelihood of WMD occurrence (Leviton & Dammann, 2004).

Third, we have recently alluded to the idea that the innate and adaptive components of the perinatal immune system interact in WMD aetiology (Leviton *et al.*, 2005). Among the multiple original observations that have led to this suggestion are the above-mentioned association between T-cell activation and MRI-defined WMD (Duggan *et al.*, 2001) and the observation that interleukin-2 and its receptor are found in the brain lesions of infants who die with WMD (Kadhim *et al.*, 2002). Interleukin-2 is thought to be produced by activated T-cells exclusively and to be toxic to oligodendrocytes and myelin.

Neuroprotection

The future challenge for obstetricians, neonatologists, and paediatric neurologists is defined by the charge to design feasible, safe, and effective interventions. We have recently provided an overview of potentially neuroprotective substances which might act mainly by downregulating inflammation or other immunomodulatory mechanisms (Wolfberg *et al.*, 2008). A more provocative recent suggestion is that the neuroinflammatory response might be not only prolonged but persistent, which could offer room for anti-inflammatory intervention even after the newborn period (Dammann, 2007).

Conclusions

The proposal that neonatal WMD aetiology includes exposure to antenatal infection and inflammation is complex indeed. However, current data suggest that infection/inflammation is associated with perinatal brain damage in observational and experimental settings and probably does not exert its adverse effects through hypoxia-ischaemia. Most importantly, the research summarized in this chapter offers much room for the design of anti-inflammatory strategies for neonatal and probably even post-neonatal neuroprotective intervention.

Acknowledgments: O.D. is supported by the Wilhelm Hirte Stiftung (Hannover), The European Union (LSHM-CT-2006-036534), the Susan B. Saltonstall Fund, and the Richard Saltonstall Foundation.

References

Adinolfi, M. (1993): Infectious diseases in pregnancy, cytokines and neurological impairment: an hypothesis. *Dev. Med. Child Neurol.* **35,** 549–553.

Banker, B.Q. & Larroche, J.C. (1962): Periventricular leucomalacia of infancy. *Arch. Neurol.* **7,** 386–410.

Cai, Z., Pan, Z.L., Pang, Y., Evans, O.B. & Rhodes, P.G. (2000): Cytokine induction in fetal rat brains and brain injury in neonatal rats after maternal lipopolysaccharide administration. *Pediatr. Res.* **47,** 64–72.

Dammann, O. (2007): Persistent neuro-inflammation in cerebral palsy: a therapeutic window of opportunity? *Acta Paediatr.* **96,** 6–7.

Dammann, O. & Leviton, A. (1997): Maternal intrauterine infection, cytokines, and brain damage in the preterm newborn. *Pediatr. Res.* **42,** 1–8.

Dammann, O. & Leviton, A. (1998): Infection remote from the brain, neonatal white matter damage, and cerebral palsy in the preterm infant. *Semin. Pediatr. Neurol.* **5,** 190–201.

Dammann, O. & Leviton, A. (2004): Inflammatory brain damage in preterm newborns – dry numbers, wet lab, and causal inference. *Early Hum. Dev.* **79,** 1–15.

Dammann, O., Durum, S. & Leviton, A. (2001): Do white cells matter in white matter damage? *Trends Neurosci.* **24,** 320–324.

Duggan, P.J., Maalouf, E.F., Watts, T.L., Sullivan, M.H., Counsell, S.J., Allsop, J., Al-Nakib, L., Rutherford, M.A., Battin, M., Roberts, I. & Edwards, A.D. (2001): Intrauterine T-cell activation and increased proinflammatory cytokine concentrations in preterm infants with cerebral lesions. *Lancet* **358,** 1699–1700.

Eklind, S., Mallard, C., Leverin, A.L., Gilland, E., Blomgren, K., Mattsby-Baltzer, I. & Hagberg, H. (2001): Bacterial endotoxin sensitizes the immature brain to hypoxic-ischaemic injury. *Eur. J. Neurosci.* **13,** 1101–1106.

Gilles, F.H. & Murphy, S.F. (1969): Perinatal telencephalic leucoencephalopathy. *J. Neurol. Neurosurg. Psychiatry* **32,** 404–413.

Gilles, F.H., Leviton, A. & Kerr, C.S. (1976): Endotoxin leucoencephalopathy in the telencephalon of the newborn kitten. *J. Neurol. Sci.* **27,** 183–191.

Hagberg, H., Dammann, O., Mallard, C. & Leviton, A. (2004): Preconditioning and the developing brain. *Semin. Perinatol.* **28,** 389–395.

Kadhim, H., Tabarki, B., De Prez, C., Rona, A.M. & Sébire, G. (2002): Interleukin-2 in the pathogenesis of perinatal white matter damage. *Neurology* **58,** 1125–1128.

Leviton, A. (1993): Preterm birth and cerebral palsy: is tumor necrosis factor the missing link? *Dev. Med. Child Neurol.* **35,** 553–558.

Leviton, A. & Gilles, F.H. (1973): An epidemiologic study of perinatal telencephalic leucoencephalopathy in an autopsy population. *J. Neurol. Sci.* **18,** 53–66.

Leviton, A. & Gilles, F. (1996): Ventriculomegaly, delayed myelination, white matter hypoplasia, and 'periventricular' leucomalacia: how are they related? *Pediatr. Neurol.* **15,** 127–136.

Leviton, A. & Dammann, O. (2004): Coagulation, inflammation, and the risk of neonatal white matter damage. *Pediatr. Res.* **55,** 541–545.

Leviton, A., Paneth, N., Reuss, M.L., Susser, M., Allred, E.N., Dammann, O., Kuban, K., Van Marter, L.J., Pagano, M., Hegyi, T., Hiatt, M., Sanocka, U., Shahrivar, F., Abiri, M., Disalvo, D., Doubilet, P., Kairam, R., Kazam, E., Kirpekar, M., Rosenfeld, D., Schonfeld, S., Share, J., Collins, M., Genest, D., Shen-Schwarz, S., *et al.* (1999): Maternal infection, fetal inflammatory response, and brain damage in very low birth weight infants. Developmental Epidemiology Network Investigators. *Pediatr. Res.* **46,** 566–575.

Leviton, A., Dammann, O. & Durum, S.K. (2005): The adaptive immune response in neonatal cerebral white matter damage. *Ann. Neurol.* **58,** 821–828.

Mallard, C., Welin, A.K., Peebles, D., Hagberg, H. & Kjellmer, I. (2003): White matter injury following systemic endotoxemia or asphyxia in the fetal sheep. *Neurochem. Res.* **28,** 215–223.

Peebles, D.M., Miller, S., Newman, J.P., Scott, R. & Hanson, M.A. (2003): The effect of systemic administration of lipopolysaccharide on cerebral haemodynamics and oxygenation in the 0.65 gestation ovine fetus in utero. *Br. J. Obstet. Gynaecol.* **110,** 735–743.

Wolfberg, A.J., Dammann, O. & Gressens, P. (2007): Anti-inflammatory and immunomodulatory strategies to protect the perinatal brain. *Semin. Fetal Neonat. Med.* **12,** 296–302.

Yan, E., Castillo-Melendez, M., Nicholls, T., Hirst, J. & Walker, D. (2004): Cerebrovascular responses in the fetal sheep brain to low-dose endotoxin. *Pediatr. Res.* **55,** 855–863.

Chapter 13

White matter diseases of prematurity

Mary A. Rutherford

*Robert Steiner MR Unit, MRC Clinical Sciences Centre, Imperial College, Hammersmith Hospital,
Du Cane Road, W12 OHS London, UK*
m.rutherford@imperial.ac.uk

Summary

Recent studies using magnetic resonance imaging (MRI) to assess the preterm brain have documented new appearances, adding to the spectrum of white matter disease of prematurity. Periventricular leucomalacia (PVL) and parenchymal venous infarction complicating germinal matrix/intraventricular haemorrhage have long been recognized as the two significant white matter diseases responsible for the majority of cases of cerebral palsy in survivors of preterm birth. MRI has detected two further disorders: punctate white matter lesions, and diffuse excessive high signal intensity (DEHSI). These appear to be much more common than PVL but less significant in terms of their impact on motor development. They may, however, be associated with later cognitive and behavioural disorders known to be common following preterm birth. It remains unclear whether PVL, punctate lesions, and DEHSI represent a continuum of disorders occurring as a result of injury to the developing white matter. This chapter discusses some of the similarities and differences between these three disorders in terms of imaging, pathology, and outcome.

Introduction

Traditionally, neonatologists have focused on white matter lesions in the preterm brain that have been visible on cranial ultrasound – periventricular leucomalacia (PVL) and haemorrhagic venous infarction. While there is still debate about the aetiology of these, particularly in any individual infant, their appearances are well described and the outcomes associated with them well documented (Figs. 1 and 2). They are the two major pathologies that result in motor impairment or cerebral palsy in the child born preterm. The incidence of severe haemorrhagic lesions is decreasing, although both disorders still result in significant morbidity.

The advent of neonatal magnetic resonance imaging (MRI) has stimulated much research into the effects of prematurity on the developing brain. Initially, visual analysis of conventional image sequences and more recently objective post-acquisition quantification of more sophisticated sequences such as diffusion tensor imaging have given new insights into the developing brain. MRI has provided a better understanding of the established pathologies but has also identified 'new' abnormalities such as punctate white matter lesions (Cornette *et al.*, 2002) (Fig. 3) and so-called DEHSI (diffuse excessive high signal intensity) (Maalouf *et al.*, 1999) (Fig. 3). Once again the aetiology of these abnormalities remains obscure, although it has

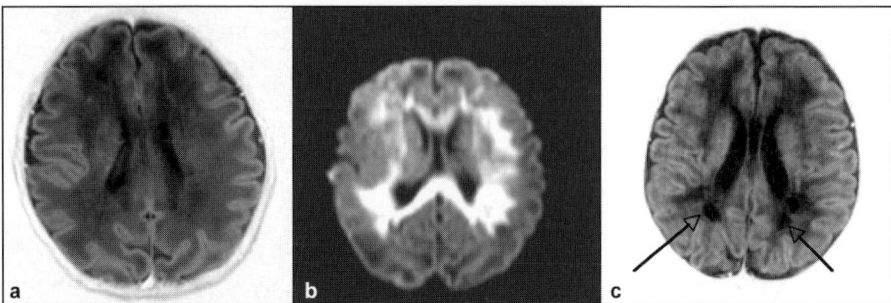

Fig. 1. Periventricular leucomalacia. Early T1-weighted (a) and diffusion-weighted imaging (b). Changes on conventional imaging are very subtle but there is marked restriction of diffusion in the periventricular white matter seen as high signal intensity (b). In T1-weighted image at term-equivalent (c), there are multiple periventricular cysts and abnormal low signal intensity in surrounding white matter (arrows).

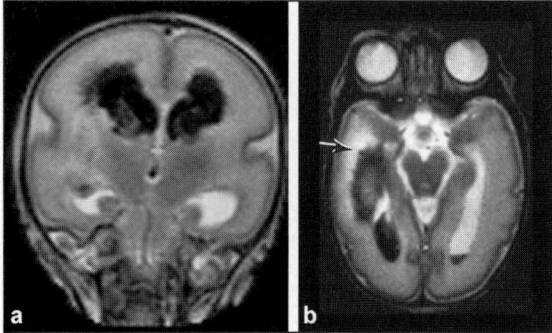

Fig. 2. Haemorrhagic periventricular infarction. T2-weighted images (a): bilateral haemorrhage with parenchymal involvement in an infant who subsequently died. (b)Venous infarction (arrow) complicating germinal matrix intraventricular haemorrhage in the right temporal lobe in a different infant.

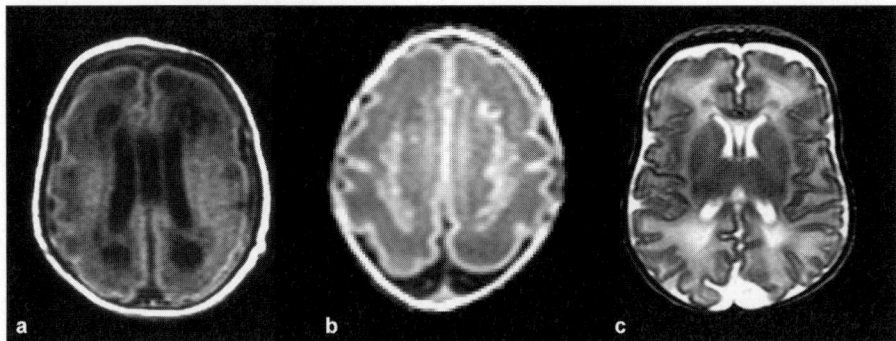

Fig. 3. A possible spectrum of white matter disease of prematurity. (a) T1-weighted image showing cystic periventricular leucomalacia. (b) T1-weighted image showing multiple high signal intensity punctate lesions in the white matter of the centrum semiovale. (c) T2-weighted imaging showing diffuse excessive signal intensity (DEHSI) at term-equivalent age. There is abnormal long T2 within the white matter.

generally been assumed that they represent milder forms of PVL (Volpe, 2003; Back et al., 2006). This, however, has not been proven and it is therefore of interest to discuss what these white matter diseases do or do not have in common.

Timing

PVL typically affects the immature brain over a limited gestational age range of 26 to 32 weeks, while punctate white matter lesions may be seen at any gestational age up to and including term (Back et al., 2006), the assumption being, perhaps incorrectly, that the aetiology of all punctate lesions is the same. Punctate lesions may be seen in term-born neonates with congenital heart disease (Miller & McQuillen, 2007) and also in term-born neonates with hypoglycaemia and in neonates with neuromuscular disorders (Fig. 4). The ultrasound evolution of early PVL is well established, with the time to cyst formation from echodensity extending from 10 days to three weeks or occasionally longer (De Vries et al., 2004). The evolution on MRI is less well established as most MR studies are done once cysts have been identified by ultrasound. Punctate lesions do not seem to evolve in appearance although their numbers decrease with time (Fig. 5). We have not confirmed their presence before 26 weeks' gestational age. If detected at a later date in an infant born before 26 weeks they cannot be assumed to have developed perinatally as they may occur during the neonatal course in a preterm infant. DEHSI is an imaging term to describe appearances within the white matter at term-equivalent age. It is unclear whether it is possible to detect imaging abnormalities within the developing white matter, either visually or more objectively, with diffusion-weighted imaging before the appearance of DEHSI, as this requires serial imaging in a large group of preterm infants.

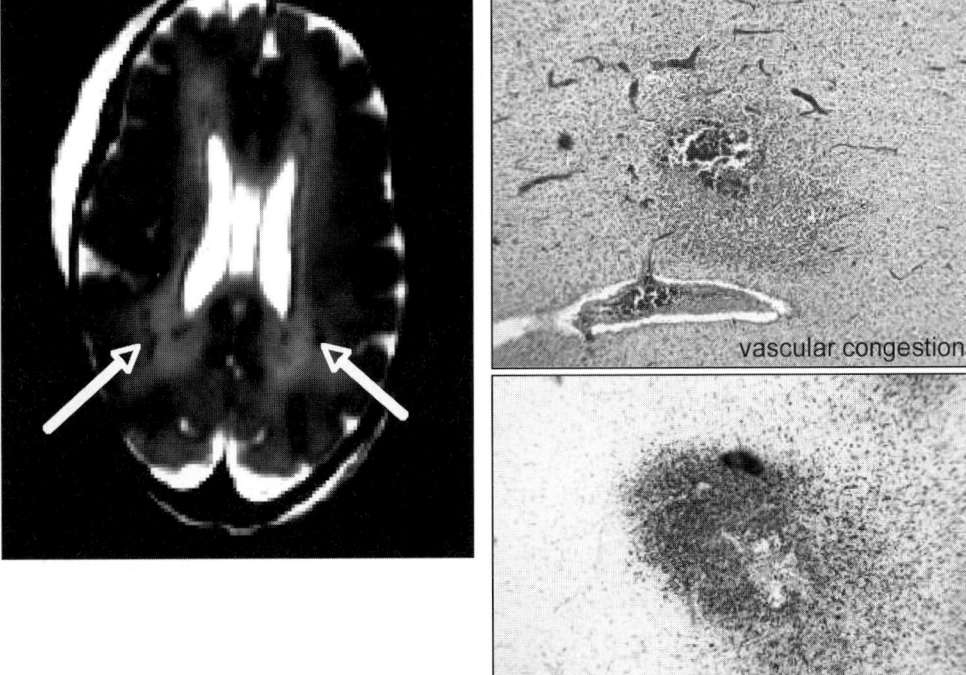

Fig. 4. Infant born at 34+6 days' gestation. Undiagnosed neuromuscular disorder. Ventilator dependent. Died at 9 days and scanned postmortem. T2-weighted images. There are multiple foci of low signal intensity within the white matter. These corresponded to areas of vascular congestion and increased activated microglia. At autopsy the abnormal foci on imaging corresponded to clusters of activated microglia (courtesy of Martin Weber).

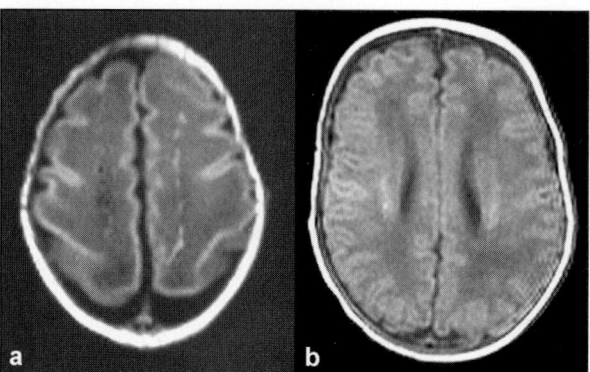

Fig. 5. Evolution of punctate white lesions; T1-weighted images. (a) 31 weeks' postmenstrual age. There are multiple high signal intensity lesions within the periventricular white matter. There are one or two low signal intensity lesions on the right that may represent small cysts. (b) Imaging at term-equivalent age shows marked decrease in the lesions. Imaging at this stage will underestimate the original number of lesions.

Aetiology

There is now a wealth of data on the aetiology of PVL, with combinations of infection, inflammation and ischaemia being major factors in animal models. High risk infants include those with severe intrauterine growth restriction (IUGR). While PVL may occur following a severe illness it can also occur in an apparently symptomless infant. In any given infant it may still be very difficult to identify which factor or combination of factors led to the development of PVL. As yet there are no consistent links between the presence of punctate lesions and signs of sepsis, chronic lung disease or IUGR but studies are relatively few. DEHSI has been shown to have an association with sepsis and with the presence of chronic lung disease (Counsell *et al.*, 2006; Dyet *et al.*, 2006).

Pathology

There are many pathological studies of human PVL. The predilection for periventricular white matter is shared by the newer white matter diseases. The vulnerability of the periventricular white matter has been extensively studied in the context of PVL and is thought to reflect a combination of the presence of a vascular watershed and an inherent susceptibility of pre-oligodendrocytes to injury. In addition, and as yet given little attention, is the presence of populations of resident microglia at these sites of periventricular white matter crossroads (Judas *et al.*, 2005) (Fig. 6). Essential for axonal guidance and white matter tract modelling, it is probable that it is these microglia that are activated abnormally in the presence of injury (Dommergues *et al.*, 2003).

In infants with PVL it is recognized that the brain may show a diffuse component around and at a distance from the focal cystic lesions (Volpe, 2003; Back *et al.*, 2006). This is confirmed by *in vivo* imaging studies where there may be both acute and chronic changes in diffusion parameters in non-cystic tissue (Counsell *et al.*, 2006) (Fig. 1). It is this 'diffuse' non-cystic change that has led to the assumption that the new white matter diseases of prematurity represent mild forms of PVL. PVL is a pathological term that does not imply a particular aetiology. Punctate lesions and DEHSI are imaging terms and therefore do not imply either a given aetiology or a given pathology. While there are many animal models of 'PVL-like' lesions, there is as yet no model that has produced injuries that are instantly recognizable as punctate lesions or DEHSI. To confirm such correlations we need either imaging studies of the animal model or human imaging and

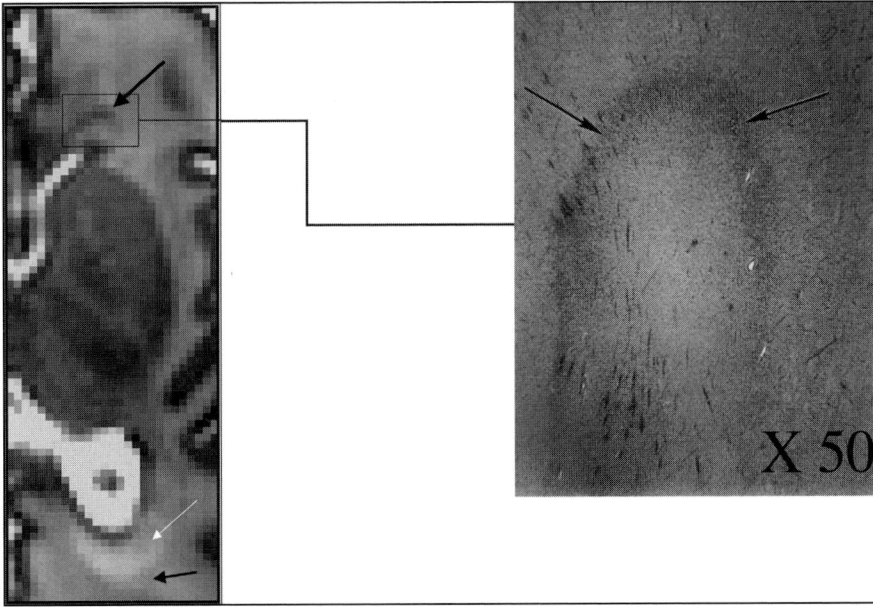

Fig. 6. T2-weighted image in the transverse plane showing periventricular white matter (left side only). There are low signal intensity regions anteriorly and posteriorly (black arrows) that correspond to areas of resident microglia (Judas et al., 2005) These can be seen in the slide (× 50 magnification) as cellular areas clustered around vessels. Regions known as white matter crossroads are seen as high signal intensity on T2-weighted images. The posterior crossroad is shown here (white arrow).

histological correlations. The latter is difficult as neonates with these milder forms of white matter disease are unlikely to die. Attempts to obtain histological correlations would be easier if a diagnosis of punctate lesions and DEHSI could be made routinely using ultrasound, the use of MRI as a routine imaging tool in neonatal intensive care being strictly limited. Florid punctate lesions are detectable with ultrasound but may be missed, and there is not as yet an ultrasound correlation for DEHSI. An easier approach would be to develop animal models for these milder white matter diseases. In a recent study using a rat model of a milder white matter injury (Baud et al., 2004), in vivo imaging of the brain showed an increase in apparent diffusion coefficient (ADC) values, as found in both DEHSI and diffuse PVL (Counsell et al., 2006), and at histology this white matter showed increased numbers of activated microglia. It has often been assumed that short T1, short T2 punctate lesions represent haemorrhage. Against this is the fact that the signal intensity on T1-weighted images is usually more pronounced than on T2-weighted images and is not enhanced by gradient echo imaging. In an isolated correlation we have found that these punctate lesions represented clusters of activated microglia (Fig. 4).

Incidence

Periventricular leucomalacia is a major cause of cerebral palsy in the child born preterm but in the spectrum of white matter diseases it is relatively uncommon. In a cohort of 119 infants born before 30 weeks' gestation at our hospital, two had PVL and nine had punctate lesions, and of the 87 scanned at term equivalent age, 70 had DEHSI (Dyet et al., 2006).

Later imaging: term-equivalent age

When preterm infants are imaged at term-equivalent age, the secondary effects of the white matter disease on various brain structures can be visualized and quantified. Infants with PVL characteristically show thalamic atrophy and abnormal delayed myelination within the posterior limb of the internal capsule (PLIC) (Cowan & De Vries, 2005; Ricci *et al.*, 2006) (Fig. 7). These findings can be used to determine whether the child will achieve independent walking. Quantitative studies have also demonstrated a reduction in cortical volume at term-equivalent age in infants with PVL (Inder *et al.*, 1999). Pathological studies have shown an increase in both cortical and central grey matter abnormalities in infants with PVL (Pierson *et al.*, 2007).

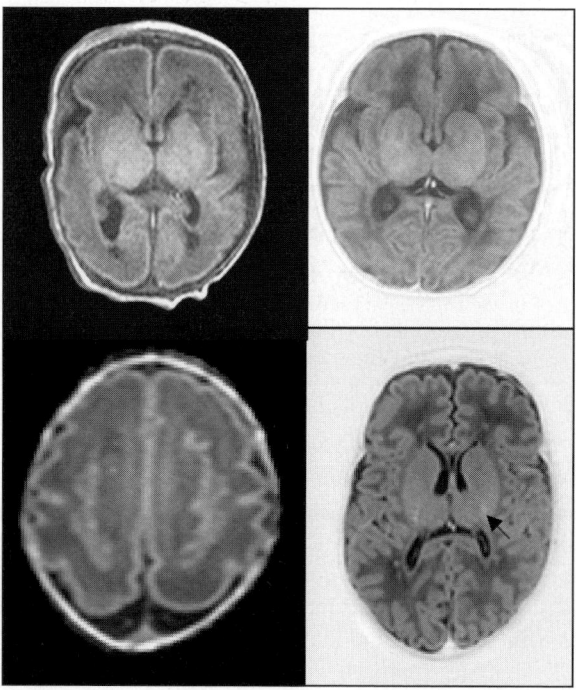

Fig. 7. Initial (left column) and term-equivalent (right column) images in periventricular leucomalacia (PVL) (top row) and punctate white matter lesions (bottom row). The images at term-equivalent age show thalamic atrophy and absent (top row) myelin in the posterior limb of the internal capsule (PLIC) in the infant with PVL. The myelin in the PLIC is reduced (arrow) in the infant with widespread punctate lesions. Both infants have developed a motor impairment.

Infants with punctate lesions that are sufficiently widespread can show similar changes to infants with PVL. A study at term-equivalent age showed that infants with punctate lesions had reduced myelin and decreased cortical folding on visual analysis (Ramenghi *et al.*, 2007). Infants with fewer lesions may show relatively normal imaging with a reduction in the original number of lesions identified (Fig. 5). Punctate lesions that are within the PLIC may result in altered myelination and may then increase the risk of motor impairment (Figs. 8 and 9). By definition DEHSI is diagnosed at term-equivalent age as regions of long T1 and long T2 within the white matter. In infants with DEHSI, the appearances of the PLIC are normally appropriate for age. On quantitative analysis, DEHSI is associated with a reduction in central grey matter volume (Boardman *et al.*, 2006).

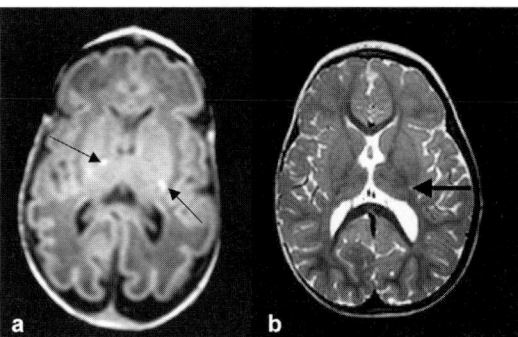

Fig. 8. Punctate white matter lesions within the central grey matter and posterior limb of the internal capsule (PLIC) in an infant born at 31 weeks' gestation. T1-weighted image at 3 weeks (a) show high signal intensity regions within the PLIC. T2-weighted image at 14 months (b) shows abnormal high signal intensity consistent with gliosis on the left. This infant has a mild diplegia.

Later imaging: infant and childhood

On later imaging, children with PVL show the classic triad of reduction in white matter, reduction in myelination, and angular dilatation of the posterior lateral ventricles (Fig. 9). Infants with punctate lesions may show similar appearances if the lesions have been widespread (Fig. 9). In infants with DEHSI there is an association with increased T2 in the posterior periventricular white matter (Fig. 9).

Association with neurodevelopmental outcome

The neurodevelopmental sequelae of PVL are well recognized. Children develop abnormal tone, usually in the form of a diplegia with involvement of the upper limbs in more severe cases. Neurocognitive impairment is usual unless changes are very mild. Long term cohort studies are now under way to determine the clinical significance of these new white matter diseases – punctate white matter lesions and DEHSI – and to establish whether they represent the anatomical correlates for the neurocognitive impairments that are now recognized as the most common sequelae in children who have been born extremely preterm (Wood et al., 2005).

To date, assessment of the effect of punctate white matter lesions has been confined to the second year, where neonates with only a few lesions had a normal outcome (Cornette et al., 2002). However, more widespread lesions may give rise to a spastic diplegia (Fig. 7). In addition, punctate lesions within the PLIC may also cause motor impairment (Fig. 8). As a group, children who showed DEHSI on term-equivalent images have significant developmental impairment but no motor abnormality at 2 years of age, compared with neonates with normal appearing white matter. However, approximately 50 per cent of neonates who show DEHSI have a normal developmental outcome at 2 years. This suggests that the effects of DEHSI may be modifiable, perhaps by genetics or the home environment (Dyet et al., 2006).

Future research

Whether these white matter diseases represent a spectrum may not be the most important question for us to answer. A more important question may be whether DEHSI, the most frequent

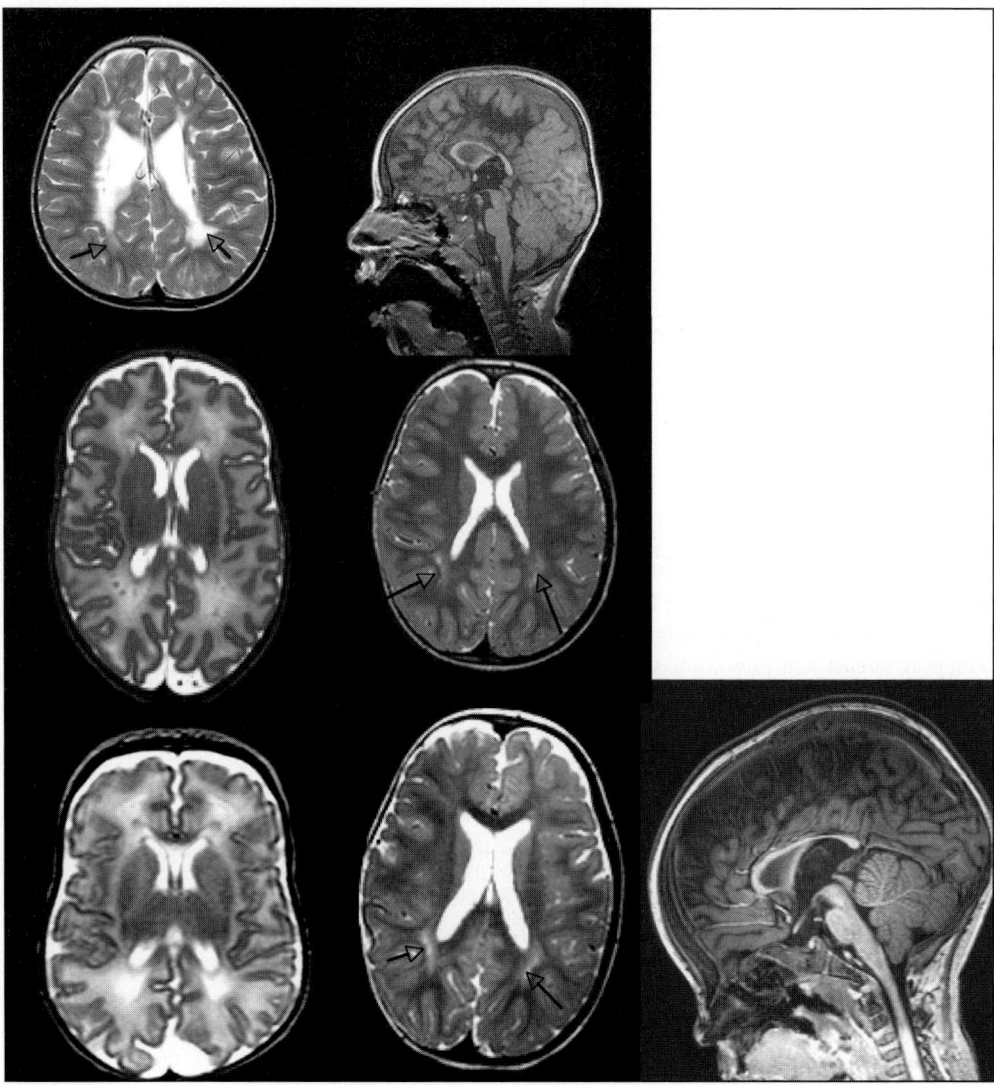

Fig. 9. Later imaging (during the second year) in the white matter disease of prematurity.
Periventricular leucomalacia (PVL) (top row): T2-weighted image in PVL showing angulated dilated ventricles, decreased myelination, and abnormal high signal intensity consistent with glial tissue in the posterior periventricular white matter (PVWM) (black arrows) and T1-weighted image in the sagittal plane showing a very thin corpus callosum.
Punctate white matter lesions (middle row): T2-weighted images in punctate white matter lesions showing early and late appearances in the white matter. Late imaging shows abnormal high signal intensity consistent with glial tissue in the posterior PVWM (arrows).
Diffuse excessive high signal intensity (DEHSI) (bottom row): T2-weighted term-equivalent imaging and later imaging showing abnormal high signal intensity consistent with glial tissue in the posterior PVWM (arrows). T1-weighted later imaging shows thinning of the corpus callosum.

abnormality, is an injurious disease or a 'deficiency' disease. The preterm infant is deprived of the normal transplacentally derived hormones and growth factors. Should we be treating to modify injury or supplementing to modify a deficiency, or possibly a combination of both?

An improved understanding of the effect of premature exposure to the *ex utero* environment and its relation with disease in the developing white matter will pave the way for interventional trials designed to modify injury (Welin *et al.*, 2007), promote normal brain development, and thereby improve long term neurological morbidity in this high risk population.

Acknowledgments: We are grateful to The Medical Research Council, The European Leucodystrophy Association, Action Medical Research, and Philips Medical Systems for supporting these studies.

References

Back, S.A., Riddle, A. & Hohimer, A.R. (2006): Role of instrumented fetal sheep preparations in defining the pathogenesis of human periventricular white-matter injury [review]. *J. Child Neurol.* **21**, 582–589.

Baud, O., Daire, J.L., Dalmaz, Y., Fontaine, R.H., Krueger, R.C., Sebag, G., Evrard, P., Gressens, P. & Verney, C. (2004): Gestational hypoxia induces white matter damage in neonatal rats: a new model of periventricular leucomalacia. *Brain Pathol.* **14**, 1–10.

Boardman, J.P., Counsell, S.J., Rueckert, D., Kapellou, O., Bhatia, K.K., Aljabar, P., Hajnal, J., Allsop, J.M., Rutherford, M.A. & Edwards, A.D. (2006): Abnormal deep grey matter development following preterm birth detected using deformation-based morphometry. *Neuroimage* **32**, 70–78.

Cornette, L.G., Tanner, S.F., Ramenghi, L.A., Miall, L.S., Childs, A.M., Arthur, R.J., Martinez, D. & Levene, M.I. (2002): Magnetic resonance imaging of the infant brain: anatomical characteristics and clinical significance of punctate lesions. *Arch. Dis. Child. Fetal Neonat. Ed.* **86**, F171–F177.

Counsell, S.J., Shen, Y., Boardman, J.P., Larkman, D.J., Kapellou, O., Ward, P., Allsop, J.M., Cowan, F.M., Hajnal, J.V., Edwards, A.D. & Rutherford, M.A. (2006): Axial and radial diffusivity in preterm infants who have diffuse white matter changes on magnetic resonance imaging at term-equivalent age. *Pediatrics* **117**, 376–386.

Counsell, S.J., Shen, Y., Boardman, J.P., Larkman, D.J., Kapellou, O., Ward, P., Allsop, J.M.,Cowan, F.M., Hajnal, J.V., Edwards, A.D. & Rutherford, M.A. (2006): Axial and radial diffusivity in preterm infants who have diffuse white matter changes on magnetic resonance imaging at term-equivalent age. *Pediatrics* **117**, 376–386.

Cowan, F. & De Vries, L. (2005): The internal capsule in neonatal imaging. *Semin. Fetal. Neonat. Med.* **10**, 461–474.

De Vries, L.S., Van Haastert, I.L., Rademaker, K.J., Koopman, C. & Groenendaal, F. (2004): Ultrasound abnormalities preceding cerebral palsy in high-risk preterm infants. *J. Pediatr.* **144**, 815–820.

Dommergues, M.A., Plaisant, F., Verney, C. & Gressens, P. (2003): Early microglial activation following neonatal excitotoxic brain damage in mice: a potential target for neuroprotection. *Neuroscience* **121**, 619–628.

Dyet, L.E., Kennea, N., Counsell, S.J., Maalouf, E.F., Ajayi-Obe, M., Duggan, P.J., Harrison, M., Allsop, J.M., Hajnal, J., Herlihy, A.H., Edwards, B., Laroche, S., Cowan, F.M., Rutherford, M.A. & Edwards, A.D. (2006): Natural history of brain lesions in extremely preterm infants studied with serial magnetic resonance imaging from birth and neurodevelopmental assessment. *Pediatrics* **118**, 536–548.

Inder, T.E., Huppi, P.S., Warfield, S., Kikinis, R., Zientara, G.P., Barnes, P.D., Jolesz, F. & Volpe, J.J. (1999): Periventricular white matter injury in the premature infant is followed by reduced cerebral cortical gray matter volume at term. *Ann. Neurol.* **46**, 755–760.

Judas, M., Rados, M., Jovanov-Milosevic, N., Hrbac, P., Stern-Padovan, R. & Kostovic, I. (2005): Structural, immunocytochemical, and MR imaging properties of periventricular crossroads of growing cortical pathways in preterm infants. *Am. J. Neuroradiol.* **26**, 2671–2684.

Maalouf, E.F., Duggan, P.J., Rutherford, M.A., Counsell, S.J., Fletcher, A.M., Battin, M., Cowan, F. & Edwards, A.D. (1999): Magnetic resonance imaging of the brain in a cohort of extremely preterm infants. *J. Pediatr.* **135**, 351–357.

Miller, S.P. & McQuillen, P.S. (2007): Neurology of congenital heart disease: insight from brain imaging. *Arch. Dis. Child. Fetal Neonat. Ed.* **92**, F435–F437.

Pierson, C.R., Folkerth, R.D., Billiards, S.S., Trachtenberg, F.L., Drinkwater, M.E., Volpe, J.J. & Kinney, H.C. (2007): Gray matter injury associated with periventricular leucomalacia in the premature infant. *Acta Neuropathol. (Berl.)* **114**, 619–631.

Ramenghi, L.A., Fumagalli, M., Righini, A., Bassi, L., Groppo, M., Parazzini, C., Bianchini, E., Triulzi, F. & Mosca, F. (2007): Magnetic resonance imaging assessment of brain maturation in preterm neonates with punctate white matter lesions. *Neuroradiology* **49**, 161–167.

Ricci, D., Anker, S., Cowan, F., Pane, M., Gallini, F., Luciano, R., Donvito, V., Baranello, G., Cesarini, L., Bianco, F., Rutherford, M., Romagnoli, C., Atkinson, J., Braddick, O., Guzzetta, F. & Mercuri, E. (2006): Thalamic atrophy in infants with PVL and cerebral visual impairment. *Early Hum. Dev.* **82,** 591–595.

Volpe, J.J. Cerebral white matter injury of the premature infant – more common than you think. *Pediatrics* **112,** 176–180.

Welin, A.K., Svedin, P., Lapatto, R., Sultan, B., Hagberg, H., Gressens, P., Kjellmer, I. & Mallard, C. (2007): Melatonin reduces inflammation and cell death in white matter in the mid-gestation fetal sheep following umbilical cord occlusion. *Pediatr. Res.* **61,** 153–115.

Wood, N.S., Costeloe, K., Gibson, A.T., Hennessy, E.M., Marlow, N. & Wilkinson, A.R. for the EPICure Study Group (2005): The EPICure study: associations and antecedents of neurological and developmental disability at 30 months of age following extremely preterm birth. *Arch. Dis. Child. Fetal Neonat. Ed.* **90,** F134–F140.

Chapter 14

Maternal and infant characteristics associated with perinatal arterial stroke in the preterm infant

Manon Benders, Floris Groenendaal, Cuno Uiterwaal *, Peter Nikkels °,
Hein Bruinse ^, Rutger-Jan Nievelstein ** and Linda de Vries

Department of Neonatology, Wilhelmina Children's Hospital, UMC Utrecht, the Netherlands;
* Julius Centre for Health Sciences and Primary Care, UMC Utrecht;
° Department of Pathology, UMC Utrecht;
^ Department of Obstetrics, Wilhelmina Children's Hospital, UMC Utrecht;
** Department of Radiology, Wilhelmina Children's Hospital, UMC Utrecht
l.s.devries@umcutrecht.nl

Summary

Most investigations of perinatal arterial stroke (PAS) have excluded preterm infants. We therefore analysed imaging findings and antenatal and perinatal risk factors in a hospital-based case-control study of preterm infants. Case infants were confirmed by reviewing brain imaging and medical records (n = 31). Three controls per case were individually matched with case infants from the study population. Gestational age (GA) ranged between 27 and 36 weeks and birth weight between 580 and 3,180 g. PAS was more common on the left (61 per cent) and 7 per cent had bilateral strokes. In most cases the stroke involved the middle cerebral artery (MCA) distribution. Involvement of one or more lenticulostriate branches was most common among the infants with a GA of 28 to 32 weeks, and main branch involvement was only seen in those with a GA of > 32 weeks. Twin-twin transfusion syndrome, fetal heart rate abnormalities, and hypoglycaemia were identified as independent risk factors for PAS. In conclusion, preterm PAS is associated with prenatal, perinatal, and postpartum risk factors. We were unable to identify any maternal risk factors. Involvement of the different branches of the MCA changed with an increase in GA.

Introduction

Perinatal arterial ischaemic stroke (PAS) is increasingly recognized with the greater use of sophisticated neuroimaging techniques (Cowan *et al.*, 2003; Miller *et al.*, 2005). In the full-term infant, PAS is the second most common underlying aetiology of neonatal seizures (Estan & Hope, 1997; Lee *et al.*, 2005). Several reports, restricted to full-term infants, have found that diverse maternal, prenatal and perinatal risk factors were independently associated with the development of PAS (Golomb *et al.*, 2001; Lee *et al.*, 2005). Infertility, preeclampsia, prolonged rupture of membranes, and chorioamnionitis were recently identified as

---

This article was originally published in *Stroke* (2007, vol. 38: 1759-65) and is reproduced here by permission of Lippincott Williams & Wilkins.

independent maternal risk factors (Lee *et al.*, 2005). Neonatal risk factors such as congenital heart disease, infection, dehydration, polycythaemia, prothrombotic factors and others have also been found to be associated with PAS (Amit & Camfield, 1980; Pellicer *et al.*, 1992; Kurnik *et al.*, 2003; Nelson & Lynch, 2004; Hunt & Inder, 2006).

There are hardly any data concerning PAS in preterm infants. A few reports included preterm infants in imaging studies (De Vries *et al.*, 1988; De Vries *et al.*, 1997; Abels *et al.*, 2006), but no studies have so far been undertaken to look at risk factors for PAS in the preterm population.

Our aim in this study was to determine antenatal and perinatal risk factors and postnatal complications in preterm infants with radiologically confirmed PAS in a hospital-based population.

Materials

This case-control study was part of a cohort of preterm infants. Infants were admitted from 1 January 1990 to 31 December 2005 to the Wilhelmina Children's Hospital. This tertiary neonatal intensive care unit takes care of a population of two million people who live in the centre of the Netherlands.

Infants with congenital anomalies, chromosomal abnormalities, or infection of the central nervous system and with PAS beyond day 28 were excluded. Cerebral ultrasonography (cUS) was part of routine clinical care. Informed parental consent was obtained for magnetic resonance imaging (MRI) in all infants. All children are seen in our follow-up clinic until at least 5 years of age.

Case ascertainment

An electronic search was undertaken in our ultrasound database (all infants were at least 9 months old when the records were searched). We retrieved all records and images of infants with a clinical diagnosis of *hemiplegia* and an imaging diagnosis of *focal infarction*, *stroke*, *MCA infarction*, and *venous infarction*.

Two study investigators (FG, RAJN) reviewed the cUS and MRI of potential cases of PAS.

cUS imaging criteria for the diagnosis of PAS were, first, the presence of a wedge-shaped area of echogenicity on coronal and parasagittal view, in the region supplied by the middle cerebral artery (MCA), anterior cerebral artery (ACA), or posterior cerebral artery (PCA) with a linear demarcation line; and second, cystic evolution of this area of increased echogenicity after 2 to 4 weeks. Echogenicity was sometimes noted to persist in the thalami/basal ganglia region despite a cystic lesion seen on MRI at term equivalent age. Diagnosis was sometimes made in the cystic phase. Taking the site, shape, and evolution into account, PAS was distinguished from cystic periventricular leucomalacia (PVL) – which is usually bilateral, although not necessarily symmetrical and is not restricted to the territory of the MCA – and from a parenchymal haemorrhage, which is unilateral but is associated with an ipsilateral haemorrhage and shows a different shape and evolution, with the formation of a porencephalic cyst which communicates with the lateral ventricle.

Neuroimaging studies showing intraventricular haemorrhage with a unilateral parenchymal haemorrhage (venous infarction), cystic PVL, or sinovenous thrombosis were excluded. One investigator (MJNLB) reviewed the medical records of children with radiologically confirmed arterial infarction.

Control selection

Three controls were randomly selected, individually matched to the infants with PAS for date of birth (< 2 weeks) and gestational age (< 3 days).

Data abstraction

One study investigator (MJNLB) reviewed prenatal, obstetric, and neonatal medical records, using a standardized protocol.

Maternal ethnicity was noted as recorded in the medical notes. Intrauterine growth restriction was defined as a birth weight less than the third centile for gestational age according to the criteria of Kloosterman (1969). The mother was considered to have a history of infertility if this was documented in a prenatal, obstetric, or neonatal record.

Pre-eclampsia was defined as either pre-eclampsia or pregnancy-induced hypertension, as diagnosed by the obstetrician. The term chorioamnionitis was used in cases where maternal temperature was at least 38° C or a diagnosis was made by the attending obstetrician according to clinical symptoms alone. Fetal heart rate abnormalities were considered present if a treating physician noted repetitive or prolonged late decelerations, fetal bradycardia, or fetal distress on electronic fetal heart rate monitoring. Decreased fetal movements were recorded if there was a maternal report of decreased movements before labour.

Placental examination

During the period from 1990 until December 1996 placentas arrived in the pathology department fixed in formalin. Routine histological examination was done using at least three samples from the placenta – that is, one paraffin block from the umbilical cord and membranes, one from the insertion, and one from normal placental parenchyma; additional blocks were taken from macroscopic lesions. The angioarchitecture of monochorionic twin placentas (the vascular anastomoses) during this period was observed after fixation. From December 1996 all placentas arrived fresh and the angioarchitecture of monochorionic twin placentas was studied using different coloured dyes for the venous and arterial circulation of both twins (Umur et al., 2003). At least four paraffin blocks of the placenta were studied: one from the umbilical cord and membranes, one from the insertion, and two from normal placental parenchyma; additional blocks were taken from macroscopic lesions. Nineteen of the 31 case-study placentas (61 per cent) were sent for pathological examination and 51 of the 93 control placentas (55 per cent) were available. The following histological abnormalities were observed: chorioamnionitis, funisitis, chronic villitis, fetal thrombosis, and disturbed materno-placental perfusion (that is, placental bed pathology). In monochorionic placentas, the typical histological abnormalities in donor and recipient parenchyma were observed. The donor parenchyma showed immature large villi compared with the recipient parenchyma which had small mature villi.

Data analysis

Maternal and infant characteristics were tabulated by disease status. As patients with PAS were matched to controls, conditional logistic regression was used with disease status (PAS or not) as the dependent variable and maternal and fetal characteristics and pre- and intrapartum complications as independent variables. Univariate statistically significant predictors were included in a multivariate logistic regression analysis. All results are expressed as odds ratios and 95 per cent confidence intervals (CI), with corresponding p values. CI's not including 1 ($p < 0.05$) were considered statistically significant. SPSS for Windows, version 14, was used for all analyses.

Results

Among 3,877 preterm infants with a gestational age of ⩽ 34 weeks and 6 days, 26 cases of PAS were confirmed (0.7 per cent). A further five cases with a gestational age between 35 weeks and 36 weeks, 6 days were confirmed to have PAS.

Clinical presentation

Gestational age ranged between 27 and 36 weeks' gestational age. Birth weight ranged between 580 and 3,180 g (Table 1). One infant died in the neonatal period and one at the age of 21 months. Six infants were one of monozygous twins, with associated twin-twin transfusion syndrome. Antenatal death of the co-twin occurred in three of the six monochorionic twinning pregnancies. One was part of a dichorionic triplet (two male, one female).

Neuroimaging findings

The diagnosis was initially made with cUS in all cases and subsequently confirmed by MRI in the neonatal period (n = 25; 81 per cent) or later in infancy (n = 2). There were no infants with a diagnosis of PAS on cUS which was not confirmed by MRI (sensitivity of cUS, 100 per cent). Eleven infants had an MRI on both occasions. Four infants were diagnosed with cUS and did not have MRI. Unilateral infarction was more common on the left (61 per cent) than on the right (32 per cent), whereas seven per cent had a bilateral arterial distribution of infarcts. The majority of strokes involved the MCA (25; 81 per cent), one of which involved both MCA and PCA distribution; four infants had an ACA distribution, one had a PCA

Table 1A. Univariate predictors of PAS in preterm infants: maternal characteristics and prepartum complications

	Cases (n = 31)	Controls (n = 93)	OR (95% CI)	p Value
Maternal characteristics (yes/no)				
	13/31	40/92	0.9 (0.4 to 2.1)	0.86
History of infertility	2/31	12/91	0.5 (0.1 to 2.2)	0.34
Clomid	1	6/12	0.5 (0.06 to 4.2)	0.52
IVF/ICSI		6/12	n.e.	
Previous miscarriage	8/31	21/93 (2 EUG/4 IUVD)	1.2 (0.5 to 3.2)	0.71
Thyroid problems	0/31	1/95	n.e.	
Outborn	12/31	35/92	1.3 (0.8 to 2.2)	0.30
Prepartum complications (yes/no)				
Twins	8/31	23/93	1.1 (1.4 to 2.7)	0.91
Monozygous	7/31	17/93	1.3 (0.5 to 3.8)	0.58
TTTS	6/31	3/93	15.4 (1.8 to 130.6)	0.01*
Death of co-twin	3/6	-	-	-
IUGR BW < p3	7/31	22/93	0.9 (0.3 to 2.6)	0.90
OFC < p3	5/27	14/84	1.1 (0.2 to 3.8)	0.87
Pre-eclampsia	9/31	14/92	2.1 (0.8 to 5.3)	0.12
Reduced fetal movements	4/30	2/93	6.0 (1.1 to 32.8)	0.04*

Values are frequencies.
* Statistically significant.
BW, birth weight; CI, confidence interval; IUGR, intrauterine growth retardation; n.e., non-estimable; OFC, occipito-frontal head circumference; OR, odds ratio; p3, third percentile; TTTS, twin-twin transfusion syndrome.

Table 1B. Univariate predictors of PAS in preterm infants: intrapartum complications and infant characteristics

	Cases (n = 31)	Controls (n = 93)	OR (95% CI)	p Value
Intrapartum complications (yes/no)				
PROM	9/31	23/93	1.3 (0.5 to 3.2)	0.63
Vaginal blood loss	2/31	17/92	0.3 (0.1 to 1.3)	0.09
Oxytocin induction	2/31	1/91	6.0 (0.5 to 66.2)	0.14
Fetal heart rate abnormality	18/31	24/92	3.7 (1.6 to 8.8)	0.003*
Ventouse delivery	2/31	1/91	6.0 (0.5 to 66.2)	0.14
Breech delivery	0/31	8/93	n.e.	
Emergency CS	14/31	28/95	(0.8 to 3.9)	0.15
Infant characteristics				
Male sex	13/31	51/93	0.5 (0.2 to 1.3)	0.17
Umbilical artery pH ≤ 7.10	4/16	11/51	1.8 (0.3 to 12.2)	0.53
Apgar score 5 min ≤ 5	2/31	7/93	1.0 (0.2 to 5.3)	1.00
GA (weeks, mean ± SD)	31.7 ± 2.5	31.7 ± 2.5	1.0 (0.4 to 2.5)	0.99
BW (g, mean ± SD)	1599 ± 633	1607 ± 720	1.000 (0.999 to 1.001)	0.96
IPPV	18/31	47/93	1.4 (0.6 to 3.5)	0.43
Hypoglycaemia (< 2 mmol/l)	13/31	16/90	3.3 (1.3 to 8.3)	0.01*
Umbilical lines	21/31	71/89	1.1 (0.7 to 3.5)	0.85
Inotropic support	5/31	23/95	0.6 (0.2 to 1.7)	0.30
Ductus (indomethacin/surgery)	1/31	8/93	0.4 (0.1 to 3.0)	0.36
NEC	3/31	4/93	2.3 (0.5 to 10.1)	0.29

Values are frequencies.
* Statistically significant.
BW, birth weight; CI, confidence interval; CS, caesarean section; IPPV, intermittent positive pressure ventilation; n.e., non-estimable; NEC, necrotizing enterocolitis; OR, odds ratio; PROM, prolonged rupture of the membranes.

distribution, and one had a unilateral watershed distribution between the ACA and MCA. Involvement of the MCA main branch was seen in nine infants, a cortical branch in four, and one or more lenticulostriate branches were involved in 12. Involvement of the different branches changed with an increase in gestational age. While only one of the 14 infants with a gestational age between 28 and 32 weeks had involvement of the main branch, eight of the 11 infants with a gestational age of more than 32 weeks did have such involvement ($p = 0.02$, Fisher's exact test). Involvement of one or more lenticulostriate branches was most common among the infants with a gestational age of 28 to 32 weeks (Fig. 1). cUS and MR images illustrate the different types of lesions in Figs. 2 and 3.

Associated intracranial lesions were found in four of our cases. All four had a lenticulostriate infarct, associated with cystic periventricular leucomalacia in two and with a large intraventricular haemorrhage in the other two.

Univariate risk factor analysis

Maternal race, primiparity, and history of previous miscarriages or infertility did not differ between case and control groups. None of the case infants or controls had been exposed to cocaine during pregnancy. Being part of monozygous twins with twin-twin transfusion

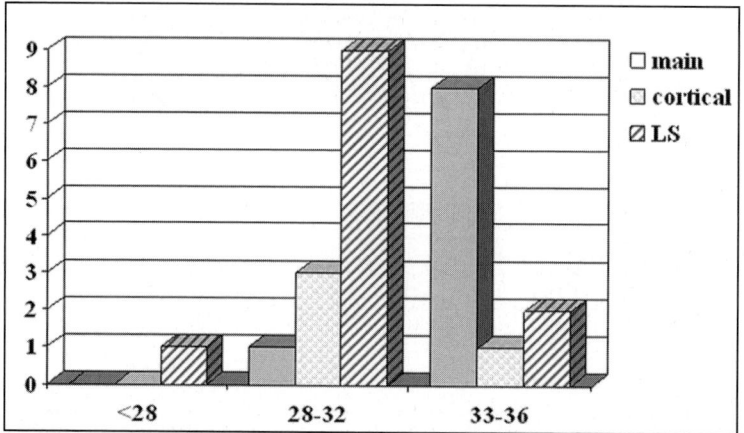

Fig. 1. Middle cerebral artery (MCA): involvement of the different branches in relation to gestational age. LS, lenticulostriate. Vertical axis, number of cases; horizontal axis, gestational age in weeks.

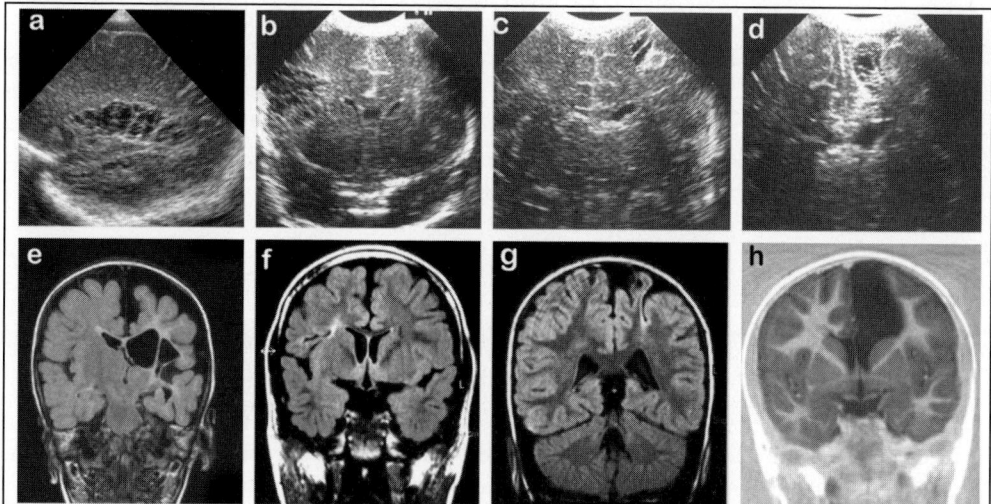

Fig. 2. (a) Cerebral ultrasound (cUS), parasagittal view, large MCA infarction, gestational age (GA), 27 weeks, twin-twin transfusion syndrome, both survived. (e) Magnetic resonance imaging (MRI), FLAIR sequence of the same child at 18 months of age, showing gliosis and extensive cavitation adjacent to the left ventricle. (b) cUS, coronal view showing right anterior MCA infarction, GA 29 weeks. (f) Corresponding MRI, FLAIR sequence at 8 years of age, gliosis adjacent to the right ventricle and a small area of cavitation. (c) cUS, coronal view, showing a left sided large MCA/ACA watershed infarction, GA 30 weeks. (g) Corresponding MRI, FLAIR sequence, at 8 years of age, a gliotic cleft and atrophy of the area involved. (d) cUS, coronal view, a left-sided terminal branch ACA infarction, GA 36 weeks. (h) Corresponding MRI, inversion recovery sequence, at 7 years of age. ACA, anterior cerebral artery; MCA, middle cerebral artery.

syndrome was associated with a 15 times greater risk of PAS. Intrauterine death of the co-twin occurred in three of the cases and none of the controls.

Pre-eclampsia was associated with a twofold greater risk of PAS, but the difference did not reach statistical significance ($p = 0.12$).

Intrapartum complications associated with PAS included the use of oxytocin, fetal heart rate abnormality, ventouse delivery, and emergency caesarean section. Reduced fetal movements

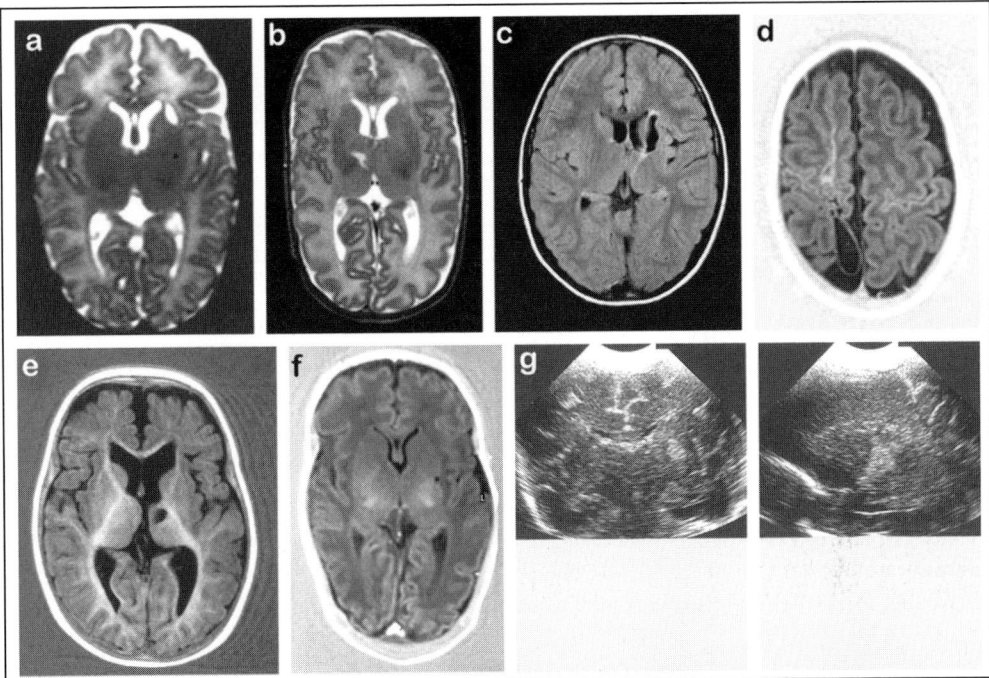

Fig. 3. (a) Magnetic resonance imaging (MRI), T2 SE sequence, term equivalent age, left sided infarction of the lateral striate MCA lesion, gestational age (GA) 30 weeks, twin-twin transfusion syndrome, both survived. (b) MRI, T2 SE sequence, term-equivalent age, right-sided lateral striate infarction, GA 28 weeks. (c) MRI, FLAIR sequence at 8 years of age, large left-sided lateral striate infarction in a male infant, GA 32 weeks. (d) MRI, inversion recovery sequence, term-equivalent age, right-sided ACA, terminal branch, GA 28 weeks. (e) MRI, inversion recovery sequence at 18 months of age, left-sided PCA thalamo-perforant branch infarction, GA 28 weeks. (f) MRI, inversion recovery sequence at term-equivalent age, small left-sided lenticulostriate infarction, GA 31 weeks. (g) The corresponding coronal and parasagittal ultrasound abnormality of this infant, preceding the cystic phase. ACA, anterior cerebral artery; MCA, middle cerebral artery; PCA, posterior cerebral artery.

were associated with a sixfold increased risk of PAS ($p = 0.04$) and fetal heart rate abnormalities with a fourfold increased risk ($p = 0.003$).

At delivery, the umbilical artery pH was less than 7.10 in four of 16 infants (25 per cent) with PAS, compared with 11 of 51 controls (22 per cent) for whom a cord blood gas result was available ($p = 0.53$).

In the neonatal period, there was no difference with respect to ventilation, the use of inotropic support, the presence of a ductus arteriosus requiring treatment, polycythaemia, umbilical catheters, or peripheral arterial lines. Hypoglycaemia resulted in a 3.3-fold increased risk of PAS than controls ($p = 0.01$). Eight case infants developed seizures (26 per cent) compared with four controls ($p = 0.007$).

Multivariate risk factor analysis

The following variables were entered to the main logistic regression model: twin-twin transfusion syndrome, decreased fetal movements, abnormal heart rate pattern, and hypoglycaemia (Table 2). The risk factors that remained independently associated with PAS were: twin-twin transfusion syndrome (odds ratio (OR) = 31.2; 95 per cent CI, 2.9 to 340.0); abnormal heart rate pattern (OR = 5.2; 95 per cent CI, 1.5 to 17.6); and hypoglycaemia (OR = 3.9; 95 per cent CI, 1.2 to 12.6).

Table 2. Multivariate odds ratios for PAS in preterm infants

	OR (95% CI)	p Value
TTTS (yes/no)	31.2 (2.9 to 340.0)	0.005*
Reduced fetal movements (yes/no)	1.6 (0.2 to 12.8)	0.64
Abnormal fetal heart rate (yes/no)	5.2 (1.5 to 17.6)	0.008*
Hypoglycaemia (< 2 mmol/l)	3.9 (1.2 to 12.6)	0.02*

CI, confidence interval; OR, odds ratio; TTTS, twin-twin transfusion syndrome; *, statistically significant.

Placental pathology

Nineteen placental pathological examinations were carried out among the 31 cases (Table 3). Extensive placental thrombosis was noted in one case. This infant showed lack of flow in the internal carotid artery on neonatal MR angiography and infarction in both the MCA and PCA distribution. Fifty-one control placentas were available for pathological examination.

Table 3. Placental examination in a subgroup of cases and controls

	Cases (n = 19)	Controls (n = 51)	OR (95% CI)	p Value
Placental pathology				
Chorioamnionitis	1/19	13/51	0.1 (0.02 to 1.2)	0.07
Infarct/hypoxia	7/19	19/51	1.5 (0.4 to 5.4)	0.49
Normal	5/19	18/51	0.5 (0.2 to 1.9)	0.35
Vascular anastomoses	6/19	1/51	n.e.	

CI, confidence interval; n.e., non-estimable; OR, odds ratio.

Comparison between case infants and controls could be done for placentas of 18 cases and 33 controls. One case infant could not be included in the statistical analysis as there was no matched control. No significant differences were found between case infants and controls.

Thrombophilia

Only 11 cases have so far been tested for presence of a genetic thrombophilia, because the remaining infants were born before these tests became routinely available in our institution. Seven infants were diagnosed with a genetic thrombophilia, including two with factor V Leiden heterozygosity, five had an MTHFR mutation (two homozygous, three heterozygous), and one had an increased Lp(a) (Lynch et al., 2005).

Preterm infants of ≤ 32 weeks gestational age

As preterm infants of ≤ 32 weeks gestational age are a more homogeneous group, as most will be inborn following *in utero* transfer, this subgroup was also analysed separately.

In the univariate risk factor analysis, case infants were also noted to have fetal heart rate abnormalities and hypoglycaemia significantly more often. Twin-twin transfusion syndrome could no longer be estimated as a risk factor as this problem was present in two of 19 case infants compared with none of 57 controls (Fisher exact test, $p = 0.06$). For the multivariate analysis abnormal heart rate pattern (OR = 11.7; 95 per cent CI, 2.2 to 61.6; $p = 0.004$) and hypoglycaemia (OR = 8.6; 95 per cent CI, 1.7 to 43.9; $p = 0.01$) remained independently associated with PAS.

Preterm singletons

Following exclusion of all case infants and controls belonging to multiple births, 23 case infants and 69 controls could be compared for the risk factors mentioned above. As reduced fetal movements were more often present among the case infants in the univariate risk factor analysis (OR = 3.8; 95 per cent CI, 0.7 to 21.6, $p = 0.03$), this variable was also entered to the main logistic regression model, together with abnormal heart rate pattern and hypoglycaemia. Only the latter two remained independently associated with PAS (respectively, OR = 6.2; 95 per cent CI, 1.7 to 22.1; $p = 0.005$; and OR = 3.6; 95 per cent CI, 1.0 to 12.9; $p = 0.05$).

Discussion

Studies on PAS in preterm infants are scarce, usually including only a few preterm infants reported as part of a group consisting mainly of term infants (Lee *et al.*, 2005). To our knowledge this is the first controlled study of risk factors for PAS in preterm infants. Except for the presence of twin-twin transfusion syndrome, antenatal risk factors such as a history of infertility, pre-eclampsia, and chorioamnionitis could not be identified as significant risk factors. Decreased fetal movements, abnormalities of fetal heart rate, and an emergency caesarean section were more often present among the cases than among the controls, but only fetal heart rate abnormalities were identified as an independent risk factor. Hypoglycaemia was the only independent risk factor identified in the neonatal period.

As preterm infants of ≤ 32 weeks' gestational age are a more homogeneous group, this subgroup was analysed separately. Abnormal heart rate pattern and hypoglycaemia were both independently associated with PAS.

We found that PAS is not uncommon in preterm infants with a gestational age of ≤ 34 weeks, with an incidence of 7/1,000, compared with an incidence of 1/4,000 in full-term infants. This incidence is similar to our incidence of 0.9 per cent for c-PVL (unpublished data) and higher than the incidence for c-PVL reported by Hamrick *et al.* (2004). The higher incidence of PAS in our cohort of preterm infants may be explained by the use of routine cUS in *all* preterm infants, many of whom did not present with clinical symptoms, while only those full-term infants who present with (hemi)convulsions will have neuroimaging. Furthermore, preterm infants are more often exposed to invasive procedures during their stay in the neonatal intensive care unit (for example, umbilical lines) than infants born at term. As suspected parenchymal lesions detected by cUS examination are always verified by MRI in both preterm and term infants, it is unlikely that varying diagnostic criteria are a reason for the discrepancy in incidence between preterm and term infants. Our PAS data are hospital-based, obtained from a level-3 neonatal intensive care unit serving a population of two million people. The incidence for the preterm infants born at 35 to 36 weeks was not calculated as these represent a selected population of very sick infants.

Lenticulostriate infarcts appeared to be especially common in this preterm population and can be well visualized using cUS as they are well within the field of view. As sequential ultrasound examinations were performed till term-equivalent age, it is unlikely that infarcts in this region were missed. Cortical infarcts were not common in our cohort. As cUS is known to miss smaller cortical infarcts, it is likely that some cases with cortical PAS were missed over the years, especially as they do not necessarily lead to neurological symptoms later in infancy (Estan & Hope, 1997; Golomb et al., 2003; Cowan et al., 2005).

In our cerebral palsy register a total of six infants were diagnosed during this 16-year period as having mild hemiplegia, which could not be explained by a unilateral parenchymal haemorrhage. Five of these six infants were not from the group of infants described here. They had an MRI in infancy and did not have a lesion which could be attributed to PAS. Instead they were noted to have mild, predominantly unilateral periventricular leucomalacia, not detected in the neonatal period with cUS. In the other infant, cUS was normal and the parents did not give permission for MRI. As the child was one of monozygous twins and the co-twin died before birth, it is likely that this infant had unconfirmed PAS.

Clinical presentation was very different from that in previously published reports on term infants. While presentation with hemiconvulsions was the presenting symptom in 75 per cent of the term infants studied by Kurnik et al. (2003), seizures or apnoeas, or both, were only seen in eight of our 31 cases, and five of these had main branch involvement and a gestational age of > 32 weeks. Identification of the preterm infant with PAS will therefore be mostly based on dedicated sequential cUS. In contrast to the data of Golomb et al. (2004), we did not find boys to be more commonly affected than girls.

Placental examination was undertaken in about half of both the cases and the controls. There was no difference in the presence of chorioamnionitis (Leistra-Leistra et al., 2004). Monochorionic placentation with vascular interconnections was more common among the case infants. This has been reported to lead to antenatal brain injury, such as antenatal cystic-PVL and porencephaly (Jung et al., 1984; Szymonowicz et al., 1986; Bernischke, 1995). There are two case reports showing PAS following death of a co-twin (Cole-Beuglet et al., 1987; de Laveaucoupet et al., 1995). The case reported by de Laveaucoupet et al., however, was of an infant with cystic-PVL and not focal infarction. Death of a co-twin may further lead to redistribution of thromboplastic material or to emboli in the circulation of the surviving twin, or lead to a sudden fall in blood pressure because of the lack of resistance of the circulation of the demised twin (Weig et al., 1995; Lopriore et al., 2006). Increased use of antenatal laser therapy appears to be associated with a reduced risk of brain injury associated with twin-twin transfusion syndrome and may therefore also reduce the risk of PAS in this subgroup of preterm infants (Senat et al., 2004). In a recent study by Golomb et al. (2006), four of 35 children diagnosed with presumed PAS were one of twins. There was no death of the co-twin and two were known to be dizygotic twins.

The neonatal problems were evenly distributed among both groups, except for the presence of hypoglycaemia, which was significantly more common among the cases. Owing to the delay in visualising ultrasound abnormalities in infants who develop PAS, it is uncertain whether the hypoglycaemia did indeed precede PAS. Bilateral occipital infarction has been noted to be associated with occipital infarction in full-term infants with symptomatic hypoglycaemia (Barkovich et al., 1998; Filan et al., 2006). Indirect evidence for occipital regional vulnerability has been studied in a newborn dog model (Mujsce et al., 1989). That study showed increased regional cerebral blood flow (to 250 per cent in the thalamus) during hypoglycaemia. Regional glucose utilization was relatively unchanged or even reduced compared with a normoglycaemic situation in the brain. This is likely to make this region more vulnerable.

Furthermore, it is not uncommon to visualize small air bubbles on cUS shortly after insertion of an umbilical venous catheter, which might pass the heart through the foramen ovale to the arterial circulation. It has been shown that these small, 'silent' air bubbles do not immediately cause obstruction of arterioles or capillaries; however, decrease in cerebral blood flow has been described because of the effects that gases have on the vascular endothelial cells. This may cause a reduction in regional perfusion and an exaggerated response to vasoconstrictor agents (Helps *et al.*, 1990).

The role of prothrombotic disorders in preterm infants with PAS still needs to be determined. Only one-third of our cases had mutation analysis performed, and these data were not available for the controls. It was of interest that seven of the 11 infants tested had a mutation, with the MTHFR mutation being especially prominent. Permission for performing mutation analysis is sought when cases visit the follow-up clinic. Retrospective analysis, using DNA obtained from Guthrie cards, will also be undertaken in the controls in the near future and will help to clarify the potential role of these prothrombotic factors. Our findings suggest that prothrombotic disorders are relatively more common in preterm neonates with PAS and therefore they should undergo extensive testing.

Conclusions

Fetal heart rate abnormalities, and especially the presence of twin-twin transfusion syndrome, were independent risk factors for preterm PAS. Hypoglycaemia was the only independent risk factor identified in the immediate neonatal period. In contrast to full-term PAS, we were unable to identify any maternal risk factors. Involvement of the different branches of the MCA changed with an increase in gestational age.

References

Abels, L., Lequin, M. & Govaert, P. (2006): Sonographic templates of newborn perforator stroke. *Pediatr. Radiol.* **36**, 663–669.

Amit, M. & Camfield, P.R. (1980): Neonatal polycythemia causing multiple cerebral infarcts. *Arch. Neurol.* **37**, 109–110.

Barkovich, A.J., Ali, F.A., Rowley, H.A. & Bass, N. (1998): Imaging patterns of neonatal hypoglycemia. *Am. J. Neuroradiol.* **19**, 523–528.

Bernischke, K. (1995): The biology of the twinning process: how placentation influences outcome. *Semin. Perinatol.* **19**, 342–350.

Cole-Beuglet, C., Aufrichtig, D., Cohen, A., Harrison, L., Miller, E.I. & Crade, M. (1987): Ultrasound case of the day. Twin pregnancy, intrauterine death of one twin with disseminated intravascular coagulation resulting in the development of a cerebral infarct in the surviving twin. *Radiographics* **7**, 389–394.

Cowan, F., Mercuri, E., Groenendaal, F., Bassi, L., Ricci, D., Rutherford, M. & de Vries, L.S. (2005): Does cranial ultrasound imaging identify arterial cerebral infarction in term neonates? *Arch. Dis. Child. Fetal Neonat. Ed.* **90**, F252–F256.

Cowan, F., Rutherford, M., Groenendaal, F., Eken, P., Mercuri, E., Bydder, G.M., Meiners, L.C., Dubowitz, L.M.S. & de Vries, L.S. (2003): Origin and timing of brain lesions in term infants with neonatal encephalopathy. *Lancet* **361**, 736–742.

de Laveaucoupet, J., Ciorascu, R., Lacaze, T., Roset, F., Musset, D. & Labrune, M. (1995): Hepatic and cerebral infarction in the survivor after the in utero death of a co-twin: sonographic pattern. *Pediatr. Radiol.* **25**, 211–213.

De Vries, L.S., Groenendaal, F., Eken, P., van Haastert, I.C., Rademaker, K.J. & Meiners, L.C. (1997): Infarcts in the vascular distribution of the middle cerebral artery in preterm and fullterm infants. *Neuropediatrics* **28**, 88–96.

De Vries, L.S., Regev, R., Connell, J.A., Pennock, J.M. & Dubowitz, L.M.S. (1988): Localised cerebral infarction in the premature infant: ultrasound diagnosis and correlation with CT and MRI. *Pediatrics* **81**, 31–34.

Estan, J. & Hope, P. (1997): Unilateral neonatal cerebral infarction in full term infants. *Arch. Dis. Child. Fetal Neonat. Ed.* **76**, F88–F93.

Filan, P.M., Inder, T.E., Cameron, F.J., Kean, M.J. & Hunt, R.W. (2006): Neonatal hypoglycemia and occipital cerebral injury. *J. Pediatr.* **148**, 552–555.

Golomb, M.R., Dick, P.T., MacGregor, D.L., Armstrong, D.C. & DeVeber, G.A. (2003): Cranial ultrasonography has a low sensitivity for detecting arterial ischemic stroke in term neonates. *J. Child Neurol.* **18**, 98–103.

Golomb, M.R., Dick, P.T., MacGregor, D.L., Curtis, R., Sofronas, M. & deVeber, G.A. (2004): Neonatal arterial ischemic stroke and cerebral sinovenous thrombosis are more commonly diagnosed in boys. *J. Child Neurol.* **19**, 493–497.

Golomb, M.R., MacGregor, D.L., Domi, T., Armstrong, D.C., McCrindle, B.W., Mayank, S. & deVeber, G.A. (2001): Presumed pre- or perinatal arterial ischemic stroke: risk factors and outcomes. *Ann. Neurol.* **50**, 163–168.

Golomb, M.R., Williams, L.S. & Garg, B.P. (2006): Perinatal stroke in twins without co-twin demise. *Pediatr. Neurol.* **35**, 75–77.

Hamrick, S.E., Miller, S.P., Leonard, C., Glidden, D.V., Goldstein, R., Ramaswamy, V., Piecuch, R. & Ferriero, D.M. (2004): Trends in severe brain injury and neurodevelopmental outcome in premature newborn infants: the role of cystic periventricular leucomalacia. *J. Pediatr.* **145**, 593–599.

Helps, S.C., Parsons, D.W., Reilly, P.L. & Gorman, D.F. (1990): The effect of gas emboli on rabbit cerebral blood flow. *Stroke* **21**, 94–99.

Hunt, R.W. & Inder, T.E. (2006): Perinatal and neonatal ischaemic stroke: a review. *Thromb. Res.* **118**, 39–48.

Jung, J.H., Graham, J.M., Schultz, N. & Smith, D.W. (1984): Congenital hydranencephaly/porencephaly due to vascular disruption in monozygotic twins. *Pediatrics* **73**, 467–469.

Kloosterman, G. (1969): [Intra-uterine growth and the intra-uterine growth curves.] *Maandschr. v Kindergeneesk.* **37**, 209–225.

Kurnik, K., Kosch, A., Strater, R., Schobess, R., Heller, C. & Nowak-Gottl, U. (2003): Childhood Stroke Study Group. Recurrent thromboembolism in infants and children suffering from symptomatic neonatal arterial stroke: a prospective follow-up study. *Stroke* **34**, 2887–2892.

Lee, J., Croen, L.A., Backstrand, K.H., Yoshida, C.K., Henning, L.H., Lindan, C., Ferriero, D.M., Fullerton, H.J., Barkovich, A.J. & Wu, Y.W. (2005): Maternal and infant characteristics associated with perinatal arterial stroke in the infant. *JAMA* **293**, 723–729.

Leistra-Leistra, M.J., Timmer, A., van Spronsen, F.J., Geven, W.B., van der Meer, J. & Erwich, J.J. (2004): Fetal thrombotic vasculopathy in the placenta: a thrombophilic connection between pregnancy complications and neonatal thrombosis? *Placenta* **25**, S102–S105.

Lopriore, E., van Wezel-Meijler, G., Middeldorp, J.M., Sueters, M., Vandenbussche, F.P. & Walther, F.J. (2006): Incidence, origin, and character of cerebral injury in twin-to-twin transfusion syndrome treated with fetoscopic laser surgery. *Am. J. Obstet. Gynecol.* **194**, 1215–1220.

Lynch, J.K., Han, C.J., Nee, L.E. & Nelson, K.B. (2005): Prothrombotic factors in children with stroke or porencephaly. *Pediatrics* **116**, 447–453.

Miller, S.P., Ramaswamy, V., Michelson, D., Barkovich, A.J., Holshouser, B., Wycliffe, N., Glidden, D.V., Deming, D., Partridge, J.C., Wu, Y.W., Ashwal, S. & Ferriero, D.M. (2005): Patterns of brain injury in term neonatal encephalopathy. *J. Pediatr.* **146**, 453–460.

Mujsce, D.J., Christensen, M.A. & Vannucci, R.C. (1989): Regional cerebral blood flow and glucose utilization during hypoglycemia in newborn dogs. *Am. J. Physiol.* **256**, H1659–H1666.

Nelson, K.B. & Lynch, J.K. Stroke in newborn infants. *Lancet Neurol.* **3**, 150–158.

Pellicer, A., Cabanas, F., Garcia-Alix, A., Perez-Higueras, A. & Quero, J. (1992): Stroke in neonates with cardiac right-to-left shunt. *Brain Dev.* **14**, 381–385.

Senat, M.V., Deprest, J., Boulvain, M., Paupe, A., Winer, N. & Ville, Y. (2004): Endoscopic laser surgery versus serial amnioreduction for severe twin-to-twin transfusion syndrome. *N. Engl. J. Med.* **351**, 136–144.

Szymonowicz, W., Preston, H. & Yu, V.Y.H. (1986): The surviving monozygotic twin. *Arch. Dis. Child.* **61**, 454–458.

Umur, A., van Gemert, M.J.C. & Nikkels, P.G.J. (2003): Monoamniotic-versus diamniotic monochorionic twin placentas: anastomoses and twin-twin transfusion syndrome. *Am. J. Obstet. Gynecol.* **189**, 1325–1329.

Weig, S.G., Marshall, P.C., Abroms, I.F. & Gauthier, N.S. (1995): Patterns of cerebral injury and clinical presentation in the vascular disruptive syndrome of monozygotic twins. *Pediatr. Neurol.* **13**, 279–285.

Chapter 15

Neonatal arterial ischaemic stroke

Paul Govaert

Sophia Children's Hospital, Erasmus MC, dr Molewaterplein 60, 3015 GJ Rotterdam, The Netherlands
paul.govaert3@pandora.be

Summary

Focal infarction in the newborn brain is a common event. Arterial ischaemic stroke can occur *in utero* before labour, during the first or second stage of labour and in the early as well as late perinatal period. Many instances present with seizures or apnoea, some are picked up following routine brain ultrasound scanning or following diagnostic imaging after recognition of focal EEG changes. Infants may present with presumed perinatal stroke if the original insult was not recognized. Some instances of arterial infarction can be prevented by avoiding embolism. This chapter is written as a guide for the neonatologist challenged by: recognition of stroke, correct nomination of the vessel affected, search for the most likely mechanism and for means of prevention in sibs or of recurrence in the propositus, prediction of outcome from within the neonatal period.

Introduction

This chapter deals with occluded artery ischaemia in the newborn brain (NAIS). Other causes of stroke are venous infarction and primary haemorrhage, in which the ruptured vessel is not known. Aspects developed here are those of interest to the practising neonatologist facing an infant with a suspicion of neonatal focal brain infarction. Different aspects of NAIS were recently reviewed (Allan & Riviello, 1992; deVeber *et al.*, 2000a, 2000b; Scher *et al.*, 2002; Nelson & Lynch, 2004; deVeber, 2005; Chalmers, 2005; Hunt & Inder, 2006).

On rare occasions one may observe hyperechoic change in an arterial territory, confirm 'stroke' with hyperacute magnetic resonance imaging (MRI), and later be surprised by the absence of tissue loss: in such instances ischaemia was reversible in the entire area. Some disease entities in the newborn result from small artery or arteriole occlusion and they enter the differential diagnosis of NAIS, although the anatomical feature of an affected large artery is absent; these include incontinentia pigmenti (Maingay-de Groof *et al.*, 2007), air embolism, infectious fetopathy, and Aicardi-Goutières syndrome (Barth *et al.*, 1999; Barth, 2002).

A myriad of focal brain lesions have to be differentiated from NAIS and sinovenous thrombosis: kernicterus, hypoglycaemia, encephalitis (bacterial and viral), mitochondrial disorders, posterior reversible encephalopathy, subarachnoid haematoma, tumour, vascular anomaly, multicystic encephalopathy, watershed injury, and lobar cerebral haematoma. Even non-accidental injury may feature in this list (McLellan et al., 1986, Jaspan et al., 1992; Bonnier et al., 2003; Jaspan et al., 2003).

The end result of arterial ischaemia depends on many variables: the degree and duration of occlusion, flow in the leptomeningeal collaterals (itself depending on cardiac output, blood pressure, and blood rheology), and the presence of seizures. The core of an affected area will develop infarction – that is, death of all cell types in the tissue, ending in cavitation. Some cells in the penumbra of an infarct may be dysfunctional but survive the insult, leaving an area of selective cell death around the infarcted core; it must be added that there is no evidence of the existence of penumbra in human neonatal imaging of NAIS. Studies of perinatal stroke (20 weeks of gestational age to 28 days after term) would have to include the cold stroke cases presenting in early childhood with hemiplegia, ophthalmoplegia, or epilepsy associated with cavitation within an arterial territory (Claeys et al., 1983; Jung et al., 1984; Weig et al., 1995; Debus et al., 1998; Golomb et al., 2001; Lynch et al., 2005; Golomb et al., 2006). The term infantile porencephaly covers arterial as well as venous cold stroke cases and is therefore not a denominator of perinatal arterial stroke (Scher et al., 1991; Dudink et al., 2007).

Clinical presentation

Some epidemiological data

It has been estimated at least one in 4,000 liveborn infants presents with NAIS and one in 10 of such patients dies (Lynch et al., 2001). A majority of neonatal stroke patients are male. Given that these data are almost exclusively based on cortical (pial) stroke and that in our own experience perforator stroke is about as common as pial arterial stroke, the incidence is higher than that, although perforator stroke is commonly observed in sick infants and has an unknown prevalence in the general population. As about half of pial strokes end in a contralateral motor hemisyndrome, the expected incidence of hemiplegia from perinatal arterial stroke is at least one in 10,000 live births (Uvebrant, 1988). Between 10 and 15 per cent of term infants with neonatal seizures suffer from acute cerebral infarction (Billard et al., 1982; Hill et al., 1983; Mannino & Trauner, 1983; Ment et al., 1984; Clancy et al., 1985; Levy et al., 1985; Aso et al., 1990; Estan & Hope, 1997; Jan & Camfield, 1998; Govaert et al., 2000; Ramaswamy et al., 2004), preceded in frequency by asphyxia only. Sonographic vigilance (Govaert & de Vries, 1996; Wang et al., 2004) and the availability of MRI have an impact on the perceived prevalence of stroke. Subcortical stroke, predominantly subclinical, is not uncommon in preterm infants (Abels et al., 2006; de Vries et al., this volume, chapter 15).

Seizures are the usual presentation of NAIS (Balcom & Redmond, 1997; Sreenan et al., 2000). The interval to clinical presentation and an additional time lag to diagnosis explain why paediatric stroke is often diagnosed around 36 hours after onset (Gabis et al., 2002). A similar or even larger interval is probably characteristic of NAIS. Focal seizures are a more common first sign of NAIS than general seizures (Filipek et al., 1987). Onset is divided 50/50 between day 1 and later in the first week, rarely beyond day 3 (Jan & Camfield, 1998). Because the interval insult to seizures may be short (less than 1 hour) but also add up to several hours, the timing in hours of an arterial insult in relation to birth is often unknown. Acute embolic stroke may cause seizures within an hour of the event (Pellicer et al., 1992) or their onset may be delayed for several hours (Fischer *et al.*, 1988). Typical are seizures contralateral to the infarct (Mannino & Trauner, 1983; Mantovani & Gerber, 1984; Clancy *et al.*, 1985; Fujimoto *et al.*, 1992). Both the middle cerebral artery (MCA) (complete or partial) and the posterior cerebral artery (PCA) can be involved in hemisomatic seizures, whereas involvement of the anterior cerebral artery (ACA) can present with arm and face convulsions only (Billard *et al.*, 1982). Isolated leg seizures were mentioned in a case of infarction of the anterior part of the region supplied by the MCA (Billard *et al.*, 1982). These findings make sense if we think of the penumbra as a partially functional area excited by waves of depolarization (Fig. 1). Starting off with general seizures is not rare (Levy *et al.*, 1985; Roodhooft *et al.*, 1987). The clonic type of seizure prevails (preliminary results of the French multicentre study on NAIS, courtesy of Drs. Saliba and Chabrier). From most reports it appeared that seizure control within the neonatal period was not unduly difficult (Fujimoto *et al.*, 1992). On occasion conjugated movement of the eyes away from the affected cerebral side has been described (Mantovani & Gerber, 1984). Subtle seizures were reported in association with MCA involvement: these included hiccups, eye blinking, staring, chewing, sucking, eye fluttering, vertical nystagmus, and thumb adduction (Mantovani & Gerber, 1984; Levy *et al.*, 1985; Klesh *et al.*, 1987; Raine *et al.*, 1989). These were rarely the only recognized form of convulsive activity. Several neonates presented with apnoeic spells or cyanotic attacks, again possibly of epileptic nature (Hill *et al.*, 1983; Mantovani & Gerber, 1984; Raine *et al.*, 1989; Fujimoto *et al.*, 1992; Jan & Camfield, 1998).

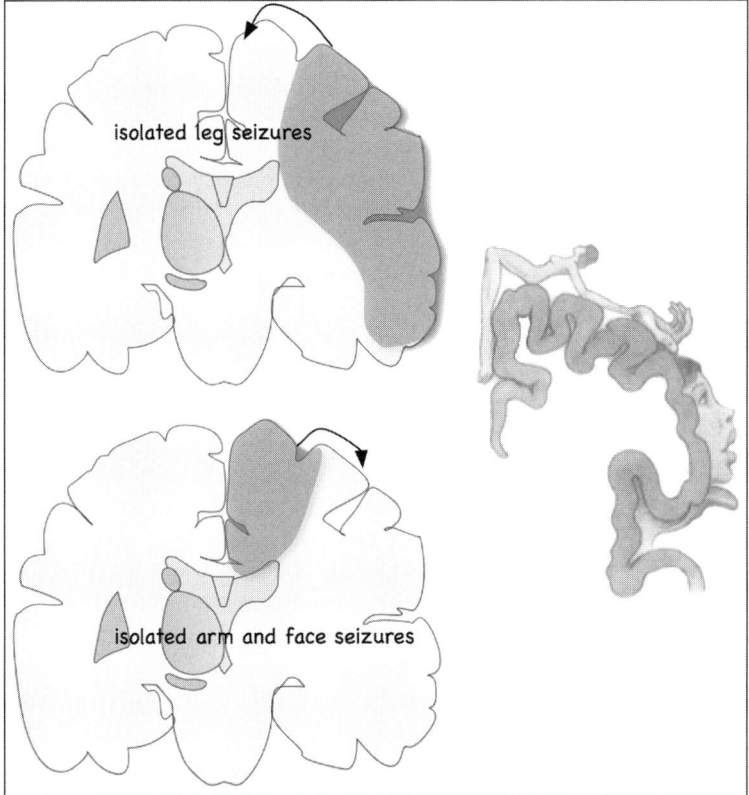

Fig. 1. Focal seizures around an infarct area may relate to the motor homunculus.

Most children seem to be alert between seizures and even accept oral feeding, although some are lethargic and do not suck well (Levy et al., 1985; Roodhooft et al., 1987). Intracranial hypertension is exceptional (Raine et al., 1989). Some present with temperature instability (Roodhooft et al., 1987), others with bouts of hypertension or hypotension caused by hypothalamic injury (personal observation). In a subgroup of infants, later hemiplegia can be predicted from neonatal appreciation of asymmetrical general movements (Guzzetta et al., 2003), but most often future hemiplegia is inconspicuous in the neonatal period. Neurological alarm signs are usually lacking in the preterm, where stroke is often a surprise finding at brain ultrasound scanning.

In the context of NAIS an alarming event is acute pallor and loss of pulsation of (part of) a limb caused by arterial embolism (or spasm?), as reported by several investigators (Asindi et al., 1988; Raine et al., 1989; Gudinchet et al., 1991; Silver et al., 1992; Guajardo et al., 1994; Broxterman et al., 2000 with factor V Leiden; Beattie et al., 2006 with subclavian steal; and one personal observation). Most of these limb-brain strokes present with limb pallor within minutes of delivery, strongly suggesting that embolic stroke may precede delivery by hours. In at least three cases antiphospholipid antibodies in neonatal serum were also present (Silver et al., 1992; Beattie et al., 2006; personal observation).

EEG findings in the acute stage

The area of infarction is the focus of epileptic discharge (Jan & Camfield, 1998; Mercuri et al., 1999), but in exceptional cases the epileptic focus occurs contralateral to the infarct. Clinical status epilepticus is always correlated with abnormal EEG findings. EEG monitoring may be an aid in detecting stroke in ventilated and sedated infants – for example, with pulmonary hypertension (Klesh et al., 1987; Scher & Beggarly, 1989; Koelfen et al., 1995; Evans & Levene, 1998; Clancy, 2006). Stroke types with subclinical seizures, escaping detection on routine serial ultrasound – such as NAIS caused by to PCA occlusion – may be suspected through EEG monitoring. The best EEG predictor of hemiplegia is not neonatal epileptic activity but a disturbed background (Mercuri et al., 1999; Mercuri, 2001), though agreement on this is not unanimous (Sreenan et al., 2000). Children with later cerebral palsy may have persisting numerous unilateral post-ictal positive rolandic slow sharp waves (Selton et al., 2003).

Vessels

The slight predilection for left hemisphere stroke remains unexplained. In our experience MCA stroke covers more than 50 per cent of the pial strokes, complete and posterior truncal stroke being most common (Govaert et al., 2000). The order of occurrence for the other arteries is internal carotid artery (ICA), PCA, ACA, and anterior choroidal artery (AChA) (Figs. 2 and 3). Templates for the sonographic diagnosis of perforator stroke have been published (de Vries et al., 1992 for thalamic focal infarction, Abels et al., 2006 for the other perforator stroke types, Garg & DeMyer, 1995 for paediatric thalamic stroke). It is not exceptional for different arteries to be involved in the same infant: infarction from thrombophilia, vasculopathy, or breakdown of a large thrombus into several emboli can all lead to multiple separate strokes in the same infant. There is insufficient knowledge of large artery stroke caused by neonatal air embolism, but multiple infarction is very likely in that condition as well. The arterial system mimics the mature end stage by the end of the embryonic period (Gillilan, 1972). It is not surprising, therefore, that viable preterm infants of any gestational age may suffer from stroke. In our experience major artery occlusion is not common in the small preterm infant, for reasons not

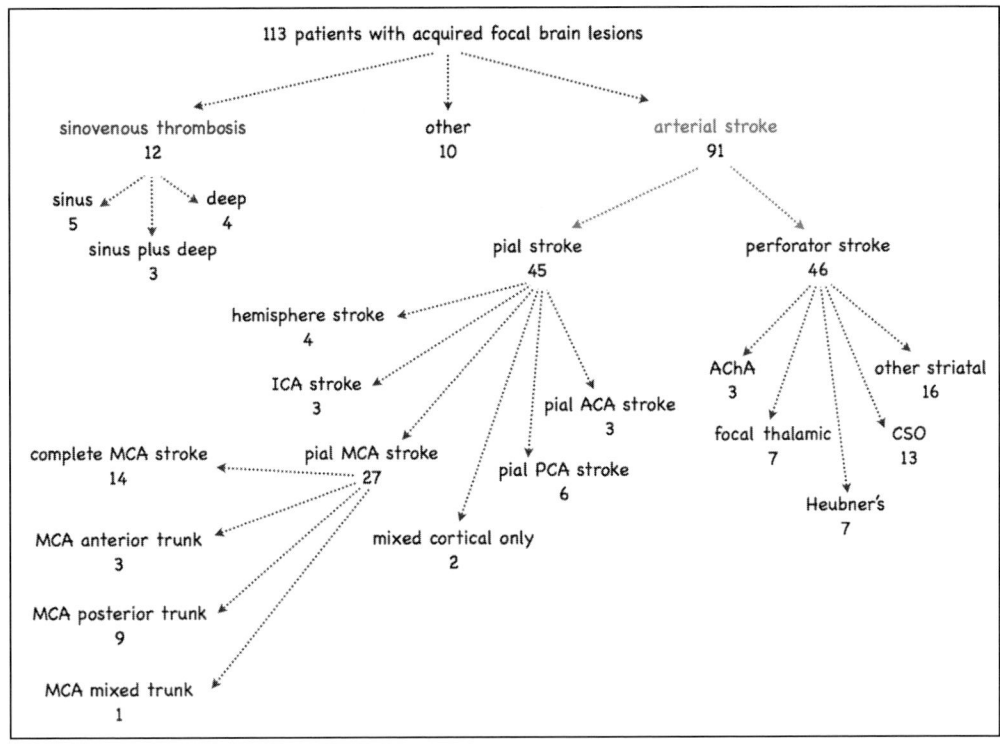

Fig. 2. Cohort of neonatal arterial ischaemic stroke (NAIS) in Sophia Children's Hospital, 2000–2006. Every child is entered only once, although many infants presented with more than one focal lesion. The sequence of classification is from most to least extensive: ICA over MCA, PCA and ACA to perforator stroke. 'Other' includes lobar bleeding and extensive watershed infarction outside the context of birth asphyxia. ACA, anterior cerebral artery; AChA, anterior chroroidal artery; CSO, centrum semi-ovale; ICA, internal carotid artery; MCA, middle cerebral artery; PCA, posterior cerebral artery.

really clear. Part of the explanation may be that preterm infants of around 24 weeks' gestation still have a preferential perfusion to basal ganglia and germinal matrix, with strong leptomeningeal loops interconnecting adjacent pial arteries (Vander Eecken, 1959). More attenuated anastomoses remain around term, shifted from the convexity near the superior sagittal sinus to the parasagittal watershed areas (Fig. 4). There are no collaterals between perforators, between corticofugal arteries, or between pial branches of the same artery.

Neonatal recognition of cerebellar stroke is only mentioned in an autopsy case report of pontocerebellar stroke following coarctectomy (Pollack et al., 1983), and paediatric cases are also scarce (Mitra et al., 2001). Specific neonatal clinical cerebellar signs are unreported in the acute phase, as are acute imaging sequences. A boy we observed presented with symptoms of cerebellar dysfunction in the first days of life in the form of massive subcortical myoclonia (Govaert, P. et al., submitted for publication). The cause of infarction was most likely *in utero* embolism, given the association with inferior vena cava thrombosis and seizure onset at 3 hours of age. The clinical context of most neonatal cerebellar strokes is probably dominated by associated cerebral injury or systemic disease. It would therefore be of interest to have further reports of acute clinical signs associated with isolated neonatal cerebellar infarction, along with the imaging presentation and outcome. Some issues of brain stem stroke are discussed with antenatal lesions below.

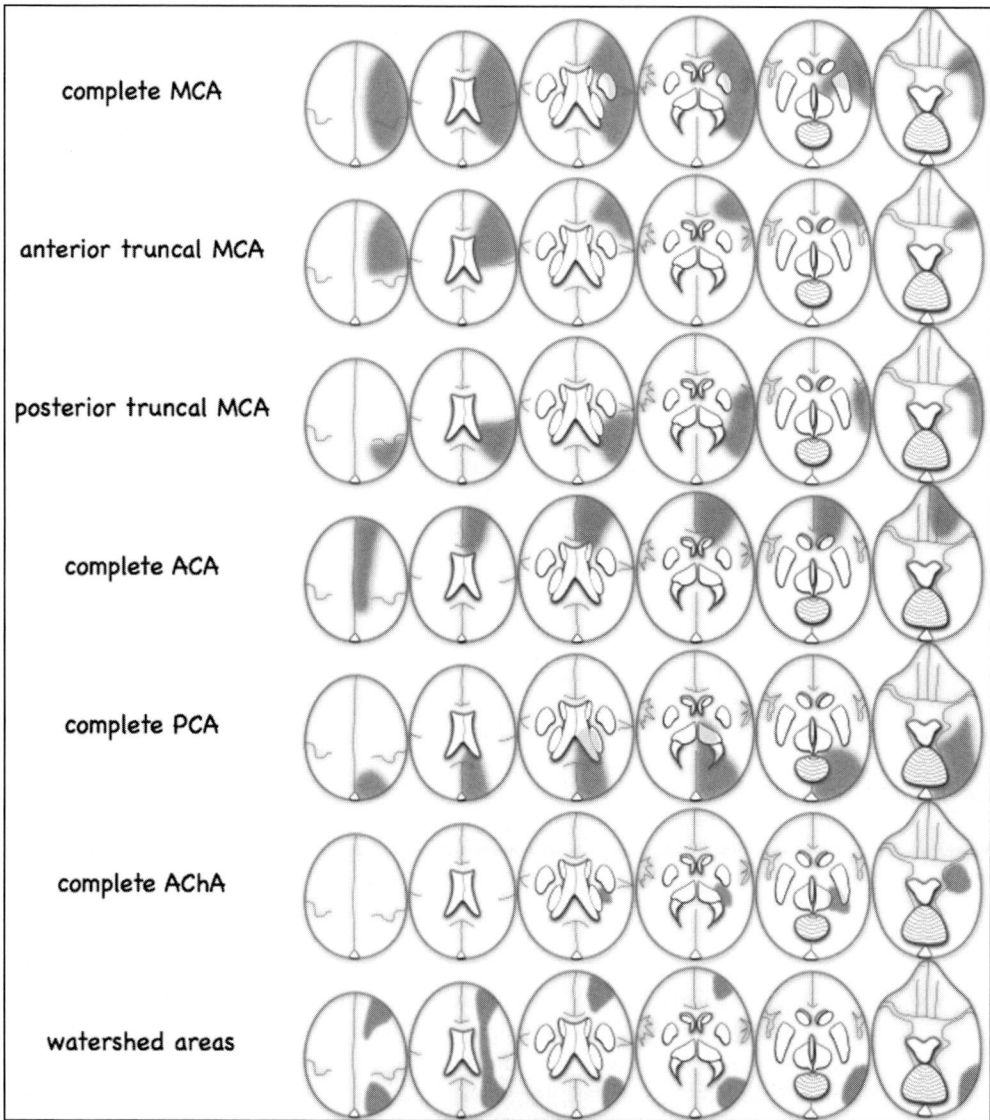

Fig. 3. Cortical arterial territories and watershed areas between them. ACA, anterior cerebral artery; AChA, anterior choroidal artery; MCA, middle cerebral artery; PCA, posterior cerebral artery.

Mechanisms and risk factors

In essence only five mechanisms can lead to arterial occlusion: local thrombosis, embolism, spasm, compression/direct trauma, and obliteration by storage or inflammation. In order to link these mechanisms to risk factors a more complex pathogenetic scheme is needed (Fig. 5). We will discuss these risk factors and mechanisms serially. In a no doubt biased attempt to recognize clinical phenotypes of NAIS, the Rotterdam cohort is presented in Fig. 6: notice how in our population birth asphyxia has an uncommon association with stroke, up to one third of cases are aetiologically elusive, and embolic conditions are common. Brain lesions within the

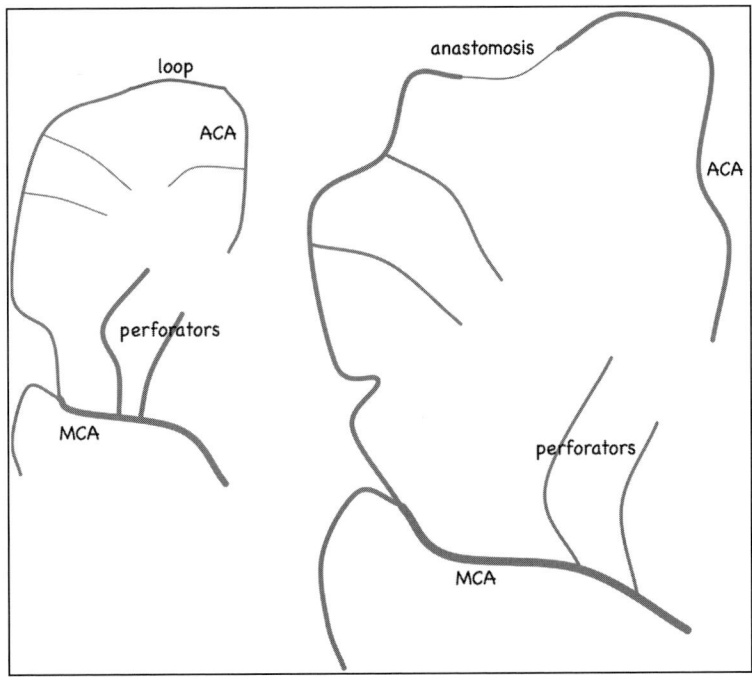

Fig. 4. Shift between 24 and 40 weeks' gestation from wide leptomeningeal loops to attenuated anastomoses between pial arteries. ACA, anterior cerebral artery; MCA, middle cerebral artery.

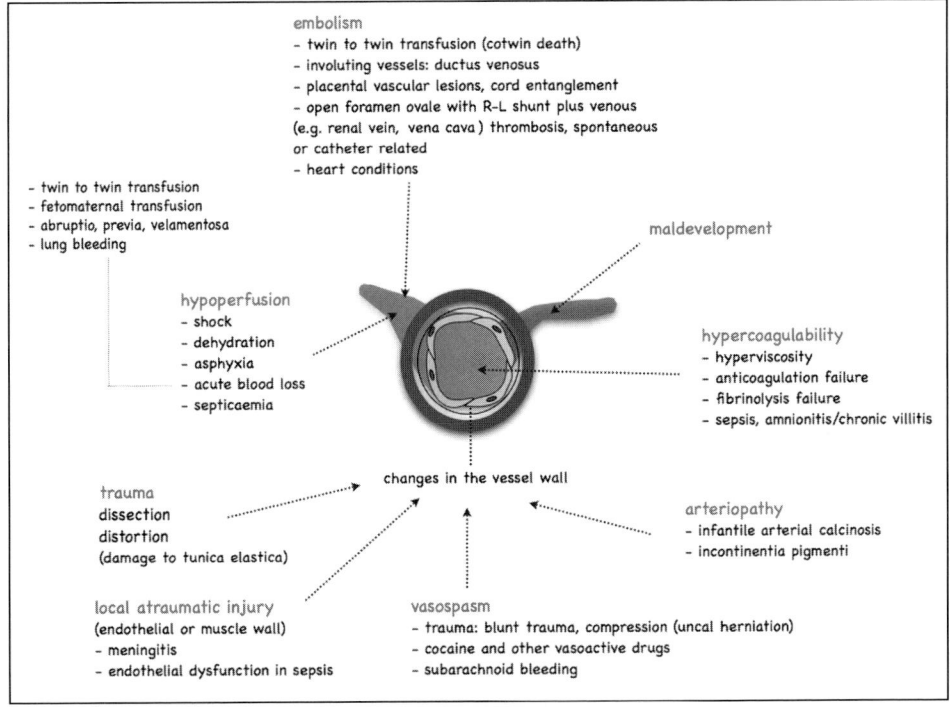

Fig. 5. Pathogenesis of neonatal arterial ischaemic stroke.

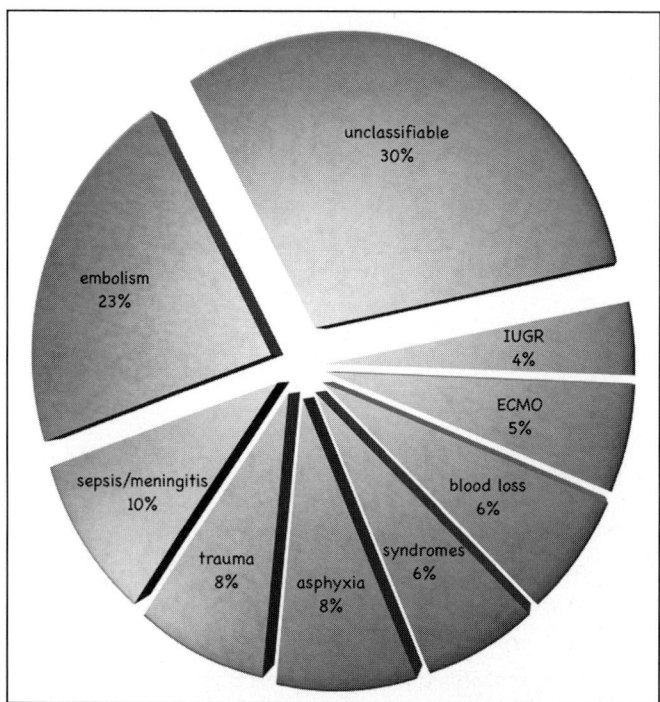

Fig. 6. Clinical phenotypes in the cohort presented in Fig. 2. ECMO, extracorporeal membrane oxygenation; IUGR, intrauterine growth retardation.

context of extracorporeal membrane oxygenation (ECMO) are complex and will not be detailed here, but NAIS is an important one of these (Taylor *et al.*, 1989).

Antenatal stroke and vascular maldevelopment

Following perinatal stroke, affected arteries wither. It is therefore impossible to differentiate between primary arterial maldevelopment and secondary atrophy in a newborn infant with longstanding stroke and arterial calibre loss (Halsey *et al.*, 1971; Koelfen *et al.*, 1993). Both at autopsy and during Doppler ultrasound of recent NAIS cases, it is most often recorded that affected arteries are without thrombus and are patent (Barmada *et al.*, 1979; Messer *et al.*, 1991; Perlman *et al.*, 1994). To designate an instance of perinatal arterial stroke, the anatomical considerations mentioned above must be taken into account, and care is needed to separate venous from arterial templates.

Circle of Willis

In adults, anomalies of the circle of Willis are not uncommon: absence of the anterior or posterior communicating artery, or of the A1 part of the ACA, are for instance observed in around five per cent of all adults (Vander Eecken, 1959; Lee, 1995; Vasovic *et al.*, 2002; Eftekhar *et al.*, 2006). Differences in anatomy are supported by haemodynamic changes (Hillen, 1986; Van Laar *et al.*, 2006) and may be relevant in clinical stroke studies (Schomer *et al.*, 1994; Emsley *et al.*, 2006). Perfusion territories of similar vessels differ between individuals (Van Der Zwan *et al.*, 1992). Leptomeningeal anastomoses are variable and important (Brozici *et al.*, 2003). Regional perfusion characteristics in different circle of Willis arteries can be found in the newborn (Lui *et al.*, 1990), indicating that anomalies of circle anatomy may be studied with Doppler ultrasound (Taylor, 1994; Harps & Helmke, 1998).

Carotid artery hypoplasia/absence

There have been several descriptions of carotid artery hypoplasia or absence and brain injury in children (Stewart *et al.*, 1978; Afifi *et al.*, 1987; Harps & Helmke, 1998; Yokochi & Iwase, 1996; Lee *et al.*, 2003); to diagnose primary hypoplasia the ICA has to be small or absent, the ICA canal has to be hypoplastic, and often there are persistent embryonic arteries and peculiar collaterals. An example of ventral porencephaly associated with carotid hypoplasia, similar to the case reported by Stewart *et al.* (1978), is presented in Fig. 7. Many individuals with carotid artery hypoplasia are asymptomatic.

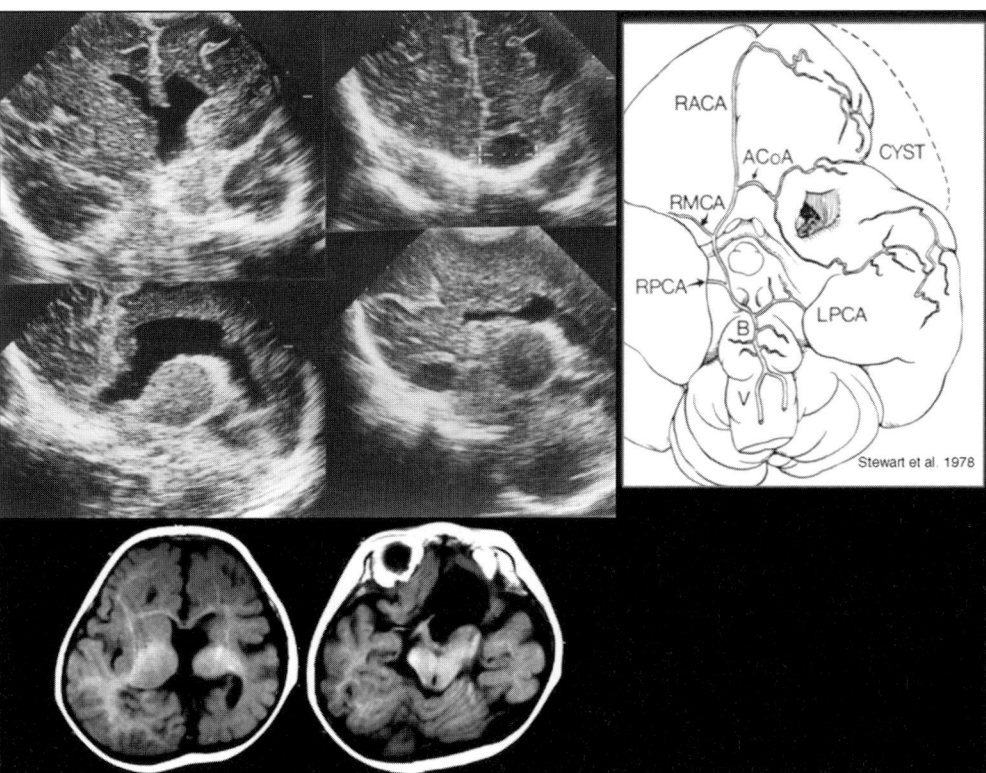

Fig. 7. Term infant with focal right clonic seizures in the neonatal period, with left microphthalmia and left anterior rhinostenosis: 7.5 MHz views (top, coronal; bottom, parasagittal); and (below) two axial magnetic resonance images (T1-weighted). In association with a dilated left lateral and third ventricle, a tubular hypodense trajectory can be seen projecting underneath the left frontal lobe to reach the orbital roof (arrows). Dilatation of the lateral ventricle is irregular, suggesting the presence of heterotopic tissue in the margins of the cleft (ventral porencephaly? ventral schizencephaly?). During neurosurgical intervention at 1.5 years for intractable seizures, the presence of a supraorbital arachnoid cyst was confirmed. The entire left hemisphere was clearly underdeveloped from birth. The drawing is adapted from Stewart et al. (1978) representing a very similar case (courtesy of Govaert & de Vries, 1996). ACoA, anterior communicating artery; LPCA, left posterior cerebral artery; RACA, right anterior cerebral artery; RMCA, right main cerebral artery; RPCA, right posterior cerebral artery.

Arterial infarction with different morphological presentations

Arterial infarction can occur – at different stages and thus with different morphological presentations – in the fetal period, days or weeks before parturition (Larroche & Amiel, 1966; Barmada *et al.*, 1979; Ong *et al.*, 1983; Ment *et al.*, 1984; Scher *et al.*, 1991; Ozduman *et al.*, 2004; de Haan *et al.*, 2006). One historical description of perinatal arterial stroke (Larroche & Amiel, 1966) gives details of a cavitated left MCA stroke, with ipsilateral corticospinal tract atrophy and ipsilateral thalamic gliosis and cell death, in an infant who died on the first day of life. Ment *et al.* (1984) reported haemorrhagic stroke within the left MCA following *in utero* seizures starting one week before delivery without birth asphyxia. Such *in utero* infarcts can be picked up in any stage of evolution, often in the end stage of porencephaly (extension of the ventricle via a porus into a white matter cavity) and (sub)cortical cavitation in an arterial field (Thorarensen *et al.*, 1997; Debus *et al.*, 1998; Lynch *et al.*, 2005), in some of them in association with the factor V Leiden prothrombotic condition.

Berg and colleagues provided the first description of *familial porencephaly* (MIM 175780) (Berg *et al.*, 1983; Mancini *et al.*, 2004; Aguglia *et al.*, 2004). The end stage of this condition is porencephaly sparing the (sub)cortex, presenting as contralateral hemiparesis, accompanied in some cases by migraine and seizures. Brain imaging shows unilateral enlargement of the lateral ventricle, although a few had bilateral involvement. The frontal horn usually shows most enlargement, making previous arterial infarction unlikely. Venous infarction is the probable mode of injury (Mancini *et al.*, 2004).

Schizencephaly may be a sequel of arterial occlusion (Fernandez-Bouzas *et al.*, 2006). *Supratentorial hydranencephaly* is the result of bilateral MCA or ICA stroke in the second trimester (Halsey *et al.*, 1971; Govaert *et al.*, 1989b: related to anticonception throughout pregnancy; causes in Table 1). A well documented range of infectious fetopathies causing stroke is known, even including parvovirus (Craze *et al.*, 1996). Extreme swelling with bilateral carotid occlusion may induce partial PCA occlusion, sparing the proximal part and the perforators, explaining why the thalamus is preserved, if atrophied. Isolated vertebro-basilar hydranencephaly is a curiosity, possibly caused by haemorrhagic infarction with cerebellar destruction from *in utero* basilar and PCA occlusion (Roessmann & Parks, 1978). Möbius syndrome can be a clinical phenotype following focal pontine ischaemia (Govaert *et al.*, 1989a; Sarnat, 2004). Focal brain stem defects can be of genetic but also focal ischaemic nature (Norman, 1974: preterm with basilar artery thrombosis and infarction of one oculomotor nucleus; Prats *et al.*, 1993: wedge-shaped infarct of the left cerebral peduncle, left cerebral hemiatrophy presenting as neonatal ptosis and ophthalmoplegia, later with right hemiparesis; Robinson *et al.*, 1993: late fetal pontine destruction; Bode *et al.*, 1994: almost absence of the medulla at olivary level, with convoluted abnormal vessels around the defect at endoscopy, and angiographically normal basilar and vertebral arteries and branches).

Table 1. Causes of hydranencephaly

- Infectious fetopathy: *Toxoplasma gondii*, cytomegalovirus, herpes simplex virus, varicella zoster virus, rubella virus, *Listeria monocytogenes*, *Treponema pallidum* and equine virus, parvo virus
- Forebrain hypoperfusion/stroke
- Maternal hypotension/hypoxia
- Cocaine use
- Smoking
- Anticonception during pregnancy
- Extensive haemorrhagic venous infarction
- Genetic: vasculopathy (Fowler syndrome), other

Focal antepartum brain injury linked to fetal conditions

Focal antepartum brain injury – intraventricular haemorrhage and periventricular venous infarction excluded – has been linked to several fetal conditions. Porencephaly and multicystic encephalopathy are among the consequences of vascular disruption in monozygous twins (Jung et al., 1984; Larroche et al., 1990; Larroche et al., 1994; Rehan & Menticoglou, 1995; Weig et al., 1995). Hypovolaemia caused by fetomaternal transfusion can lead to ischaemic brain injury in watershed areas (Boyce et al., 1994). Genuine NAIS has not been reported in such instances. Cocaine abuse by the mother may have complex effects on the fetal brain, including focal infarction – instances of Poland-Möbius syndrome, schizencephaly, porencephaly, germinolysis, and perinatal stroke have been related to the use of cocaine and its vasoconstrictive effects (Chasnoff et al., 1986; Dominguez et al., 1991; Heier et al., 1991; Volpe, 1992; Cohen et al., 1994; Puvabanditsin et al., 2005). There are concerns about blue cohosh (a medicinal herb for native Americans) used by mothers as a risk factor for NAIS (Chan & Nelson, 2004; Finkel & Zarlengo, 2004).

Trauma during delivery

Typical instances of trauma as a cause of NAIS are on record. Ischaemia within the region of the middle or posterior cerebral artery following mechanical birth trauma has been reported to be followed by temporal lobe epilepsy, homonymous hemi- or quadranopsia, and enlargement of the temporo-occipital lateral ventricle area (Hoyt, 1960; Remillard et al., 1974). The observation of difficult birth in some of these patients, one with forceps extraction, and the angiographic demonstration of occlusion of the PCA or its calcarine and parieto-occipital branches were suggestive of a perinatal insult. A different and well documented neonatal stretch injury of the MCA was reported in a full-term girl delivered by caesarean section following a failed high forceps extraction attempt (Roessman & Miller, 1980). Lumbar CSF in this child was blood stained, while computed tomography suggested bleeding in the falx and brain oedema. She died on day 4. Postmortem examination revealed subarachnoid haemorrhage, a swollen right cerebrum in the distribution of the MCA with central haemorrhagic necrosis, right uncal herniation, and bilateral cerebellar coning. The MCA carried a thrombus 0.8 cm from its origin. Light and electron microscopy detailed disruption of the lamina elastica interna near the occlusion. It was the author's conviction that this lesion followed stretching of the vessel during difficult delivery.

Several mechanisms between trauma and NAIS have thus been described (Table 2). In a case-control study of risk factors for NAIS, Wu et al. (2004) isolated intrauterine growth retardation and pre-eclampsia, emergency caesarean section, and resuscitation at birth as significant associated factors. The intermediary between 'dystocia' without obvious cranial injury and later NAIS is still elusive (example in Fig. 8).

Propagated thrombosis from an injured superior sagittal sinus into deep cerebral veins is a venous paradigm of trauma-induced infarction.

Embolism

There are two solid reasons for suspecting embolism as the mechanism of NAIS. One is finding a thrombus that is a source of embolism (Table 3 and Fig. 9). The other is to detect NAIS in combination with arterial infarction in another organ or (part of) a limb (Asindi et al., 1988;

Table 2. Trauma and stroke

Direct trauma	Ballance & Balance (1922): rupture of the middle meningeal artery due to cranial fracture during forceps delivery; Krauland (1952): rupture of the basilar artery in a preterm infant.
Vasospasm in pial arteries due to subarachnoid blood	Meyer (1951), Fullerton et al. (2001) (older children).
Stretch injury of the internal carotid artery or vertebro-basilar arteries	Mann et al. (2001), Lequin et al. (2004): neck rotation may be the cause of the dissection below the skull base, due to an intimal tear through compression against the transverse processes of cervical vertebra (Mokri, 1987); 'spontaneous' dissection of cervicocephalic arteries due to minor trauma (e.g., during easy delivery) can also occur; the most common site of dissection is between the carotid bulb and skull base or in the supraclinoid portion; disruption of the intimal layer results in an intramural haematoma which narrows the lumen and impedes flow; this causes thrombosis and embolization. Yates (1959): searching for traumatic neck lesions, this investigator reported haemorrhages in the adventitial coat of one or both vertebral arteries, sometimes up to 1 cm in length, occluding part or whole of the lumen; some arose from torn arterial branches near their origin; it was suggested that obstruction of one vertebral artery was sufficient to produce bilateral lesions in brain stem, cerebellum, and occipito-temporal cerebral cortex.
Compression and vasospasm by mass lesion	Govaert et al. (1992) suggested this mechanism as a cause for arterial stroke following basal convexity subdural haematoma; in some cases the mechanism was supratentorial intracranial hypertension → uncal herniation → occlusion of the ipsilateral PCA; for others the mechanism was different: basal convexity subdural bleeding → occlusion of the ipsilateral MCA or its branches; the association was confirmed by others [Hanigan et al. (1993), Steinbok et al. (1995)].
Blunt skull trauma	Not yet reported in the newborn, but a case is on record of a 12-year-old boy with isolated double lenticulostriate and Heubner's artery stroke following a simple fall on the head, from a fence [Erbayraktar et al. (2001)]; in the absence of bleeding, carotid thrombosis and herniation, the authors felt spasm was the mechanism involved.
Embolism following trauma	One term boy we recently observed (Fig. 8) suffered from two strokes in the context of fatal mechanical birth injury to the brain stem.

MCA, middle cerebral artery; PCA, posterior cerebral artery.

Raine et al., 1989; Gudinchet et al., 1991; Silver et al., 1992; Guajardo et al., 1994; Broxterman et al., 2000; Beattie et al., 2006). All reported NAIS cases have been ipsilateral to the affected limb.

Table 3. Sources of neonatal brain embolism

From the heart	TGV with or without Rashkind [McQuillen et al. (2006)], cardiac surgery [Monagle (2003), Chun et al. (2004)], arrhythmia, myocardial infarction, tumour (e.g., tuberous sclerosis)
Through the heart, paradoxical	The principle: Scher et al. (1986), Klesh et al. (1987), Mohr & Homma (2003), Kupari & Roine (2005), Beattie et al. (2006) From placenta [tumour embolism, Chandra et al. (1990)] From umbilical vein, portal vein [Ruff et al. (1979), Parker et al. (2002)] From femoral vein (catheter related) or (inferior) caval vein (Fig. 9) Air embolism: may lead to large stroke areas [Sivan et al. (1990), Temesvari (2000), Temesvari (2002)]
During ECMO	Luisiri et al. (1988), Campbell et al. (1988), Jarjour & Ahdab-Barmada (1994)
From a temporal artery catheter	Prian et al. (1978), Bull et al. (1980)
From the internal carotid artery or vertebral artery	Garg & Edwards-Brown (1995), Alfonso et al. (2001)

ECMO, extracorporeal membrane oxygenation; TGV, transposition of the great vessels.

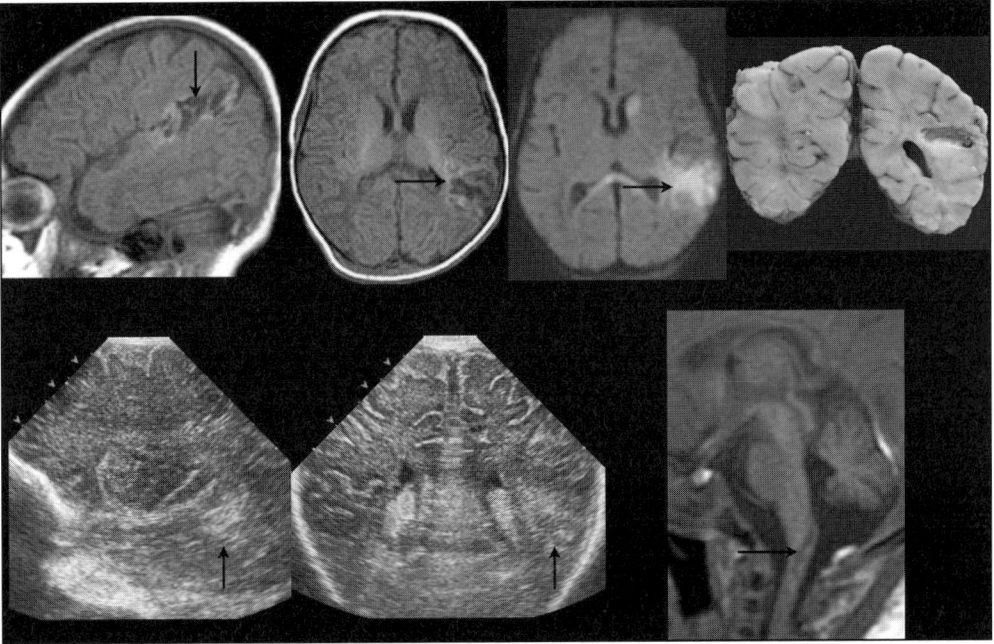

Fig. 8. This boy was born by caesarean section following failed vacuum and forceps traction. He died one month later with quadriplegia and apnoea due to medullary infarction, together with left medial striate and posterior truncal MCA stroke: though the brain stem lesion may have been the result of direct contusion, the cerebral strokes must have been the result of embolism because the affected arteries were distal from the circle of Willis and therefore unlikely to have undergone vasospasm or direct trauma.

Prothombotic conditions

The balance of neonatal haemostasis can be disturbed in the direction of thrombosis along several pathways (Fig. 10): reduced fibrinolytic activity, enhanced generation or function of thrombin, enhanced platelet aggregation, or endothelial dysfunction promoting platelet adhesion/aggregation. The extent of testing needed in clinical practice is not determined. Prothrombotic conditions are risk factors that readily find partners in the perinatal period and together these cause NAIS, as reported by many investigators (Table 4).

Maternal anticardiolipin antibodies can cause thrombosis within the fetoplacental vasculature resulting in paradoxical embolus from the placenta, or IgG antibodies may cross the placenta and cause thrombosis within the fetal cerebral vasculature (Kurnik *et al.*, 2003). Familial activated protein C resistance is caused by factor V Leiden mutation (Thorarensen *et al.*, 1997; Debus *et al.*, 1998; Broxterman *et al.*, 2000). One multicentre case-control study of stroke at term found that none of 91 instances was associated with protein S deficiency (Gunther *et al.*, 2000). The prothrombotic factors detected included increased serum lipoprotein A, factor V Leiden mutation, homozygous C677T polymorphism in methylene tetrahydrofolate reductase (MTHFR), protein C deficiency, and prothrombin mutation. Case reports suggest antithrombin deficiency may be part of the list (Brenner *et al.*, 1988). Multiple heterozygosity or other associations may enhance prothrombotic tendencies. Hyperviscosity (in practice, polycythaemia) was, in an exceptional instance, referred to as a risk factor for lateral striate infarction

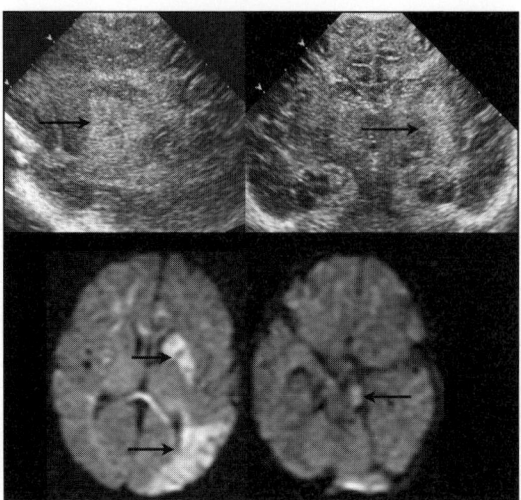

Fig. 9. Term infant with seizures due to posterior truncal left middle cerebral artery stroke and ipsilateral lenticulostriate stroke; the plausible source of embolism was renal vein thrombosis with limited thrombus formation in the inferior caval vein. Observe hypersignal in corticospinal fibres predicting a motor hemisyndrome.

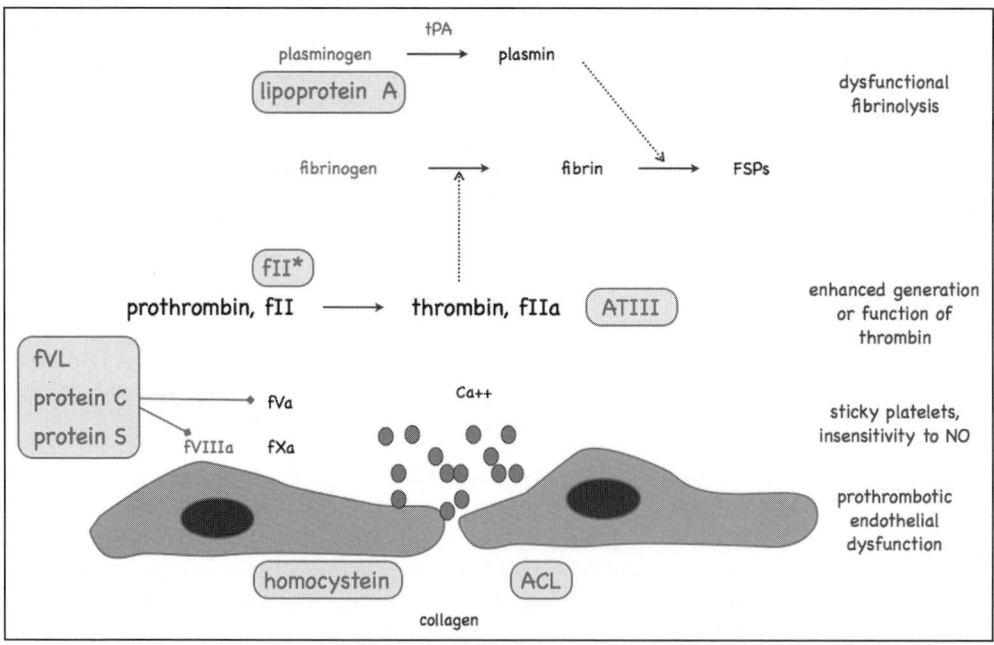

Fig. 10. Simplified scheme of coagulation and fibrinolysis, with prothrombotic entry points. Lipoprotein A interferes with plasminogen activity; increased activity of tPA inhibition reduces fibrinolytic activity, as may dysfibrinogenaemia; factor II mutation and ATIII deficiency enhance thrombin generation; factor V mutations (fVLeiden) as well as protein C and S deficiency reduce the curtailment of factor V, X, and VIII activity; platelet dysfunctions may increase aggregation; endothelial dysfunction (by high homocysteine levels or the presence of phospholipid antibodies) may do the same. ACL, anticardiolipin; FSP, fibrin split product; fVL, factor V Leiden; NO, nitrous oxide; tPA, tissue plasminogen activator.

Table 4. Prothrombotic conditions as risk factors for neonatal arterial ischaemic stroke

fV Leiden ARG506GLN	DNA, neonatal	Very likely risk factor in child, ? in neonate	Thorarensen et al. (1997), Debus et al. (1998), Harum et al. (1999), Broxterman et al. (2000), Lynch et al. (2001)
fII mutation	DNA, neonatal	Risk factor in venous thrombosis only?	Swarte et al. (2004)
Hyperlipoproteinaemia A	Neonatal and at 12 months	Increasing values postnatally role in recurrence?	Gunther et al. (2000)
Antithrombin III	Neonatal and at 12 months	Rare risk factor	Brenner et al. (1988), Volpe (1995), Kuhle et al. (2001)
Protein C	Neonatal and at 12 months	Role in recurrence?	Gould et al. (1996), Koh & Chen (1997), Gunther et al. (2000), Kurnik et al. (2003)
Protein S	Neonatal and at 12 months		No neonatal cases
Plasminogen activator inhibitor	Neonatal and at 12 months		Lynch et al. (2005), paediatric stroke and porencephaly: tPAI1 mutation in 15/56
Hyperhomocysteinaemia	Neonatal and at 12 months MTHFR: DNA, neonatal	Role in recurrence?	Gunther et al. (2000)
Antiphospholipid syndrome	Neonatal and at 12 months		Silver et al. (1992), Tabbutt et al. (1994), de Klerk et al. (1997), Akanli et al. (1998), Niemann et al. (1999), Carrilho et al. (2001), Scher et al. (2002), Kurnik et al. (2003)

MTHFR, methylene-tetrahydrofolate reductase.

(Amit & Camfield, 1980): the possible link between hyperviscosity and stroke is not well documented. The significance of fetal thrombotic vasculopathy in relation to NAIS is still not clear (Kraus & Acheen, 1999).

Syndromes

NAIS in association with other clinical findings can point to syndromal conditions (Figs. 11 and 12). Such associations are of further interest because some of these syndromes may help our understanding of the genetic predisposition to stroke and in elucidating the biochemical pathways involved. Examples are the pro-inflammatory mutation in the NEMO gene underlying incontinentia pigmenti which induces an eosinophilic arteritis causing occlusion of medium and small arteries (Maingay-de Groof et al., 2007), or hypoperfusion with infantile arterial calcinosis.

Bacterial infection

Both meningitis and ventriculitis can lead to inflammation and occlusion of arteries and veins. Periventricular or (sub)cortical infarction then follows (Berman & Banker, 1966). Large vessel

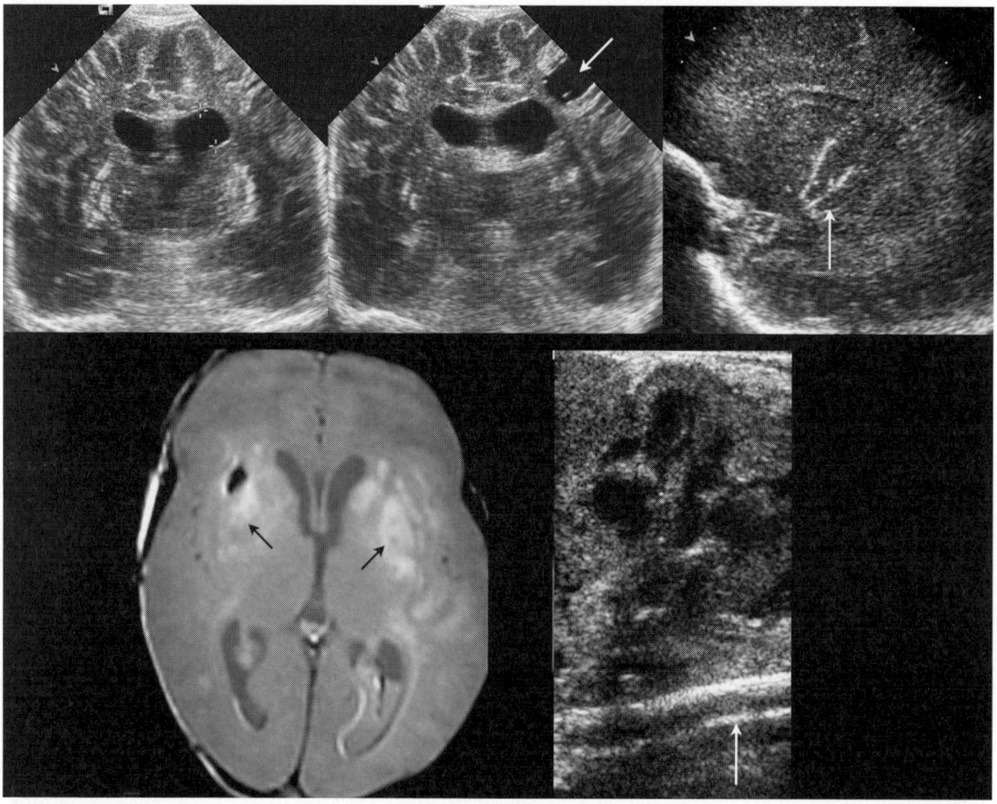

Fig. 11. Near-term premature infant with hypertension, seizures, and raised serum C-reactive protein in the absence of positive blood and cerebrospinal fluid cultures. Calcification of aorta and branches (bottom right) as well as tendons and ligaments was typical of infantile arterial calcinosis. The top right scan is from day 2 and displays arteriopathy not surrounded by infiltrates. Second week scans (top left, coronal) confirmed arteriopathy but evolving fluffy hyperechoic changes were seen around still-patent arteries. The diffuse nature of these changes are well depicted in the proton magnetic resonance as hyperintense (white areas) in the striatum and insular cortex. Haemorrhage is seen at some vessel lesions and in the ventricles. At the end of the neonatal period striatal arteriopathy had further increased, and cavitating watershed injury was seen in the left parasagittal cerebral (sub)cortex (top middle, coronal) (van der Sluis et al., 2006).

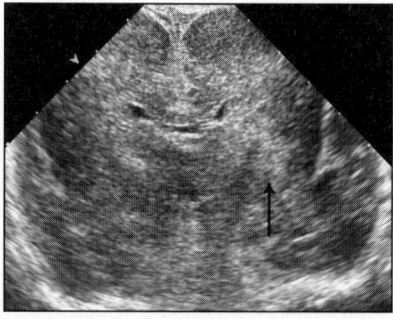

Fig. 12. Term infant with Miller-Dieker lissencephaly: second day hyperechoic left lateral striate infarction of prenatal origin (coronal ultrasound).

NAIS has been reported infrequently, sometimes with exotic organisms (Snyder et al., 1981; Ment et al., 1986; Larnaout et al., 1992: syphilis; Ries et al., 1994: enterobacter; Chiu et al., 1995: meningococcus; Harris, 1997: listeria; Wade et al., 1999: *Pasteurella multocida*; Kay's Kayemba et al., 2003: salmonella). The role of imaging of neonatal infectious brain lesions is discussed elsewhere (Jan et al., 2003; de Vries et al., 2006).

Table 5. Syndromes with stroke in newborn or infant

Gruppo et al. (1998)	Cutis marmorata telangiectatica congenita (and factor V Leiden)
Nordborg et al. (1997)	Galactosialidosis
Soper et al. (1995), Wollack et al. (1996)	Williams syndrome
van der Sluis et al. (2006)	Infantile arterial calcinosis (Fig. 11)
Van Geet & Jaeken (1993)	Carbohydrate-deficient glycoprotein syndrome (phosphomannomutase deficiency, OMIM 212065: reduced function of ATIII, protein C) Fibromuscular dysplasia of arteries (OMIM 135580)
Tjoelker & Stafforini (2000)	Miller-Dieker syndrome: platelet-activating factor acetylhydrolase mutation (OMIM 601690) may lead to increased levels of PAF (Fig. 12)
Kaplan (2007)	Placental chorangiosis with fetal hypoperfusion and thrombophilia
Butrum et al. (2003)	Diamond-Blackfan anaemia and MTHFR deficiency Aicardi-Goutières syndrome
Maingay-De Groof et al. (2007)	Incontinentia pigmenti (eosinophilic vasculopathy)
Rossi & Tortori-Donati (2006), Drolet et al. (2006)	Cervicofacial angioma and progressive cerebrovascular stenoses (PHACE syndrome, stroke in infancy)
Thompson et al. (1975)	Carotid elastin hyperplasia

MTHFR, methylene-tetrahydrofolate reductase.

Staging using imaging

Staging using imaging is discussed by Hill et al., 1983; Raybaud et al., 1985; Bode et al., 1986; Hernanz-Schulman et al., 1988; Pellicer et al., 1992; Taylor et al., 1993; Koelfen et al., 1995; Govaert & de Vries, 1996; Mader et al., 2002; and Cowan et al., 2005.

Swelling

From 30 minutes to a few hours, cytotoxic oedema increases the water content by up to five per cent. Changes in water diffusion occur within minutes (seen on diffusion-weighted imaging (DWI)); the nadir of the apparent diffusion coefficient (ADC) is on average around 33 hours after the ictus and it takes 4 to 10 days before the ADC normalizes and in fact overshoots the normal. Changes in diffusion are not specific and are seen with encephalitis, venous ischaemia, and even seizures *per se*. On day 1, decreased pulsatility in the affected vessel and mild hyperechogenicity are inconspicuous. In the vessel flow, void is lost in the affected artery for hours: this dampening disappears within 24 hours (D'Orey et al., 1999). Magnetic resonance angiography may not depict the length of thrombosis well in a large artery and may fail to show occlusion of small arteries. Most neonatal strokes present with reopened vessels.

Necrosis

From 6 hours to about 6 days, vasogenic oedema and coagulation necrosis are associated with damage to the endothelium and breakdown of the blood-brain barrier. Maturation of the infarct occurs following reperfusion of a pressure-passive vascular bed, either through the recanalized artery or through anastomotic arteries. The peak of events is between 2 and 4 days following acute infarction. Invading macrophages and glial cells make the infarct macroscopically visible at postmortem and on images (ultrasound or MRI) between 24 and 72 hours after onset (Fig. 13). If very large, swelling may produce signs of a mass effect. There is a gradual increase in echogenicity in the core and penumbra, and bleeding increases inhomogeneity. Swelling continues for about a week. In our experience NAIS can nearly always be visualized with ultrasound (de Vries et al., 1997; Govaert et al., 2000), except for small cortical infarcts far away from the transducer, although even in cases of temporal or occipital infarction insonation from asterion or posterior fontanelle can depict the lesion (Fig. 14). On recuperation, discrepant high flow velocities may be recorded up to 160 cm/s; this is regional luxury perfusion and may persist for over a week (Donaldson, 1987; Taylor, 1994; Steventon & John, 1997) (Fig. 15).

As measured on DWI, large strokes grow to maximum size at around 70 hours after onset. In adults the penumbra shows restricted diffusion; consequently the final T2 lesion is smaller than the volume of diffusion restriction. Changes on T2 and proton density images probably repre-

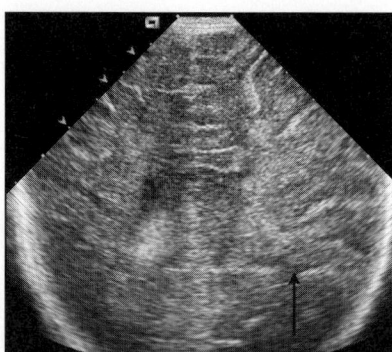

Fig. 13. Hyperechoic stage of complete left middle cerebral artery stroke in coronal ultrasound.

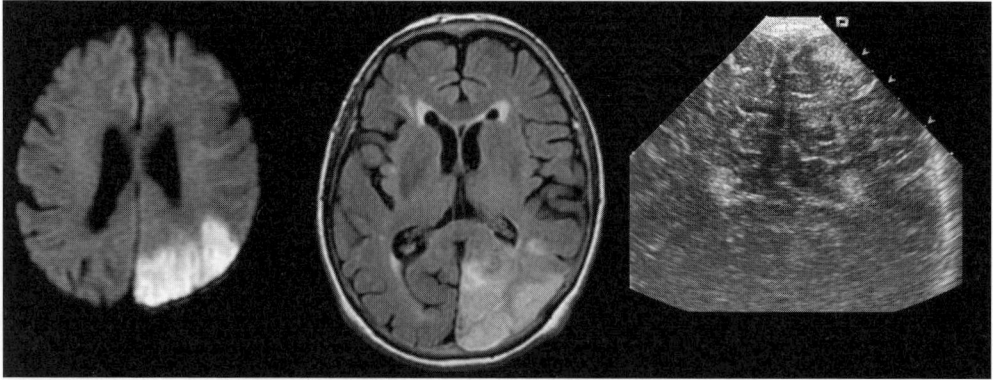

Fig. 14. Difficult vacuum extraction at term, presenting with subgaleal bleeding and pulmonary hypertension. Left posterior cerebral artery stroke on DWI, axial FLAIR, and coronal ultrasound through posterior fontanelle.

Chapter 15 Neonatal arterial ischaemic stroke

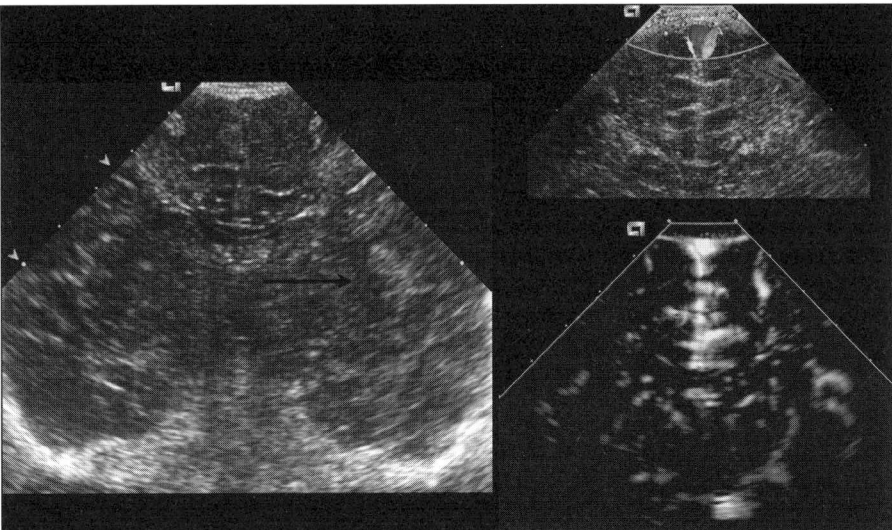

Fig. 15. Luxury perfusion in the branches of the left middle cerebral artery in coronal ultrasound 5 days following presentation: observe larger signals from affected side, including vessels near the superior sagittal sinus.

sent definitive damage. In the absence of haemorrhage, disappearance of the cortical ribbon in the affected pial area is typical. In the acute stage intensity changes are seen on DWI along the pyramidal tract; this phenomenon has prognostic value, especially at a mesencephalic and pontine level (Krishnamoorthy *et al.*, 2000; Miller *et al.*, 2000; Mazumdar *et al.*, 2003; de Vries *et al.*, 2005; Kirton & deVeber, 2006) (Fig. 16). Restricted diffusion is seen within the infarcted area for several days and up to a week; the changes in the axons involved begin after one or a few days and persist into the second week. Connected nuclei – like pulvinar – may also suffer secondarily from cell injury with restriction of water diffusion in the acute phase (Govaert *et al.*, 2008).

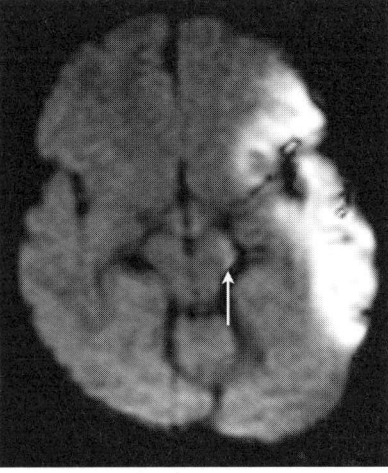

Fig. 16. Hypersignal along the left corticospinal tract in DWI sequence on day 6 of a term infant with left middle cerebral artery stroke.

Limited data are available about magnetic resonance spectroscopy in NAIS: lactate resonances, which are not present in normal brain after term, were demonstrated in two patients tested at 7 and 10 days of age, respectively, and in one of these lactate was still present at 2 months; in four neonates a decrease in the N-acetylaspartate/choline (NAA/Cho) ratio was seen within the area of infarction (Groenendaal et al., 1995).

Organization

From 3 days to 6 weeks, the infarct organizes and this involves gliosis, breakdown of myelin, microcyst formation, and neovascularization. Total necrosis may lead to central liquefaction with ensuing cavitation. Ingrowth of new vessels is most marked in grey matter, although young infants and neonates produce important vascular reactions in white matter. The hyperechoic stage persists for 3 to 4 weeks. Cavitation follows an intermediate checkerboard pattern. A CSF cavity is fully developed after 6 to 10 weeks. Compensatory neuropil growth around the infarct may create the impression that the defect has shrunk.

Tissue loss

From the second month on, infarction within a major cortical vessel is recognized as an area of cortico-subcortical tissue loss, based against the skull. Wallerian degeneration of the ipsilateral pyramidal tract and trans-synaptic degeneration of ipsilateral thalamus and contralateral cerebellar hemisphere (diaschisis) proceed for several months after the initial injury. The thalamus on the side of extensive frontoparietal (sub)cortical tissue loss will have shrunk by 20 to 40 per cent in 3 to 6 months.

Prognosis

Many strokes lead to hemiplegia or contralateral motor dysfunction (Table 6; Fig. 17). Some details on outcome are summarized in Table 7.

Cerebral palsy is predicted by large stroke size, but specific regional injury (to Broca's or Wernicke's areas and to the posterior limb of the internal capsule) (PLIC) is helpful in predicting motor outcome (Boardman et al., 2005; Wu et al., 2005). Only large strokes involve

Table 6. Prognosis of neonatal arterial ischaemic stroke

Study	N	Details	Normal (%)	CP (%)	MDI < 70 (%)	Epilepsy (%)	Other
Wulfeck et al. (1991)	14	CT or MR; all < 2 years follow-up	14	79	21	50	All walk independently
Sreenan et al. (2000)	46	CT diagnoses; follow-up on average 42 months	33	48	41	46	
Mercuri et al. (2003)	22	MR diagnoses; school age	40	30	14	0	
Lee et al. (2005)	36	MR diagnoses; follow-up > 12 months	32	58		39	Language delay 25%; behavioural changes 22%

CP, cerebral palsy; CT, computed tomography; MDI, Bayley mental developmental index; MR, magnetic resonance.

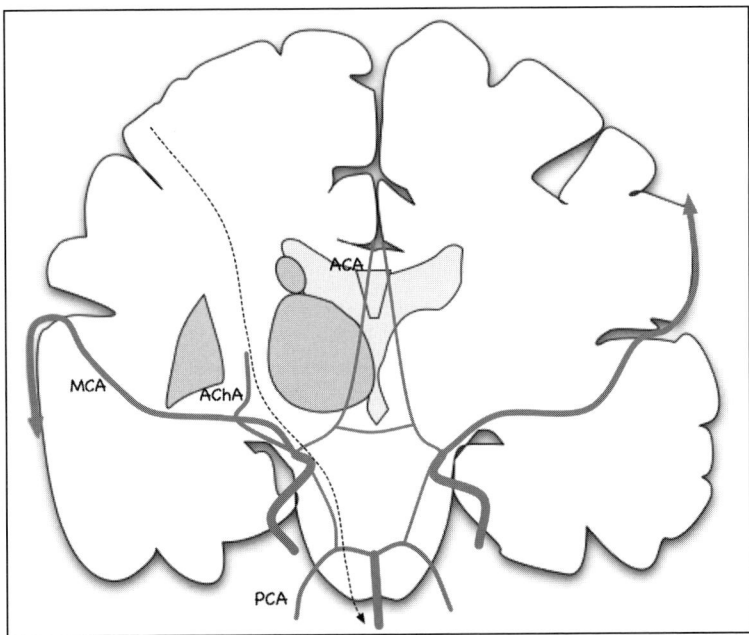

Fig. 17. Hemimotor syndrome from stroke: corticospinal, corticobulbar, and corticopontine fibres can be injured by stroke at the level of the cortex in middle cerebral artery (MCA) and anterior cerebral artery territory, at the level of the internal capsule in MCA and anterior choroidal artery territory, and at mesencephalic level in posterior cerebral artery territory. ACA, anterior cerebral artery; AChA, anterior choroidal artery; PCA, posterior cerebral artery.

damage to basal nuclei, PLIC, and cortex and more readily predict hemiplegia. Spasticity develops only when at cortical level both the primary and the premotor/supplementary motor cortices are affected, not with pure M1 lesions. The extent of infarction influences the outcome. In adult patients with hemiplegia following perinatal injury, the lateral extent of the periventricular injury has been correlated with motor dysfunction of the upper and lower limbs (Staudt et al., 2000). Upper limb corticospinal fibres are injured more by lesions lateral and anterior to sites where lower limb fibres are injured. Hemimotor symptoms are subtle before 3 to 6 months of age (Bouza et al., 1994; Govaert, 1994b; Guzzetta et al., 2003). This timing agrees with the transition from bimanual skills to single hand preference in normal infants. The earlier hemimotor signs become apparent, the more severe the ultimate disability. In some, deterioration may seem to be present because of loss of pre-existing skills, without any correlation with seizure onset. Impaired dexterity seems to be the result of an inability to ensure a precise synergy between fingertip forces while manipulating objects (Duque et al., 2003). The long-term effect of right hemisphere lesions on drawing were studied by Stiles et al. (1997). The presence of increased signal intensity on DWI at the level of the PLIC and the cerebral peduncles in newborn infants with arterial ischaemic stroke is often followed by Wallerian degeneration and subsequent development of hemiplegia, although measurement of the extent of signal change may refine the strength of this indicator (Kirton & deVeber, 2006). Complete MCA stroke (including cortical areas and the striatum) causes residual contralateral spasticity which tends to cause more upper limb involvement. Depending on whether there is direct involvement of the M1 and premotor area, truncal infarction within the MCA may or may not lead to hemiplegia. ACA stroke may cause contralateral leg monoplegia. PCA stroke leads to the

Table 7. Details about outcome following neonatal arterial ischaemic stroke

Outcome	Study	Findings
Motor	Wulfeck et al. (1991)	Most hemiplegics walk alone by 2 years of age.
	Bouza et al. (1994a)	Obvious left-right differences are present by 6 months.
	Staudt et al. (2000)	MRI lesion measurement correlates with functional deficit.
	Eyre et al. (2000)	Window between ingrowth of CST fibres in spinal motor centres around 26 weeks GA and development of fine motor control at 6–12 months after birth: window for cortical to spinal influence.
Language	Varga-Khadem et al. (1985)	Persistent dysphasia if right hemiplegic, expressive more than receptive [Hecaen et al. (1976)]; not all left hemiplegics have language deficit.
	Wulfeck et al. (1991)	Language delay already in earliest communicative efforts (babbling).
	Fair et al. (2006)	Cortical language areas may differ transiently from normal in perinatal posterior truncal MCA stroke.
Plasticity	Maegaki et al. (1997)	Axonal sprouting from unlesioned CST to ipsilateral proximal and distal arm muscles of hemiplegic side.
	Staudt et al. (2005)	Small lesions permit ipsilateral use of cortex as M1, premotor reorganization in unaffected cortex; severe lesions do not permit ipsilateral cortical use, primary motor reorganization happens in unaffected cortex.
	Duque et al. (2003)	Competition in unaffected cortex leads to impaired dexterity of unaffected hand; dysfunction of paretic hand is due to differences in fingertip force and time shifts between muscle activations.
Epilepsy	Kolk et al. (2001)	Epilepsy in congenital hemiplegia affects cognition in children with normal IQ; cognitive dysfunction more severe in contralateral to lesion handedness (absence of interhemispheric transfer).
	Gaggero et al. (2001)	Epilepsy in 25–50% of congenital hemiplegics; severe epilepsy correlates with cortical lesions and onset before 2 years; mental retardation in 14/34 hemiplegics with epilepsy; first epileptic insult after 3 years or more in 16/34.
	Selton et al. (2003)	Serial EEG changes may help to predict outcome: positive Rolandic slow sharp waves can be associated with contralateral motor sequelae, while positive left temporal fast sharp waves can be associated with behavioural problems.
	Squier et al. (2003)	Hippocampal sclerosis is uncommon in children with early onset strokes but develops in many children whose strokes are of later origin.

CST, corticospinal tract; EEG, electroencephalography; GA, gestational age; MRI, magnetic resonance imaging.

classical residual triad: temporal lobe epilepsy, homonymous hemi- or quadranopia, and enlargement of the occipital horn; oculomotor palsy may be part of this spectrum. Following perinatal lenticulostriate stroke some children escape hemisyndrome (especially if the caudate is not involved and infarction is limited to the putamen); other infants (usually with complete lenticulostriate injury to the putamen and caudate all the way up to the lateral ventricle) develop hemiplegia (Abels et al., 2006).

Thalamic shrinkage from transneuronal atrophy is associated with a reduction in somatosensory evoked potential amplitude, suggesting a clinical effect on sensory perception (Giroud et al.,

1995). The substrate for facial recognition in the parietal lobe may be affected by perinatal stroke (Ballantyne & Trauner, 1999). Motor performance is usually worse than mental, but side-specific language problems are common (Wulfeck et al., 1991; Schulzke et al., 2005; Lee et al., 2005). Serial study (clinically and with functional magnetic resonance imaging) (fMRI) of language development may be very instructive about plasticity following perinatal stroke (Fair et al., 2006). The psychomotor development index is below 90 in many children with severe or moderate hemiplegia (Table 6). Motor impairment tends to correlate with lower mental development. Visual dysfunction originating in cortex injured by NAIS has been described by Mercuri and colleagues (Mercuri et al., 1996; 2003): it is more common in children with complete than truncal MCA stroke. Visual dysfunction is often but not always associated with involvement of the optic radiations or of the occipital primary visual cortex. Recuperation of visual function after a stroke can be followed with fMRI (Seghier et al., 2004).

Epilepsy following stroke may be of late onset (after 2 years or more) and affects cognitive function. The contrasting low incidence of epilepsy in cohorts gathered from the neonatal period onwards could reflect a short follow-up period. In the long run, epilepsy affects 25 to 50 per cent of those affected by stroke. Pharmacoresistance (epilepsy failing response to treatment with at least three first-choice antiepileptics) is expected in cases with mixed and frequent seizures in infancy and early childhood. Cognitive dysfunction is worse in children with partial epilepsy and hemiplegia than in those with partial epilepsy only. The association of stroke with neonatal presentation and later infantile spasms carries a bad prognosis (Golomb et al., 2006).

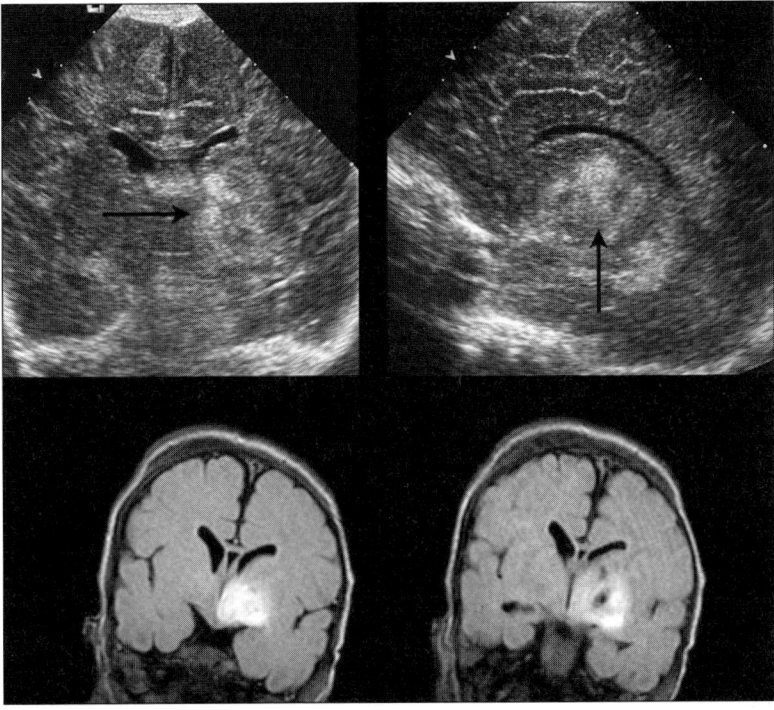

Fig. 18. Left anterior choroidal artery stroke leading to cognitive dysfunction (top ultrasound, bottom coronal FLAIR) at 2 years of age.

The outcome of stroke related to vessels other than the MCA needs better description, particularly for AChA, Heubner's artery, ACA, and PCA pial stroke. Contralateral upper extremity athetosis has been reported following paediatric Heubner's artery stroke (Miller et al., 2000). Two instances of AChA stroke we have observed were both followed not only by predictable hemiplegia but also by a surprising degree of cognitive dysfunction at 2 years of age (Fig. 18). ACA stroke is rare and, in the few occasions we have observed it, not isolated, making it difficult to relate the outcome to ACA stroke alone (Fig. 19).

Management

There are no treatment options of proven value in NAIS. Heparinization is proposed in instances with ongoing thrombosis in the heart or a large systemic vein (Nowak-Göttl et al., 2003; Monagle et al., 2004; Chalmers, 2005). A heparinization protocol following cardiac catheterization may be useful (Weissman et al., 1985).

A synthesis of suggestions for pharmacological intervention from animal stroke experiments is beyond our scope (Ashwal & Pearce, 2001; Ashwal et al., 2007). Easily applicable candidates could be albumin or hypothermia (Ginsberg, 2003). Beyond doubt it is clear that insight is needed in many areas of NAIS to arrive at treatment options. Theoretically this may in the end facilitate intervention at five levels (Fig. 20). Prevention of risk factors (like vaginal breech delivery, difficult instrumental traction, catheter-related embolism), reopening of an occluded vessel with fibrinolytics, protecting cells in the penumbra from secondary excitotoxic or apoptotic death (by maintaining perfusion and metabolic homeostasis), and preventing recurrence (in children with recognized risk factors or ongoing cardiac or venous thrombosis) are several modes of possible intervention. Treatment or rehabilitation strategies will have to be tested in

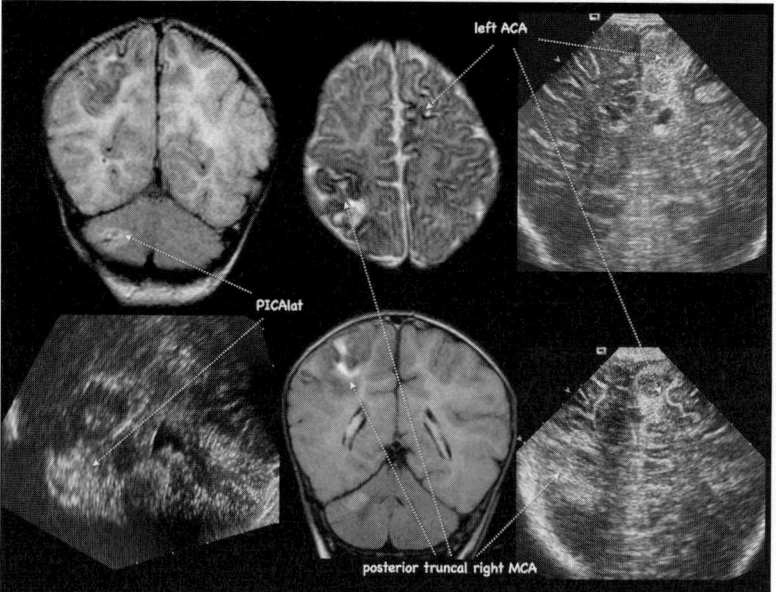

Fig. 19. *Left anterior cerebral artery stroke associated with right posterior truncal middle cerebral artery and right lateral posterior inferior cerebellar artery (PICAlat) cerebellar stroke, in an infant with ventricular septal defect, resulting from paradoxic multiple embolism. The lower left is a coronal sonogram through the left asterion. ACA, anterior cerebral artery; MCA, middle cerebral artery.*

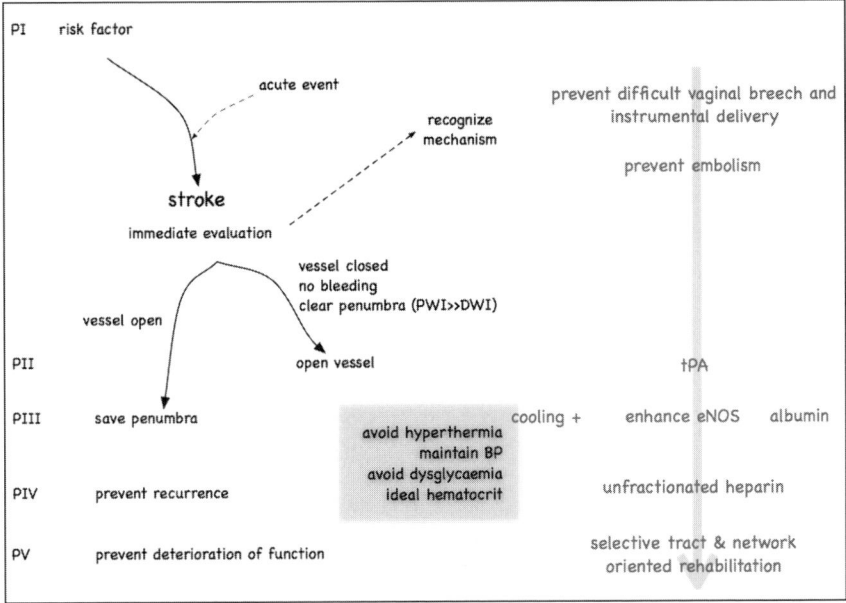

Fig. 20. Hypothetical opportunities for prevention of permanent injury from neonatal arterial ischaemic stroke (NAIS). BP, blood pressure; DWI, diffusion-weighted imaging; eNOS, endothelial nitric oxide synthase; PWI, perfusion-weighted imaging; tPA, tissue plasminogen activator.

randomized trials following inclusion of anatomically identical strokes – for example, complete MCA stroke – to avoid the confounding influence of stroke type on outcome (Fehlings *et al.*, 2000; Boyd *et al.*, 2001; Eliasson *et al.*, 2003). Once the damage is done, intervention studies with normal rehabilitation *versus* targeted overtraining, with prior knowledge of lesioned structures and tracts, may be needed to guide ideal post-stroke rehabilitation. In the near future efforts will have to be combined for further study of the phenotypes and causes of the complex panel of perinatal strokes we are confronted with.

A guide to assessment of perinatal stroke (drawn on several reviews and the data presented in this article) is presented in Table 8.

Table 8. Investigations to be considered in neonatal arterial ischaemic stroke

History*	Family	Neurological disorders (epilepsy, hemiplegia, migraine, stroke); thrombosis below 40–50 years of age.
	Obstetric	Previous pregnancies: (recurrent) fetal loss, (pre)eclampsia, IUGR. This pregnancy: fetal ultrasound pathology, twinning, IUGR, maternal diseases (SLE...) and accidents (hypotension, hypoxia, trauma), drug (ab)use. Delivery: arguments in support of asphyxia and trauma (CTG, cord pH, Apgar scores, resuscitation, early postnatal lactate, clinical recuperation within first hour; cord problems; details about breech vaginal or instrumental delivery).
	Neonatal (serial consultation with the child neurologist is inherent)	Neurological presentation: onset, type, time and response to treatment of clinical and subclinical seizures; other presenting signs, including detailed examination of motor dysfunction and staging of encephalopathy; description of recovery of feeding behaviour and cranial nerve function; details about interventions within the cardiovascular system, including catheter position and serial platelet count; description of visceral and limb thrombosis (kidney, gut, lung, adrenals); description of severe adverse events: septicaemia, NEC, shock.
Imaging	Brain	Serial ultrasound to stage evolution of infarct.* Serial Doppler examination of affected arteries to document dampening or luxury perfusion (compare with normal surrounding arteries). Early MRI* to describe arterial stroke territory, with MRA to document patency or anomalies of arteries, with DWI or DTI to document tract lesions; perfusion studies with very acute imaging to detect penumbra. Neonatal evolution MRI (near end of first week following insult): to study network injury (projection tracts at brain stem level, thalamic subnuclei) and definite lesion extent. Follow-up MRI later in infancy or childhood: to study thalamic and cortical end-stage atrophy, with fMRI to study functional plasticity serially.
	Other	Heart*: status of foramen ovale, presence of thrombus or tumour, endocarditis. Abdomen*: inferior vena cava or femoro-iliac thrombosis, renal vein thrombosis, arterial calcification, thrombus in ductus venosus; location of catheter tips. Arteries: patency of cervical internal carotids and vertebral arteries; visualization of circle of Willis (anomalies), flow velocities in affected vessels. Limbs and skull: document birth trauma. Document air embolism in acute stage.
Neurophysiology	EEG*	sEEG and/or aEEG: describe evolution of background stages and localization as well as severity of seizures.
	Other	Targeted (serial) use of SSEP (perforator or MCA stroke), VEP (perforator, AChA or PCA stroke), ABR (vertebrobasilar stroke) to evaluate dysfunctions within an area of injury; EMG for documentation of plexus injury due to trauma.
Biochemistry	Blood (consult with paediatric haematologist)†	Indicators of inflammation, serial glucose measurements, platelets and haematocrit.* Maternal fetopathy status and Kleihauer test of appropriate. Functional prothrombotic screen, including antiphospholipid testing (repeat after > 6 months and expand testing to parents if appropriate). Genetic prothrombotic screen: fVL, fII mutation, MTHFR deficiency.
	Other	Exclude meningitis if needed. Urine toxicology screen (drugs, herbal components).
Miscellaneous	Placenta	Fetal thrombotic vasculopathy, per cent of infarction, chorioamnionitis, villitis of unknown aetiology, tumour or vascular anomaly, cord anomaly.
	ECG	Document arrhythmia.
Subspecialties	Syndrome?	Consult with ophthalmologist, geneticist, paediatric dermatologist or metabolic specialist depending on associated clinical features.
Follow-up*	Multidisciplinary	Focus on cerebral palsy, cognition, behaviour, language, vision and hearing, epilepsy; expand clinical findings with appropriate fMRI or neurophysiological testing; document effect of rehabilitation.

* Mandatory investigations are marked with an asterisk.
† In many centres an extensive prothrombotic screen is advised, but the extent of testing needed is not known; minimally one would investigate infants in families with early thrombosis, with associated limb or visceral infarction, and with multiple unexplained brain infarcts.
ABR, auditory brain stem responses; AChA, anterior choroidal artery; aEEG, amplitude integrated encephalography; CTG, cardiotography; EMG, electromyography; IUGR, intrauterine growth retardation; MRA, magnetic resonance angiography; MTHFR, methylene-tetrahydrofolate reductase; NEC, necrotising enterocolitis; PCA, posterior cerebral artery; sEEG, standard encephalography; SSEP, somatosensory evoked potentials; VEP, visual evoked potentials.

References

Abels, L., Lequin, M. & Govaert, P. (2006): Sonographic templates of newborn perforator stroke. *Pediatr. Radiol.* **36**, 663–669.

Afifi, A.K., Godersky, J.C., Menezes, A., Smoker, W.R., Bell, W.E. & Jacoby, C.G. (1987): Cerebral hemiatrophy, hypoplasia of internal carotid artery, and intracranial aneurysm. A rare association occurring in an infant. *Arch. Neurol.* **44**, 232–235.

Aguglia, U., Gambardella, A., Breedveld, G.J., Oliveri, R.L., Le Piane, E., Messina, D., Quattrone, A. & Heutink, P. (2004): Suggestive evidence for linkage to chromosome 13qter for autosomal dominant type 1 porencephaly. *Neurology* **62**, 1613–1615.

Akanli, L.F., Trasi, S.S., Thuraisamy, K., Bergtraum, M.P., Thantu, A., Fischer, R.F. & Cohen-Addad, N. (1998): Neonatal middle cerebral artery infarction: association with elevated maternal anticardiolipin antibodies. *Am. J. Perinatol.* **15**, 399–402.

Alfonso, I., Prieto, G., Vasconcellos, E., Aref, K., Pacheco, E. & Yelin, K. (2001): Internal carotid artery thrombus: an underdiagnosed source of brain emboli in neonates? *J. Child Neurol.* **16**, 446–447.

Allan, W.C. & Riviello, J.J. (1992): Perinatal cerebrovascular disease in the neonate. Parenchymal ischemic lesions in term and preterm infants. *Pediatr. Clin. North Am.* **39**, 621–650.

Amit, M. & Camfield, P.R. (1980): Neonatal polycythemia causing multiple cerebral infarcts. *Arch. Neurol.* **37**, 109–110.

Ashwal, S. & Pearce, W.J. (2001): Animal models of neonatal stroke. *Curr. Opin. Pediatr.* **13**, 506–516.

Ashwal, S., Tone, B., Tian, H.R., Chong, S. & Obenaus, A. (2007): Comparison of two neonatal ischemic injury models using magnetic resonance imaging. *Pediatr. Res.* **61**, 9–14.

Asindi, A.A., Stephenson, J.B. & Young, D.G. (1988): Spastic hemiparesis and presumed prenatal embolisation. *Arch. Dis. Child.* **63**, 68–69.

Aso, K., Scher, M.S. & Barmada, M.A. (1990): Cerebral infarcts and seizures in the neonate. *J. Child Neurol.* **5**, 224–228.

Balcom, T.A. & Redmond, B.G. (1997): Cerebral infarction as multifocal clonic seizures in a term neonate. *J. Am. Board Fam. Pract.* **10**, 43–49.

Ballance, A.C. & Ballance, C.A. (1922): Intracranial hemorrhage in the newborn with observations on fracture of the skull of the infant. *Lancet* **203**, 1109.

Ballantyne, A.O. & Trauner, D.A. (1999): Facial recognition in children after perinatal stroke. *Neuropsychiatry Neuropsychol. Behav. Neurol.* **12**, 82–87.

Barmada, M.A., Moossy, J. & Shuman, R.M. (1979): Cerebral infarcts with arterial occlusion in neonates. *Ann. Neurol.* **6**, 495–502.

Barth, P.G., Walter, A. & van Gelderen, I. (1999): Aicardi-Goutieres syndrome: a genetic microangiopathy? *Acta Neuropathol. (Berl.)* **98**, 212–216.

Barth, P.G. (2002): The neuropathology of Aicardi-Goutieres syndrome. *Eur. J. Paediatr. Neurol.* **6** (Suppl. A), A27–A31; discussion A37–A39, A77–A86.

Beattie, L.M., Butler, S.J. & Goudie, D.E. (2006): Pathways of neonatal stroke and subclavian steal syndrome. *Arch. Dis. Child. Fetal Neonat. Ed.* **91**, F204–F207.

Berg, R.A., Aleck, K.A. & Kaplan, A.M. (1983): Familial porencephaly. *Arch. Neurol.* **40**, 567–569.

Berman, P.H. & Banker, B.Q. (1966): Neonatal meningitis. A clinical and pathological study of 29 cases. *Pediatrics* **38**, 6–24.

Billard, C., Dulac, O. & Diebler, C. (1982): [Ischemic cerebral softening in newborn infants. Possible etiology of neonatal convulsive states]. *Arch. Fr. Pediatr.* **39**, 677–683.

Boardman, J.P., Ganesan, V., Rutherford, M.A., Saunders, D.E., Mercuri, E. & Cowan, F. (2005): Magnetic resonance image correlates of hemiparesis after neonatal and childhood middle cerebral artery stroke. *Pediatrics* **115**, 321–326.

Bode, H., Strassburg, H.M., Pringsheim, W. & Kunzer, W. (1986): Cerebral infarction in term neonates: diagnosis by cerebral ultrasound. *Childs Nerv. Syst.* **2**, 195–199.

Bode, H., Bubl, R., Rutishauser, M. & Nars, P.W. (1994): Congenital tetraplegia, respiratory insufficiency, and hypoplasia of medulla oblongata. *Pediatr. Neurol.* **10**, 161–163.

Bonnier, C., Nassogne, M.C., Saint-Martin, C., Mesples, B., Kadhim, H. & Sébire, G. (2003): Neuroimaging of intraparenchymal lesions predicts outcome in shaken baby syndrome. *Pediatrics* **112**, 808–814.

Bouza, H., Dubowitz, L.M., Rutherford, M. & Pennock, J.M. (1994a): Prediction of outcome in children with congenital hemiplegia: a magnetic resonance imaging study. *Neuropediatrics* **25**, 60–66.

Bouza, H., Rutherford, M., Acolet, D., Pennock, J.M. & Dubowitz, L.M. (1994b): Evolution of early hemiplegic signs in full-term infants with unilateral brain lesions in the neonatal period: a prospective study. *Neuropediatrics* **25**, 201–207.

Boyce, L.H., Khandji, A.G., DeKlerk, A.M. & Nordli, D.R. (1994): Fetomaternal hemorrhage as an etiology of neonatal stroke. *Pediatr. Neurol.* **11**, 255–257.

Boyd, R.N., Morris, M.E. & Graham, H.K. (2001): Management of upper limb dysfunction in children with cerebral palsy: a systematic review. *Eur. J. Neurol.* **8** (Suppl. 5), 150–166.

Brenner, B., Fishman, A., Goldsher, D., Schreibman, D. & Tavory, S. (1988): Cerebral thrombosis in a newborn with a congenital deficiency of antithrombin III. *Am. J. Hematol.* **27**, 209–211.

Broxterman, K.J., Mathew, P. & Chicoine, L. (2000): Left brachial artery thrombus, left axillary vein thrombus, and stroke in a neonate with factor V Leiden mutation. *J. Pediatr. Hematol. Oncol.* **22**, 472–475.

Brozici, M., van der Zwan, A. & Hillen, B. (2003): Anatomy and functionality of leptomeningeal anastomoses: a review. *Stroke* **34**, 2750–2762.

Bull, M.J., Schreiner, R.L., Garg, B.P., Hutton, N.M., Lemons, J.A. & Gresham, E.L. (1980): Neurologic complications following temporal artery catheterization. *J. Pediatr.* **96**, 1071–1073.

Butrum, M.W., Williams, L.S. & Golomb, M.R. (2003): A child with Diamond-Blackfan anemia, methylenetetrahydrofolate reductase mutation, and perinatal stroke. *J. Child. Neurol.* **18**, 800–802.

Campbell, L.R., Bunyapen, C., Holmes, G.L., Howell, C.G., & Kanto, W.P. (1988): Right common carotid artery ligation in extracorporeal membrane oxygenation. *J. Pediatr.* **113**, 110–113.

Carrilho, I., Costa, E., Barreirinho, M.S., Santos, M., Barbot, C. & Barbot, J. (2001): Prothrombotic study in full term neonates with arterial stroke. *Haematologica* **86**, E16.

Chalmers, E.A. (2005): Perinatal stroke – risk factors and management. *Br. J. Haematol.* **130**, 333–343.

Chan, G.M. & Nelson, L.S. (2004): More on blue cohosh and perinatal stroke. *N. Engl. J. Med.* **351**, 2239–2241; author reply: 2241.

Chandra, S.A., Gilbert, E.F., Viseskul, C., Strother, C.M., Haning, R.V. & Javid, M.J. (1990): Neonatal intracranial choriocarcinoma. *Arch. Pathol. Lab. Med.* **114**, 1079–1082.

Chasnoff, I.J., Bussey, M.E., Savich, R. & Stack, C.M. (1986): Perinatal cerebral infarction and maternal cocaine use. *J. Pediatr.* **108**, 456–459.

Chiu, C.H., Lin, T.Y. & Huang, Y.C. (1995): Cranial nerve palsies and cerebral infarction in a young infant with meningococcal meningitis. *Scand. J. Infect. Dis.* **27**, 75–76.

Chun, D.S., Schamberger, M.S., Flaspohler, T., Turrentine, M.W., Brown, J.W., Farrell, A.G. & Girod, D.A. (2004): Incidence, outcome, and risk factors for stroke after the Fontan procedure. *Am. J. Cardiol.* **93**, 117–119.

Claeys, V., Deonna, T. & Chrzanowski, R. (1983): Congenital hemiparesis: the spectrum of lesions. A clinical and computerized tomographic study of 37 cases. *Helv. Paediatr. Acta* **38**, 439–455.

Clancy, R.R. (2006): Summary proceedings from the neurology group on neonatal seizures. *Pediatrics* **117**, S23–S27.

Clancy, R., Malin, S., Laraque, D., Baumgart, S. & Younkin, D. (1985): Focal motor seizures heralding stroke in full-term neonates. *Am. J. Dis. Child.* **139**, 601–606.

Cohen, H.L., Sloves, J.H., Laungani, S., Glass, L. & DeMarinis, P. (1994): Neurosonographic findings in full-term infants born to maternal cocaine abusers: visualization of subependymal and periventricular cysts. *J. Clin. Ultrasound* **22**, 327–333.

Cowan, F., Mercuri, E., Groenendaal, F., Bassi, L., Ricci, D., Rutherford, M. & de Vries, L. (2005): Does cranial ultrasound imaging identify arterial cerebral infarction in term neonates? *Arch. Dis. Child. Fetal Neonat. Ed.* **90**, F252–F256.

Craze, J.L., Salisbury, A.J. & Pike, M.G. (1996): Prenatal stroke associated with maternal parvovirus infection. *Dev. Med. Child Neurol.* **38**, 84–85.

Debus, O., Koch, H.G., Kurlemann, G., Strater, R., Vielhaber, H., Weber, P. & Nowak-Gottl, U. (1998): Factor V Leiden and genetic defects of thrombophilia in childhood porencephaly. *Arch. Dis. Child. Fetal Neonat. Ed.* **78**, F121–124.

De Haan, T.R., Van Wezel-Meijler, G., Beersma, M.F., Von Lindern, J.S., Van Duinen, S.G. & Walther, F.J. (2006): Fetal stroke and congenital parvovirus B19 infection complicated by activated protein C resistance. *Acta Paediatr.* **95**, 863–867.

deVeber, G., Roach, E.S., Riela, A.R. & Wiznitzer, M. (2000a): Stroke in children: recognition, treatment, and future directions. *Semin. Pediatr. Neurol.* **7**, 309–317.

deVeber, G.A., MacGregor, D., Curtis, R. & Mayank, S. (2000b): Neurologic outcome in survivors of childhood arterial ischemic stroke and sinovenous thrombosis. *J. Child Neurol.* **15**, 316–324.

deVeber, G. (2005): In pursuit of evidence-based treatments for paediatric stroke: the UK and Chest guidelines. *Lancet Neurol.* **4**, 432–436.

de Vries, L.S., Smet, M., Goemans, N., Wilms, G., Devlieger, H. & Casaer, P. (1992): Unilateral thalamic haemorrhage in the pre-term and full-term newborn. *Neuropediatrics* **23**, 153–156.

de Vries, L.S., Groenendaal, F., Eken, P., van Haastert, I.C., Rademaker, K.J. & Meiners, L.C. (1997): Infarcts in the vascular distribution of the middle cerebral artery in preterm and fullterm infants. *Neuropediatrics* **28**, 88–96.

de Vries, L.S., Van der Grond, J., Van Haastert, I.C. & Groenendaal, F. (2005): Prediction of outcome in new-born infants with arterial ischaemic stroke using diffusion-weighted magnetic resonance imaging. *Neuropediatrics* **36**, 12–20.

de Vries, L.S., Verboon-Maciolek, M.A., Cowan, F.M. & Groenendaal, F. (2006): The role of cranial ultrasound and magnetic resonance imaging in the diagnosis of infections of the central nervous system. *Early Hum. Dev.* **82**, 819–825.

Dominguez, R., Aguirre Vila-Coro, A., Slopis, J.M. & Bohan, T.P. (1991): Brain and ocular abnormalities in infants with in utero exposure to cocaine and other street drugs. *Am. J. Dis. Child.* **145**, 688–695.

Donaldson, B. (1987): Real time ultrasound, arterial pulsation and neonatal cerebral infarction. *Postgrad. Med. J.* **63**, 263–265.

D'Orey, M.C., Melo, M.J., Ramos, I., Guimaraes, H., Alves, A.R., Silva, J.S., Vasconcelos, G., Costa, A., Silva, G. & Santos, N.T. (1999): Cerebral ischemic infarction in newborn infants. Diagnosis using pulsed and color Doppler imaging. *Arch. Pediatr.* **6**, 457–459.

Drolet, B.A., Dohil, M., Golomb, M.R., Wells, R., Murowski, L., Tamburro, J., Sty, J. & Friedlander, S.F. (2006): Early stroke and cerebral vasculopathy in children with facial hemangiomas and PHACE association. *Pediatrics* **117**, 959–964.

Dudink, J., Lequin, M., Weisglas-Kuperus, N., Conneman, N., van Goudoever, J.B. & Govaert, P. (2008): Venous subtypes of preterm periventricular haemorrhagic infarction. *Arch. Dis. Child.* **93**, F201–F206.

Duque, J., Thonnard, J.L., Vandermeeren, Y., Sebire, G., Cosnard, G. & Olivier, E. (2003): Correlation between impaired dexterity and corticospinal tract dysgenesis in congenital hemiplegia. *Brain* **126**, 732–747.

Eftekhar, B., Dadmehr, M., Ansari, S., Ghodsi, M., Nazparvar, B. & Ketabchi, E. (2006): Are the distributions of variations of circle of Willis different in different populations? Results of an anatomical study and review of literature. *B.M.C. Neurol.* **6**, 22.

Eliasson, A.C., Bonnier, B. & Krumlinde-Sundholm, L. (2003): Clinical experience of constraint induced movement therapy in adolescents with hemiplegic cerebral palsy – a day camp model. *Dev. Med. Child. Neurol.* **45**, 357–359.

Emsley, H.C., Young, C.A. & White, R.P. (2006): Circle of Willis variation in a complex stroke presentation: a case report. *B.M.C. Neurol.* **6**, 13.

Erbayraktar, S., Tekinsoy, B., Acar, F. & Acar, U. (2001): Posttraumatic isolated infarction in the territory of Heubner's and lenticulostriate arteries. *Kobe J. Med. Sci.* **47**, 113–121.

Estan, J. & Hope, P. (1997): Unilateral neonatal cerebral infarction in full term infants. *Arch. Dis. Child. Fetal Neonat. Ed.* **76**, F88–F93.

Evans, D. & Levene, M. (1998): Neonatal seizures. *Arch. Dis. Child. Fetal Neonat. Ed.* **78**, F70–F75.

Eyre, J.A., Miller, S., Clowry, G.J., Conway, E.A. & Watts, C. (2000): Functional corticospinal projections are established prenatally in the human foetus permitting involvement in the development of spinal motor centres. *Brain* **123**, 51–64.

Fair, D.A., Brown, T.T., Petersen, S.E. & Schlaggar, B.L. (2006): fMRI reveals novel functional neuroanatomy in a child with perinatal stroke. *Neurology* **67**, 2246–2249.

Fehlings, D., Rang, M., Glazier, J. & Steele, C. (2000): An evaluation of botulinum-A toxin injections to improve upper extremity function in children with hemiplegic cerebral palsy. *J. Pediatr.* **137**, 331–337.

Fernandez-Bouzas, A., Harmony, T., Santiago-Rodriguez, E., Ricardo-Garcell, J., Fernandez, T. & Avila-Acosta, D. (2006): Schizencephaly with occlusion or absence of middle cerebral artery. *Neuroradiology* **48**, 171–175.

Filipek, P.A., Krishnamoorthy, K.S., Davis, K.R. & Kuehnle, K. (1987): Focal cerebral infarction in the newborn: a distinct entity. *Pediatr. Neurol.* **3**, 141–147.

Finkel, R.S. & Zarlengo, K.M. (2004): Blue cohosh and perinatal stroke. *N. Engl. J. Med.* **351**, 302–303.

Fischer, A.Q., Anderson, J.C. & Shuman, R.M. (1988): The evolution of ischemic cerebral infarction in infancy: a sonographic evaluation. *J. Child. Neurol.* **3**, 105–109.

Fujimoto, S., Yokochi, K., Togari, H., Nishimura, Y., Inukai, K., Futamura, M., Sobajima, H., Suzuki, S. & Wada, Y. (1992): Neonatal cerebral infarction: symptoms, CT findings and prognosis. *Brain Dev.* **14**, 48–52.

Fullerton, H.J., Johnston, S.C. & Smith, W.S. (2001): Arterial dissection and stroke in children. *Neurology* **57**, 1155–1160.

Gabis, L.V., Yangala, R. & Lenn, N.J. (2002): Time lag to diagnosis of stroke in children. *Pediatrics* **110**, 924–928.

Gaggero, R., Devescovi, R., Zaccone, A. & Ravera, G. (2001): Epilepsy associated with infantile hemiparesis: predictors of long-term evolution. *Brain Dev.* **23,** 12–17.

Garg, B.P. & DeMyer, W.E. (1995): Ischemic thalamic infarction in children: clinical presentation, etiology, and outcome. *Pediatr. Neurol.* **13,** 46–49.

Garg, B.P. & Edwards-Brown, M.K. (1995): Vertebral artery compression due to head rotation in thalamic stroke. *Pediatr. Neurol.* **12,** 162–164.

Gillilan, L.A. (1972): Blood supply to primitive mammalian brains. *J. Comp. Neurol.* **145,** 209–221.

Ginsberg, M.D. (2003): Adventures in the pathophysiology of brain ischemia: penumbra, gene expression, neuroprotection: the 2002 Thomas Willis Lecture. *Stroke* **34,** 214–223.

Giroud, M., Fayolle, H., Martin, D., Baudoin, N., Andre, N., Gouyon, J.B., Nivelon, J.L. & Dumas, R. (1995): Late thalamic atrophy in infarction of the middle cerebral artery territory in neonates. A prospective clinical and radiological study in four children. *Childs Nerv. Syst.* **11,** 133–136.

Golomb, M.R., MacGregor, D.L., Domi, T., Armstrong, D.C., McCrindle, B.W., Mayank, S. & deVeber, G.A. (2001): Presumed pre- or perinatal arterial ischemic stroke: risk factors and outcomes. *Ann. Neurol.* **50,** 163–168.

Golomb, M.R., Garg, B.P. & Williams, L.S. (2006): Outcomes of children with infantile spasms after perinatal stroke. *Pediatr. Neurol.* **34,** 291–295.

Gould, R.J., Black, K. & Pavlakis, S.G. (1996): Neonatal cerebral arterial thrombosis: protein C deficiency. *J. Child Neurol.* **11,** 250–252.

Govaert, P. & de Vries, L. (1996): An atlas of neonatal brain sonography. *Clin. Dev. Med.* **141/142.**

Govaert, P., Vanhaesebrouck, P., De Praeter, C., Frankel, U. & Leroy, J. (1989a): Moebius sequence and prenatal brainstem ischemia. *Pediatrics* **84,** 570–573.

Govaert, P., Vanhaesebrouck, P., De Praeter, C. & Leroy, J. (1989b): Hydranencéphalie et prise d'oestrogènes pendant la grossesse. *Arch. Franc. Pediatr.* **46,** 235.

Govaert, P., Vanhaesebrouck, P. & de Praeter, C. (1992): Traumatic neonatal intracranial bleeding and stroke. *Arch. Dis. Child.* **67,** 840–845.

Govaert, P., Matthys, E., Zecic, A., Roelens, F., Oostra, A. & Vanzieleghem, B. (2000): Perinatal cortical infarction within middle cerebral artery trunks. *Arch. Dis. Child. Fetal Neonat. Ed.* **82,** F59–F63.

Govaert, P., Zingman, A., Jung, Y.H., Dudink, J., Swarte, R., Zecic, A., Meersschaut, V., van Engelen, S. & Lequin, M. (2007): Network injury to pulvinar with neonatal arterial ischemic stroke. *Neuroimage* **39,** 1850–1857.

Groenendaal, F., van der Grond, J., Witkamp, T.D. & de Vries, L.S. (1995): Proton magnetic resonance spectroscopic imaging in neonatal stroke. *Neuropediatrics* **26,** 243–248.

Gruppo, R.A., DeGrauw, T.J., Palasis, S., Kalinyak, K.A. & Bofinger, M.K. (1998): Strokes, cutis marmorata telangiectatica congenita, and factor V Leiden. *Pediatr. Neurol.* **18,** 342–345.

Guajardo, L., Strauss, A. & Amster, J. (1994): Idiopathic cerebral infarction and upper limb ischemia in neonates. *Am. J. Perinatol.* **11,** 119–122.

Gudinchet, F., Dreyer, J.L., Payot, M., Duvoisin, B. & Laurini, R. (1991): Imaging of neonatal arterial thrombosis. *Arch. Dis. Child.* **66,** 1158–1159.

Gunther, G., Junker, R., Strater, R., Schobess, R., Kurnik, K., Heller, C., Kosch, A. & Nowak-Gottl, U. (2000): Symptomatic ischemic stroke in full-term neonates: role of acquired and genetic prothrombotic risk factors. *Stroke* **31,** 2437–2441.

Guzzetta, A., Mercuri, E., Rapisardi, G., Ferrari, F., Roversi, M.F., Cowan, F., Rutherford, M., Paolicelli, P.B., Einspieler, C., Boldrini, A., Dubowitz, L., Prechtl, H.F. & Cioni, G. (2003): General movements detect early signs of hemiplegia in term infants with neonatal cerebral infarction. *Neuropediatrics* **34,** 61–66.

Halsey, J.H., Allen, N. & Chamberlin, H.R. (1971): The morphogenesis of hydranencephaly. *J. Neurol. Sci.* **12,** 187–217.

Hanigan, W.C., Olivero, W.C. & Miller, T.C. (1993): Traumatic neonatal intracranial bleeding and stroke. *Arch. Dis. Child.* **68,** 339–340.

Harps, E. & Helmke, K. (1998): Diagnosis of congenital absence of internal carotid artery by power angio sonography. *Eur. Radiol.* **8,** 1245–1247.

Harris, N.L. (1997): Respiratory distress and seizure in a neonate. *N. Engl. J. Med.* **336,** 1439–1446.

Harum, K.H., Hoon, A.H., Kato, G.J., Casella, J.F., Breiter, S.N. & Johnston, M.V. (1999): Homozygous factor-V mutation as a genetic cause of perinatal thrombosis and cerebral palsy. *Dev. Med. Child Neurol.* **41,** 777–780.

Heier, L.A., Carpanzano, C.R., Mast, J., Brill, P.W., Winchester, P. & Deck, M.D. (1991): Maternal cocaine abuse: the spectrum of radiologic abnormalities in the neonatal CNS. *Am. J. Neuroradiol.* **12,** 951–956.

Hernanz-Schulman, M., Cohen, W. & Genieser, N.B. (1988): Sonography of cerebral infarction in infancy. *Am. J. Roentgenol.* **150,** 897–902.

Hill, A., Martin, D.J., Daneman, A. & Fitz, C.R. (1983): Focal ischemic cerebral injury in the newborn: diagnosis by ultrasound and correlation with computed tomographic scan. *Pediatrics* **71,** 790–793.

Hillen, B. (1986): The variability of the circle of Willis: univariate and bivariate analysis. *Acta Morphol. Neerl. Scand.* **24,** 87–101.

Hoyt, W.F. (1960): Vascular lesions of the visual cortex with brain herniation through the tentorial incisura. Neuro-ophthalmologic considerations. *Arch. Ophthalmol.* **64,** 44–57.

Hunt, R.W. & Inder, T.E. (2006): Perinatal and neonatal ischaemic stroke: a review. *Thromb. Res.* **118,** 39–48.

Jan, M.M. & Camfield, P.R. (1998): Outcome of neonatal stroke in full-term infants without significant birth asphyxia. *Eur. J. Pediatr.* **157,** 846–848.

Jan, W., Zimmerman, R.A., Bilaniuk, L.T., Hunter, J.V., Simon, E.M. & Haselgrove, J. (2003): Diffusion-weighted imaging in acute bacterial meningitis in infancy. *Neuroradiology* **45,** 634–639.

Jarjour, I.T. & Ahdab-Barmada, M. (1994): Cerebrovascular lesions in infants and children dying after extracorporeal membrane oxygenation. *Pediatr. Neurol.* **10,** 13–19.

Jaspan, T., Narborough, G., Punt, J.A. & Lowe, J. (1992): Cerebral contusional tears as a marker of child abuse – detection by cranial sonography. *Pediatr. Radiol.* **22,** 237–245.

Jaspan, T., Griffiths, P.D., McConachie, N.S. & Punt, J.A. (2003): Neuroimaging for non-accidental head injury in childhood: a proposed protocol. *Clin. Radiol.* **58,** 44–53.

Jung, J.H., Graham, J.M., Schultz, N. & Smith, D.W. (1984): Congenital hydranencephaly/porencephaly due to vascular disruption in monozygotic twins. *Pediatrics* **73,** 467–469.

Kaplan, C.G. (2007): Fetal and maternal vascular lesions. *Semin. Diagn. Pathol.* **24,** 14–22.

Kay's Kayemba, S., Raobijoana, H., Francois, P., Croize, J. & Bost-Bru, C. (2000): [Acute Salmonella typhi meningitis in a 25-day-old newborn infant complicated by obstruction of the sylvian artery]. *Arch. Pediatr.* **7,** 154–157.

Kirton, A. & deVeber, G. (2006): Cerebral palsy secondary to perinatal ischemic stroke. *Clin. Perinatol.* **33,** 367–386.

Klesh, K.W., Murphy, T.F., Scher, M.S., Buchanan, D.E., Maxwell, E.P. & Guthrie, R.D. (1987): Cerebral infarction in persistent pulmonary hypertension of the newborn. *Am. J. Dis. Child.* **141,** 852–857.

Koelfen, W., Freund, M., Konig, S., Varnholt, V., Rohr, H. & Schultze, C. (1993): Results of parenchymal and angiographic magnetic resonance imaging and neuropsychological testing of children after stroke as neonates. *Eur. J. Pediatr.* **152,** 1030–1035.

Koelfen, W., Freund, M. & Varnholt, V. (1995): Neonatal stroke involving the middle cerebral artery in term infants: clinical presentation, EEG and imaging studies, and outcome. *Dev. Med. Child Neurol.* **37,** 204–212.

Koh, S. & Chen, L.S. (1997): Protein C and S deficiency in children with ischemic cerebrovascular accident. *Pediatr. Neurol.* **17,** 319–321.

Kolk, A., Beilmann, A., Tomberg, T., Napa, A. & Talvik, T. (2001): Neurocognitive development of children with congenital unilateral brain lesion and epilepsy. *Brain Dev.* **23,** 88–96.

Krauland, W. (1952): Riss der Art. basilaris als Geburtzverletzung. *Beitr. Gerichtl. Med.* **19,** 82.

Kraus, F.T. & Acheen, V.I. (1999): Fetal thrombotic vasculopathy in the placenta: cerebral thrombi and infarcts, coagulopathies, and cerebral palsy. *Hum. Pathol.* **30,** 759–769.

Krishnamoorthy, K.S., Soman, T.B., Takeoka, M. & Schaefer, P.W. (2000): Diffusion-weighted imaging in neonatal cerebral infarction: clinical utility and follow-up. *J. Child Neurol.* **15,** 592–602.

Kuhle, S., Lane, D.A., Jochmanns, K., Male, C., Quehenberger, P., Lechner, K. & Pabinger, I. (2001): Homozygous antithrombin deficiency type II (99 Leu to Phe mutation): and childhood thromboembolism. *Thromb. Haemost.* **86,** 1007–1011.

Kupari, M. & Roine, R.O. (2005): [Stroke and foramen ovale. The hypothesis of paradoxal embolization is still without proof]. *Duodecim* **121,** 1203–1205.

Kurnik, K., Kosch, A., Strater, R., Schobess, R., Heller, C. & Nowak-Gottl, U. (2003): Recurrent thromboembolism in infants and children suffering from symptomatic neonatal arterial stroke: a prospective follow-up study. *Stroke* **34,** 2887–2892.

Larnaout, A., Mongalgi, M.A., Ben Ameur, H., Hentati, F., Debbabi, A. & Ben Hamida, M. (1992): [Antenatal bilateral sylvian infarction and congenital syphilis]. *Arch. Fr. Pediatr.* **49,** 895–897.

Larroche, J.C. & Amiel, C. (1966): [Thrombosis of the sylvian artery during the neonatal period. Anatomical study and pathogenic discussion of so-called congenital hemiplegia]. *Arch. Fr. Pediatr.* **23,** 257–274.

Larroche, J.C., Droullé, P., Delezoide, A.L., Narcy, F. & Nessmann, C. (1990): Brain damage in monozygous twins. *Biol. Neonat.* **57,** 261–278.

Larroche, J.C., Girard, N., Narcy, F. & Fallet, C. (1994): Abnormal cortical plate (polymicrogyria), heterotopias and brain damage in monozygous twins. *Biol. Neonat.* **65,** 343–352.

Lee, R.M. (1995): Morphology of cerebral arteries. *Pharmacol. Ther.* **66,** 149–173.

Lee, J.H., Oh, C.W., Lee, S.H. & Han, D.H. (2003): Aplasia of the internal carotid artery. *Acta Neurochir. (Wien)* **145,** 117–125.

Lee, J., Croen, L.A., Lindan, C., Nash, K.B., Yoshida, C.K., Ferriero, D.M., Barkovich, A.J. & Wu, Y.W. (2005): Predictors of outcome in perinatal arterial stroke: a population-based study. *Ann. Neurol.* **58,** 303–308.

Lequin, M.H., Peeters, E.A., Holscher, H.C., de Krijger, R. & Govaert, P. (2004): Arterial infarction caused by carotid artery dissection in the neonate. *Eur. J. Paediatr. Neurol.* **8,** 155–160.

Levy, S.R., Abroms, I.F., Marshall, P.C. & Rosquete, E.E. (1985): Seizures and cerebral infarction in the full-term newborn. *Ann. Neurol.* **17,** 366–370.

Lui, K., Hellmann, J., Soto, G., Donoghue, V. & Daneman, A. (1990): Regional cerebral blood flow velocity patterns in newborn infants. *J. Paediatr. Child Health* **26,** 55–57.

Luisiri, A., Graviss, E.R., Weber, T., Silberstein, M.J., Tantana, S., Connors, R. & Brodeur, A.E. (1988): Neurosonographic changes in newborns treated with extracorporeal membrane oxygenation. *J. Ultrasound Med.* **7,** 429–438.

Lynch, J.K., Nelson, K.B., Curry, C.J. & Grether, J.K. (2001): Cerebrovascular disorders in children with the factor V Leiden mutation. *J. Child Neurol.* **16,** 735–744.

Lynch, J.K., Han, C.J., Nee, L.E. & Nelson, K.B. (2005): Prothrombotic factors in children with stroke or porencephaly. *Pediatrics* **116,** 447–453.

Mader, I., Schoning, M., Klose, U. & Kuker, W. (2002): Neonatal cerebral infarction diagnosed by diffusion-weighted MRI: pseudonormalization occurs early. *Stroke* **33,** 1142–1145.

Maegaki, Y., Maeoka, Y., Ishii, S., Shiota, M., Takeuchi, A., Yoshino, K. & Takeshita, K. (1997): Mechanisms of central motor reorganization in pediatric hemiplegic patients. *Neuropediatrics* **28,** 168–174.

Maingay-de Groof, F., Lequin, M., Roofthooft, D.W., Oranje, A., de Coo, I.F., Bok, L.A., Mancini, G.M., Govaert, P.P. (2007): Extensive cerebral infarction in the newborn due to incontinentia pigmenti. *Eur. J. Paediatr. Neurol.*, epub Oct 18.

Mancini, G.M., de Coo, I.F., Lequin, M.H. & Arts, W.F. (2004): Hereditary porencephaly: clinical and MRI findings in two Dutch families. *Eur. J. Paediatr. Neurol.* **8,** 45–54.

Mann, C.I. (2001): Posttraumatic carotid artery dissection in children: evaluation children. *Neurology* **57,** 1155–1160.

Mannino, F.L. & Trauner, D.A. (1983): Stroke in neonates. *J. Pediatr.* **102,** 605–610.

Mantovani, J.F. & Gerber, G.J. (1984): 'Idiopathic' neonatal cerebral infarction. *Am. J. Dis. Child.* **138,** 359–362.

Mazumdar, A., Mukherjee, P., Miller, J.H., Malde, H. & McKinstry, R.C. (2003): Diffusion-weighted imaging of acute corticospinal tract injury preceding Wallerian degeneration in the maturing human brain. *Am. J. Neuroradiol.* **24,** 1057–1066.

McLellan, N.J., Prasad, R. & Punt, J. (1986): Spontaneous subhyaloid and retinal haemorrhages in an infant. *Arch. Dis. Child.* **61,** 1130–1132.

McQuillen, P.S., Hamrick, S.E., Perez, M.J., Barkovich, A.J., Glidden, D.V., Karl, T.R., Teitel, D. & Miller, S.P. (2006): Balloon atrial septostomy is associated with preoperative stroke in neonates with transposition of the great arteries. *Circulation* **113,** 280–285.

Ment, L.R., Duncan, C.C. & Ehrenkranz, R.A. (1984): Perinatal cerebral infarction. *Ann. Neurol.* **16,** 559–568.

Ment, L.R., Ehrenkranz, R.A. & Duncan, C.C. (1986): Bacterial meningitis as an etiology of perinatal cerebral infarction. *Pediatr. Neurol.* **2,** 276–279.

Mercuri, E. (2001): Early diagnostic and prognostic indicators in full term infants with neonatal cerebral infarction: an integrated clinical, neuroradiological and EEG approach. *Minerva Pediatr.* **53,** 305–311.

Mercuri, E. & Cowan, F. (1999): Cerebral infarction in the newborn infant: review of the literature and personal experience. *Eur. J. Paediatr. Neurol.* **3,** 255–263.

Mercuri, E., Atkinson, J., Braddick, O., Anker, S., Nokes, L., Cowan, F., Rutherford, M., Pennock, J. & Dubowitz, L. (1996): Visual function and perinatal focal cerebral infarction. *Arch. Dis. Child. Fetal Neonat. Ed.* **75,** F76–F81.

Mercuri, E., Rutherford, M., Cowan, F., Pennock, J., Counsell, S., Papadimitriou, M., Azzopardi, D., Bydder, G. & Dubowitz, L. (1999): Early prognostic indicators of outcome in infants with neonatal cerebral infarction: a clinical, electroencephalogram, and magnetic resonance imaging study. *Pediatrics* **103,** 39–46.

Mercuri, E., Anker, S., Guzzetta, A., Barnett, A., Haataja, L., Rutherford, M., Cowan, F., Dubowitz, L., Braddick, O. & Atkinson, J. (2003): Neonatal cerebral infarction and visual function at school age. *Arch. Dis. Child. Fetal Neonat. Ed.* **88,** F487–F491.

Messer, J., Haddad, J. & Casanova, R. (1991): Transcranial Doppler evaluation of cerebral infarction in the neonate. *Neuropediatrics* **22,** 147–151.

Meyer, J.E. (1951): Uber Gefassveränderungen beim fetalen und frükindlichen Cerebralschaden. *Arch. Psychiatr.* **186,** 437.

Miller, S.P., O'Gorman, A.M. & Shevell, M.I. (2000): Recurrent artery of Heubner infarction in infancy. *Dev. Med. Child Neurol.* **42**, 344–346.

Mitra, S., Ghosh, D., Puri, R. & Parmar, V.R. (2001): Top-of-the-basilar-artery stroke. *Ind. Pediatr.* **38**, 83–87.

Mohr, J.P. & Homma, S. (2003): Patent cardiac foramen ovale: stroke risk and closure. *Ann. Intern. Med.* **139**, 787–788.

Mokri, B. (1987): *Dissection of cervical and cephalic arteries: diagnosis and surgical treatment, in occlusive cerebrovascular disease*, ed. T.M. Sundt, pp. 38–59. Philadelphia: W.B. Saunders.

Monagle, P. (2003): Thrombosis in pediatric cardiac patients. *Semin. Thromb. Hemost.* **29**, 547–555.

Monagle, P., Chan, A., Massicotte, P., Chalmers, E. & Michelson, A.D. (2004): Antithrombotic therapy in children: the Seventh ACCP Conference on Antithrombotic and Thrombolytic Therapy. *Chest* **126**, 645S–687S.

Nelson, K.B. & Lynch, J.K. (2004): Stroke in newborn infants. *Lancet Neurol.* **3**, 150–158.

Niemann, G., Dobler-Neumann, M., Scheel, P. & Klein, R. (1999): [Why do newborn infants already suffer from 'stroke'. Studies of focal, arterial, ischemic infarct]. *Klin. Padiatr.* **211**, 154–160.

Nordborg, C., Kyllerman, M., Conradi, N. & Mansson, J.E. (1997): Early-infantile galactosialidosis with multiple brain infarctions: morphological, neuropathological and neurochemical findings. *Acta Neuropathol. (Berl.)* **93**, 24–33.

Norman, M.G. (1974): Unilateral encephalomalacia in cranial nerve nuclei in neonates: report of two cases. *Neurology* **24**, 424–427.

Nowak-Gottl, U., Gunther, G., Kurnik, K., Strater, R. & Kirkham, F. (2003): Arterial ischemic stroke in neonates, infants, and children: an overview of underlying conditions, imaging methods, and treatment modalities. *Semin. Thromb. Hemost.* **29**, 405–414.

Ong, B.Y., Ellison, P.H. & Browning, C. (1983): Intrauterine stroke in the neonate. *Arch. Neurol.* **40**, 55–56.

Ozduman, K., Pober, B.R., Barnes, P., Copel, J.A., Ogle, E.A., Duncan, C.C. & Ment, L.R. (2004): Fetal stroke. *Pediatr. Neurol.* **30**, 151–162.

Parker, M.J., Joubert, G.I. & Levin, S.D. (2002): Portal vein thrombosis causing neonatal cerebral infarction. *Arch. Dis. Child. Fetal Neonat. Ed.* **87**, F125–F127.

Pellicer, A., Cabanas, F., Garcia-Alix, A., Perez-Higueras, A. & Quero, J. (1992): Stroke in neonates with cardiac right-to-left shunt. *Brain Dev.* **14**, 381–385.

Perlman, J.M., Rollins, N.K. & Evans, D. (1994): Neonatal stroke: clinical characteristics and cerebral blood flow velocity measurements. *Pediatr. Neurol.* **11**, 281–284.

Pollack, M.A., Llena, J.F., Fleischman, A. & Fish, B. (1983): Neonatal brainstem infarction. A case report with clinicopathologic correlation. *Arch. Neurol.* **40**, 52–53.

Prats, J.M., Monzon, M.J., Zuazo, E. & Garaizar, C. (1993): Congenital nuclear syndrome of oculomotor nerve. *Pediatr. Neurol.* **9**, 476–478.

Prian, G.W., Wright, G.B., Rumack, C.M. & O'Meara, O.P. (1978): Apparent cerebral embolization after temporal artery catheterization. *J. Pediatr.* **93**, 115–118.

Puvabanditsin, S., Garrow, E., Augustin, G., Titapiwatanakul, R. & Kuniyoshi, K.M. (2005): Poland-Moebius syndrome and cocaine abuse: a relook at vascular etiology. *Pediatr. Neurol.* **32**, 285–287.

Raine, J., Davies, H. & Gamsu, H.R. (1989): Multiple idiopathic emboli in a full term neonate. *Acta Paediatr. Scand.* **78**, 644–646.

Ramaswamy, V., Miller, S.P., Barkovich, A.J., Partridge, J.C. & Ferriero, D.M. (2004): Perinatal stroke in term infants with neonatal encephalopathy. *Neurology* **62**, 2088–2091.

Raybaud, C.A., Livet, M.O., Jiddane, M. & Pinsard, N. (1985): Radiology of ischemic strokes in children. *Neuroradiology* **27**, 567–578.

Rehan, V.K. & Menticoglou, S.M. (1995): Mechanism of visceral damage in fetofetal transfusion syndrome. *Arch. Dis. Child. Fetal Neonat. Ed.* **73**, F48–F50.

Remillard, G.M., Ethier, R. & Andermann, F. (1974): Temporal lobe epilepsy and perinatal occlusion of the posterior cerebral artery. A syndrome analogous to infantile hemiplegia and a demonstrable etiology in some patients with temporal lobe epilepsy. *Neurology* **24**, 1001–1009.

Ries, M., Harms, D. & Scharf, J. (1994): [Multiple cerebral infarcts with resulting multicystic encephalomalacia in a premature infant with Enterobacter sakazakii meningitis]. *Klin. Padiatr.* **206**, 184–186.

Robinson, R.O., Trounce, J.Q., Janota, I. & Cox, T. (1993): Late fetal pontine destruction. *Pediatr. Neurol.* **9**, 213–215.

Roessmann, U. & Parks, P.J. (1978): Hydranencephaly in vertebral-basilar territory. *Acta Neuropathol. (Berl.)* **44**, 141–143.

Roessmann, U. & Miller, R.T. (1980): Thrombosis of the middle cerebral artery associated with birth trauma. *Neurology* **30**, 889–892.

Roodhooft, A.M., Parizel, P.M., Van Acker, K.J., Deprettere, A.J. & Van Reempts, P.J. (1987): Idiopathic cerebral arterial infarction with paucity of symptoms in the full-term neonate. *Pediatrics* **80**, 381–385.

Rossi, A. & Tortori-Donati, P. (2006): Agenesis of bilateral internal carotid arteries in the PHACE syndrome. *Am. J. Neuroradiol.* **27**, 1602.

Ruff, R.L., Shaw, C.M., Beckwith, J.B. & Iozzo, R.V. (1979): Cerebral infarction complicating umbilical vein catheterization. *Ann. Neurol.* **6**, 85.

Sarnat, H.B. (2004): Watershed infarcts in the fetal and neonatal brainstem. An aetiology of central hypoventilation, dysphagia, Moebius syndrome and micrognathia. *Eur. J. Paediatr. Neurol.* **8**, 71–87.

Scher, M.S. & Beggarly, M. (1989): Clinical significance of focal periodic discharges in neonates. *J. Child. Neurol.* **4**, 175–185.

Scher, M.S., Klesh, K.W., Murphy, T.F. & Guthrie, R.D. (1986): Seizures and infarction in neonates with persistent pulmonary hypertension. *Pediatr. Neurol.* **2**, 332–339.

Scher, M.S., Belfar, H., Martin, J. & Painter, M.J. (1991): Destructive brain lesions of presumed fetal onset: antepartum causes of cerebral palsy. *Pediatrics* **88**, 898–906.

Scher, M.S., Wiznitzer, M. & Bangert, B.A. (2002): Cerebral infarctions in the fetus and neonate: maternal-placental-fetal considerations. *Clin. Perinatol.* **29**, 693–724, vi-vii.

Schomer, D.F., Marks, M.P., Steinberg, G.K., Johnstone, I.M., Boothroyd, D.B., Ross, M.R., Pelc, N.J. & Enzmann, D.R. (1994): The anatomy of the posterior communicating artery as a risk factor for ischemic cerebral infarction. *N. Engl. J. Med.* **330**, 1565–1570.

Schulzke, S., Weber, P., Luetschg, J. & Fahnenstich, H. (2005): Incidence and diagnosis of unilateral arterial cerebral infarction in newborn infants. *J. Perinat. Med.* **33**, 170–175.

Seghier, M.L., Lazeyras, F., Zimine, S., Maier, S.E., Hanquinet, S., Delavelle, J., Volpe, J.J. & Huppi, P.S. (2004): Combination of event-related fMRI and diffusion tensor imaging in an infant with perinatal stroke. *Neuroimage* **21**, 463–472.

Selton, D., Andre, M. & Hascoet, J.M. (2003): [EEG and ischemic stroke in full-term newborns]. *Neurophysiol. Clin.* **33**, 120–129.

Silver, R.K., MacGregor, S.N., Pasternak, J.F. & Neely, S.E. (1992): Fetal stroke associated with elevated maternal anticardiolipin antibodies. *Obstet. Gynecol.* **80**, 497–499.

Sivan, Y., Nelson, M.D., Lee, S. & Wood, B.P. (1990): Radiological case of the month: cerebral air embolism. *Am. J. Dis. Child.* **144**, 1351–1352.

Snyder, R.D., Stovring, J., Cushing, A.H., Davis, L.E. & Hardy, T.L. (1981): Cerebral infarction in childhood bacterial meningitis. *J. Neurol. Neurosurg. Psychiatry* **44**, 581–585.

Soper, R., Chaloupka, J.C., Fayad, P.B., Greally, J.M., Shaywitz, B.A., Awad, I.A. & Pober, B.R. (1995): Ischemic stroke and intracranial multifocal cerebral arteriopathy in Williams syndrome. *J. Pediatr.* **126**, 945–948.

Squier, W., Salisbury, H. & Sisodiya, S. (2003): Stroke in the developing brain and intractable epilepsy: effect of timing on hippocampal sclerosis. *Dev. Med. Child Neurol.* **45**, 580–585.

Sreenan, C., Bhargava, R. & Robertson, C.M. (2000): Cerebral infarction in the term newborn: clinical presentation and long-term outcome. *J. Pediatr.* **137**, 351–355.

Staudt, M., Niemann, G., Grodd, W. & Krageloh-Mann, I. (2000): The pyramidal tract in congenital hemiparesis: relationship between morphology and function in periventricular lesions. *Neuropediatrics* **31**, 257–264.

Staudt, M., Krageloh-Mann, I. & Grodd, W. (2005): Ipsilateral corticospinal pathways in congenital hemiparesis on routine magnetic resonance imaging. *Pediatr. Neurol.* **32**, 37–39.

Steinbok, P., Haw, C.S., Cochrane, D.D. & Kestle, J.R. (1995): Acute subdural hematoma associated with cerebral infarction in the full-term neonate. *Pediatr. Neurosurg.* **23**, 206–215.

Steventon, D.M. & John, P.R. (1997): Power Doppler ultrasound appearances of neonatal ischaemic brain injury. *Pediatr. Radiol.* **27**, 147–149.

Stewart, R.M., Williams, R.S., Lukl, P. & Schoenen, J. (1978): Ventral porencephaly: a cerebral defect associated with multiple congenital anomalies. *Acta Neuropathol. (Berl.)* **42**, 231–235.

Stiles, J., Trauner, D., Engel, M. & Nass, R. (1997): The development of drawing in children with congenital focal brain injury: evidence for limited functional recovery. *Neuropsychologia* **35**, 299–312.

Swarte, R., Appel, I., Lequin, M., van Mol, C. & Govaert, P. (2004): Factor II gene (prothrombin G20210A): mutation and neonatal cerebrovenous thrombosis. *Thromb. Haemost.* **92**, 719–721.

Tabbutt, S., Griswold, W.R., Ogino, M.T., Mendoza, A.E., Allen, J.B. & Reznik, V.M. (1994): Multiple thromboses in a premature infant associated with maternal phospholipid antibody syndrome. *J. Perinatol.* **14**, 66–70.

Taylor, G.A. (1994): Alterations in regional cerebral blood flow in neonatal stroke: preliminary findings with color Doppler sonography. *Pediatr. Radiol.* **24**, 111–115.

Taylor, G.A., Fitz, C.R., Kapur, S. & Short, B.L. (1989): Cerebrovascular accidents in neonates treated with extracorporeal membrane oxygenation: sonographic-pathologic correlation. *Am. J. Roentgenol.* **153,** 355–361.

Taylor, G.A., Trescher, W.A., Traystman, R.J. & Johnston, M.V. (1993): Acute experimental neuronal injury in the newborn lamb: US characterization and demonstration of hemodynamic effects. *Pediatr. Radiol.* **23,** 268–275.

Temesvari, P. (2000): Perinatal cortical infarction with no obvious cause. *Arch. Dis. Child. Fetal Neonat. Ed.* **83,** F77.

Temesvari, P. (2002): Arterial air embolization and cerebral damage. *Acta Paediatr.* **91,** 728; author's reply, 728.

Thompson, J.A., Grunnet, M.L. & Anderson, R.E. (1975): Carotid arterial elastic hyperplasia in a newborn. *Stroke* **6,** 391–394.

Thorarensen, O., Ryan, S., Hunter, J. & Younkin, D.P. (1997): Factor V Leiden mutation: an unrecognized cause of hemiplegic cerebral palsy, neonatal stroke, and placental thrombosis. *Ann. Neurol.* **42,** 372–375.

Tjoelker, L.W. & Stafforini, D.M. (2000): Platelet-activating factor acetylhydrolases in health and disease. *Biochim. Biophys. Acta* **1488,** 102–123.

Uvebrant, P. (1988): Hemiplegic cerebral palsy: aetiology and outcome. *Acta Paediatr. Scand. Suppl.* **345,** 1–100.

Vander Eecken (1959): Normal cerebral arterial anatomy. In: *The anastomoses between the leptomeningeal arteries of the brain,* pp. 7–35. Springfield: C.C. Thomas.

van der Sluis, I.M., Boot, A.M., Vernooij, M., Meradji, M. & Kroon, A.A. (2006): Idiopathic infantile arterial calcification: clinical presentation, therapy and long-term follow-up. *Eur. J. Pediatr.* **165,** 590–593.

van der Zwan, A., Hillen, B., Tulleken, C.A., Dujovny, M. & Dragovic, L. (1992): Variability of the territories of the major cerebral arteries. *J. Neurosurg.* **77,** 927–940.

Van Geet, C. & Jaeken, J. (1993): A unique pattern of coagulation abnormalities in carbohydrate-deficient glycoprotein syndrome. Pediatr. Res. **33,** 540–541.

van Laar, P.J., Hendrikse, J., Golay, X., Lu, H., van Osch, M.J. & van der Grond, J. (2006): In vivo flow territory mapping of major brain feeding arteries. *Neuroimage* **29,** 136–144.

Vasovic, L., Milenkovic, Z. & Pavlovic, S. (2002): Comparative morphological variations and abnormalities of circles of Willis: a minireview including two personal cases. *Neurosurg. Rev.* **25,** 247–251.

Volpe, J.J. (1992): Effect of cocaine use on the fetus. *N. Engl. J. Med.* **327,** 399–407.

Volpe, J.J. (1995): *Neurology of the newborn,* 3rd edition, p. 306. Philadelphia: W.B. Saunders.

Wade, T., Booy, R., Teare, E.L. & Kroll, S. (1999): Pasteurella multocida meningitis in infancy – (a lick may be as bad as a bite). *Eur. J. Pediatr.* **158,** 875–878.

Wang, L.W., Huang, C.C. & Yeh, T.F. (2004): Major brain lesions detected on sonographic screening of apparently normal term neonates. *Neuroradiology* **46,** 368–373.

Weig, S.G., Marshall, P.C., Abroms, I.F. & Gauthier, N.S. (1995): Patterns of cerebral injury and clinical presentation in the vascular disruptive syndrome of monozygotic twins. *Pediatr. Neurol.* **13,** 279–285.

Weissman, B.M., Aram, D.M., Levinsohn, M.W. & Ben-Shachar, G. (1985): Neurologic sequelae of cardiac catheterization. *Cathet. Cardiovasc. Diagn.* **11,** 577–583.

Wollack, J.B., Kaifer, M., LaMonte, M.P. & Rothman, M. (1996): Stroke in Williams syndrome. *Stroke* **27,** 143–146.

Wu, Y.W., March, W.M., Croen, L.A., Grether, J.K., Escobar, G.J. & Newman, T.B. (2004): Perinatal stroke in children with motor impairment: a population-based study. *Pediatrics* **114,** 612–619.

Wu, Y.W., Lynch, J.K. & Nelson, K.B. (2005): Perinatal arterial stroke: understanding mechanisms and outcomes. *Semin. Neurol.* **25,** 424–434.

Wulfeck, B.B., Trauner, D.A. & Tallal, P.A. (1991): Neurologic, cognitive, and linguistic features of infants after early stroke. *Pediatr. Neurol.* **7,** 266–269.

Yates, P.O. (1959): Birth trauma to the vertebral arteries. *Arch. Dis. Child.* **34,** 436–441.

Yokochi, K. & Iwase, K. (1996): Bilateral internal carotid artery agenesis in a child with psychomotor developmental delay. *Pediatr. Neurol.* **15,** 76–78.

Chapter 16

Neonatal cerebral sinovenous thrombosis

Mahendranath Moharir * and Gabrielle deVeber °

* Department of Neurology, Children's Hospital at Westmead, Locked Bag # 4001, Westmead, Sydney NSW 2145, Australia;
° Department of Neurology, The Hospital for Sick Children, 555 University Ave., Toronto, M5G1X8 Ontario, Canada
gabrielledev@cogeco.ca

Summary

Cerebral sinovenous thrombosis (CSVT) is increasingly encountered in neonates and children. CSVT in neonates differs from CSVT in older children and adults. In neonates and young children it is less easily recognized owing to the non-specific symptoms and signs and the difficult radiographic diagnosis, although advances in imaging of the intracranial venous system have improved the rate of diagnosis. Risk factors for CSVT are different in neonates from those in older children and adults. Several randomized controlled trials (RCTs) have established the usefulness and safety of anticoagulants in adult CSVT; however, only cohort studies have been conducted in neonates and children. RCTs in neonates and children are lacking, mainly because the safety of anticoagulants is not yet well established. There are significant developmental differences in haemostatic, sinovenous, and neurological systems in young children, particularly neonates; this limits the extrapolation of adult data to young children. Lastly, radiographic and clinical outcomes – which will determine the need and sample size for RCTs – have not been well characterized in neonates. Specifically, there are no data on the rate of and the time for thrombus dissolution (recanalization) and what effect this has on the ultimate outcome. This chapter focuses on neonatal CSVT, based on the current understanding and published reports on the subject.

Introduction

Stroke and cerebrovascular diseases appear to be on the rise in children, including neonates, owing to increasing awareness of these disorders and advances in neuroimaging. Stroke is defined as the sudden occlusion or rupture of cerebral arteries or veins, resulting in focal brain damage. Stroke caused by vascular occlusion is broadly divided into *arterial ischaemic stroke* (AIS) and *cerebral sinovenous thrombosis* (CSVT). In AIS, arterial occlusion caused by thromboembolism results in cerebral infarction. In CSVT, thrombotic occlusion of the cerebral veins or venous sinuses results in cerebral venous congestion with or without venous infarction. Although there is some overlap in the conditions predisposing to AIS and CSVT in neonates, the clinico-radiographic features, management, and outcome are distinct. There are important differences in CSVT in neonates compared with older children and adults. CSVT is under-recognized in neonates owing to the subtle and non-specific presentation, and the diagnosis may be delayed or even missed. The risk factors causing CSVT are different in neonates and are frequently multiple. While randomized controlled trials (RCTs) have established the usefulness of anticoagulant therapy for adults with CSVT and at least there are some cohort studies in children, there are no such data for neonatal CSVT. There are important developmental differences in the haemostatic, sinovenous, and neurological systems in neonates, which prevent the direct extrapolation of treatment data from adult research. In particular, the neonatal period comprises a unique age group which requires a specialized approach to diagnosis and treatment. In general, therefore, the diagnosis of CSVT should be considered in neonates with seizures or encephalopathy, which are the most common presenting manifestations of this condition.

Epidemiology of neonatal CSVT

The annual incidence of CSVT in adults is reported to be 0.22/100,000 (Ferro et al., 2001) and in children it is higher, at 0.67 per 100,000 (term birth to 18 years; from the Canadian Pediatric Ischemic Stroke Registry, deVeber et al., 2001). On the basis of that study, the incidence in neonates is probably much higher, as they constituted nearly half the sample in the cohort, but accurate incidence figures remain to be determined because the diagnosis may be missed (Rivkin et al., 1992). The incidence in newborn infants is likely to increase with improvements in diagnostic neuroimaging. Also, increasing survival of infants with previously lethal conditions – including prematurity, complex congenital heart disease, and multiorgan dysfunction – places them at risk for CSVT. However, there remains the potential for underestimating the true frequency of neonatal CSVT (NCSVT) so long as the diagnosis continues to be missed.

Published reports on NCSVT have consisted primarily of small case series (Wong et al., 1987; Hanigan et al., 1988; Tarras et al., 1988; Shevell et al., 1989; Barron et al., 1992; Govaert et al., 1992; Martinez-Menedez et al., 1992; Rivkin et al., 1992; Herman & Siegel, 1995; Khurana et al., 1996; Sagrera et al., 1996; Fofah & Roth, 1997; Baumeister et al., 2000; Ergenekon et al., 2000; Ibrahim et al., 2000; Moliner et al., 2000; Carvalho et al., 2001; Gebara & Everett, 2001; Tardy-Poncet et al., 2001; Abrantes et al., 2002; Ramenghi et al., 2002; Farstad et al., 2003; Friese et al., 2003; Wu et al., 2003; Ezgu et al., 2004; Fumagalli et al., 2004; Klein et al., 2004; Hanigan et al., 2005; Soman et al., 2006). Only three studies have involved a large number of neonates with CSVT (deVeber et al., 2001; Wu et al., 2002; Fitzgerald et al., 2006). The first study, although not primarily of NCSVT, reported on 69 neonates; the second on 30, and the third on 42. Boys have been found to be at greater risk of CSVT than girls in childhood (Golomb et al., 2004).

Anatomy and physiology of the cerebral venous system

The venous dural sinuses and cerebral veins consist of the superficial and deep cerebral venous systems. In the superficial venous system, cortical veins drain into the superior sagittal sinus, which in turn drains into the torcular and then predominantly into the right transverse (lateral) sinus and the right internal jugular vein. The deep system – including the inferior sagittal sinus, the basal vein of Rosenthal, and the paired internal cerebral veins – empties into the vein of Galen and the straight sinus and then into the torcular and the smaller calibre left transverse (lateral) sinus and left internal jugular vein (Woodhall, 1936). Although the internal jugular veins are the major common exit for cerebral venous drainage, extrajugular pathways such as the vertebral venous plexus are also active (Schreiber et al., 2003). The vertebral venous plexus has connections with the transverse sinus-jugular system that are poorly understood. The internal jugular veins appear to drain blood primarily in the supine position whereas vertebral venous plexus drainage occurs mainly in the upright position in humans (Valdueza et al., 2000).

The cerebral sinovenous system lacks valves and is a low-pressure, slow-velocity circuit. The dural lining of the venous sinuses is rigid and the walls are therefore non-collapsible. This results in a passive drainage of blood flow to the heart (Capra & Anderson, 1984). The flow in the sinuses is gravity- and respiration-dependent and can be bidirectional, depending on the venous pressure gradient (Mehta et al., 2000; Kudo et al., 2004). Reduction in systemic blood pressure can lead to stasis or reversal of sinus blood flow. Cerebrospinal fluid (CSF) is absorbed through the arachnoid granulations into the venous blood within the superior sagittal sinus and the transverse sinuses.

The physiology of the immature sinovenous system probably differs from that of older children and adults. It is likely that the cerebral venous system, like other bodily systems, undergoes maturational changes over time. In neonates, the presence of factors that are poorly understood but potentially important in maturational changes include the following: prematurity, persistence/involution of embryonic venous collaterals, venous pressure gradients and their effect on cerebral perfusion pressure and CSF pressure, immaturity of the arachnoid villi with respect to CSF absorption, development of venous collaterals in the wake of obstruction, and obstruction of the posterior portion of the superior sagittal sinus with compression by the mobile bony plates of the skull in supine position. This emphasizes the need to develop and study animal models of neonatal CSVT in future.

Pathophysiology of NCSVT

In the normal physiological state, the procoagulant and anticoagulant or fibrinolytic processes in the blood are balanced. Thrombosis develops when there is a relative excess of procoagulant factors or a relative deficiency of the fibrinolytic mechanisms; this is often referred to as a 'hypercoagulable state'. Thrombosis can develop in any vascular structure including the intracranial veins and the dural venous sinuses. It can result from local or regional structural or inflammatory abnormalities exerting mechanical effects on the sinovenous system, or from systemic disturbances of either a congenital or an acquired nature. The equilibrium between the procoagulant and fibrinolytic system is dynamic and is constantly changing, depending on the forces promoting, maintaining, and antagonizing these states. This often produces fluctuations in the thrombotic process that can, in turn, result in a typically fluctuating rate of thrombosis propagation and dissolution, reflected in the variability of the clinical course. Thus the severity and duration of CSVT are often dependent on how acutely a clot develops and on the extent and number of the thrombosed channels. If a collateral venous circulation develops adequately and rapidly, significant venous obstruction may be tolerated without decompensation. The brain tolerates thrombi poorly in certain sites such as the torcular or the dominant transverse sinus, as these are the final exit points for cerebral venous drainage. However, the extent to which the various factors discussed above play a role in NCSVT needs further clarification.

In CSVT, the mechanisms underlying venous infarction are initiated by the obstruction of venous drainage, resulting in retrograde venous congestion in the absence of collateral venous drainage. The venous congestion results in increased tissue and capillary hydrostatic pressure with consequent extravasation of fluid into the interstitium, producing focal or sometimes diffuse cerebral oedema. Haemorrhage results from diapedesis of red blood cells through the leaky capillaries. This explains the high rate of spontaneous haemorrhage within areas of venous infarction in CSVT. Haemorrhage has been reported at all levels: intraparenchymal, intraventricular (IVH), subdural, and subarachnoid. In a study of IVH in term neonates, about one-third were found to have had CSVT (Wu *et al.*, 2003). The cerebral oedema and congestion may be transient if venous flow is re-established, or it may be associated with permanent tissue infarction if the increased regional tissue pressure ultimately exceeds the arterial perfusion pressure. Eventually the delivery of arterial blood and glucose and oxygen are compromised and ischaemic injury with 'venous' infarction results (Ungersbrock *et al.*, 1993; Bousser & Russell, 1997). Cytotoxic oedema preceding the onset of vasogenic oedema has been documented early in acute CSVT, signifying the presence of neuronal injury early in venous infarction (Forbes *et al.*, 2001). Once the initial thrombus has formed, the ensuing obstruction and venous stasis can promote propagation of the initial thrombus. Relief of venous obstruction, even if delayed, can ease the circulatory congestion in CSVT completely, with potential improvement in the clinical outcome. Occlusion of the superior sagittal sinus or the dominant transverse sinus impairs the function of the arachnoid granulations, which interferes with the absorption of CSF. This further increases the extent of cerebral swelling and occasionally results in communicating hydrocephalus (Bousser & Russell, 1997).

Animal models of CSVT

Experimental adult animal models of CSVT have been developed to improve our understanding of the pathophysiology of CSVT and the effects of anticoagulant therapy. A study has documented the relation between local and regional blood flow and haemoglobin oxygen saturation in a rat model of CSVT (Nakase *et al.*, 1996). This study showed a critically reduced supply of blood and oxygen in the draining areas in superior sagittal sinus thrombosis. The investigators suggested monitoring cerebral blood flow (CBF), local haemoglobin saturation, and serial angiography for the early detection of perfusion abnormalities after CSVT. They also recommended treatment directed at improving perfusion pressure or reducing vascular resistance to open further therapeutic targets during CSVT progression. Another study demonstrated regional tissue recovery in CSVT, based on partial reversal of the diffusion-weighted imaging (DWI) signal in areas of venous infarction following treatment with tissue plasminogen activator (t-PA) in rats (Röther *et al.*, 1996). In yet another study, low molecular weight heparin treatment in rats with CSVT significantly improved the clinical outcome, although there was no effect on recanalization (Rottger *et al.*, 2005). These investigators also demonstrated that glycoprotein IIb/IIIa antagonists and t-PA accelerated thrombolysis and could be good alternatives in the treatment of CSVT. However, the applicability of animal model data to humans is fraught with uncertainty. Up to now, no neonatal animal models of CSVT have been developed to the best of our knowledge. Very probably, differences would be expected between the mature and the immature brain in its ability to tolerate and react to venous obstruction. In this regard, there are some preliminary data suggesting that venous congestion could interfere with myelination maturation processes in human neonates (Porto *et al.*, 2006).

Clinical features of NCSVT

NCSVT may occur in isolation but it is more common as part of a coexisting intracranial or systemic disorder. Seizures and encephalopathy are the chief clinical manifestations. These clinical signs are subtle and diffuse and often show considerable overlap with manifestations of other conditions causing brain injury such as perinatal brain insults and intracranial infection. It may not be possible in individual cases to differentiate symptoms caused by NCSVT from those caused by coexisting neurological disease. Seizures are the predominant presenting feature in neonates (Shevell *et al.*, 1989; Rivkin *et al.*, 1992; deVeber *et al.*, 1996; deVeber *et al.*, 2001; Fitzgerald *et al.*, 2006). In a recent study from our centre, nearly 70 per cent of the 68 neonates with CSVT had seizures (unpublished observations). Seizures were generalized, focal, or typical subtle neonatal seizures. In spite of the presence of focal venous infarction in many cases, focal neurological deficits are rare in neonates (Shevell *et al.*, 1989; Barron *et al.*, 1992). The second commonest manifestation of NCSVT is encephalopathy, ranging from irritability and lethargy to frank coma. Raised intracranial pressure (caused by retrograde venous congestion) – manifested by a tense, bulging, non-pulsatile fontanelle, split sutures, and dilated scalp veins – has been reported in severe NCSVT (Hartmann *et al.*, 1987). Constitutional symptoms such as vomiting and poor feeding are other features. Rarer manifestations of NCSVT include head tremor (Sagrera *et al.*, 1996) and palpebral ecchymosis (Fumagalli *et al.*, 2004). Coexistent systemic (below neck) thrombosis is highly likely in neonates with CSVT owing to the existence of a 'hypercoagulable' state. Thus neonates with CSVT should be screened for systemic thrombosis and *vice versa*. In the Toronto study, concurrent systemic thrombosis was observed in 20 per cent of neonates with CSVT (unpublished observations).

Risk factors for NCSVT

Neonates are vulnerable to CSVT for many physiological and pathological reasons. Physiological factors include the maternal hypercoagulable state of pregnancy (Delorme *et al.*, 1992; Ballem, 1998); moulding of the infant's skull bones (Newton & Gooding, 1975); instrumentation during labour, causing mechanical damage to the underlying dural sinuses; a relatively high haematocrit; venous flow that is dependent on head positioning (Cowan & Thoresen, 1985); and lower than normal levels of anticoagulant factors including protein C, protein S, and anti-thrombin III (Andrew *et al.*, 1990). Compression of the posterior superior sagittal sinus by the occipital bone because of dependent head position has been invoked as another potential mechanism predisposing to stasis and a probable increase in the risk of thrombus formation (Shroff & deVeber, 2003). Pathological disorders in the pre- or perinatal period have been reported in approximately 51 per cent of neonates with CSVT and include maternal infections, gestational diabetes, premature rupture of the membranes, abruptio placentae, and birth asphyxia (Andrew *et al.*, 1990). Other neonatal disorders associated with CSVT include dehydration, bacterial sepsis, meningitis, and congenital heart disease (deVeber *et al.*, 2001). *E. coli* meningitis was reported to be a strong risk factor in one study (Farstad *et al.*, 2003). Hypernatraemic dehydration in exclusively breast-fed neonates has also been associated with neonatal CSVT (Gebara & Everett, 2001; van Amerongen *et al.*, 2001; Soman *et al.*, 2006). Prothrombotic abnormalities have been reported in 15 to 20 per cent of neonates with CSVT (deVeber *et al.*, 1998a; Bonduel *et al.*, 1999; deVeber *et al.*, 2001). These have included protein C deficiency (Tarras *et al.*, 1988; Ridley *et al.*, 1990; Ibrahim *et al.*, 2000; Tardy-Poncet *et al.*, 2001), protein S deficiency (Burneo *et al.*, 2002), factor V Leiden mutation (Moliner *et al.*, 2000; Abrantes *et al.*, 2002; Ramenghi *et al.*, 2002), plasminogen activator inhibitor-1 deficiency (Baumeister *et al.*, 2000), prothrombin gene mutation (Klein *et al.*, 2004), raised lipoprotein-a levels (Friese *et al.*, 2003), homozygous MTHFR gene mutation (Grow *et al.*, 2002), and anti-thrombin-III gene mutation (Baud *et al.*, 2001). Wu *et al.* (2002) reported genetic thrombophilia in four of seven tested neonates. In another report, low carnitine levels were found in two neonates with CSVT in association with hypoxic-ischaemic encephalopathy (Ezgu *et al.*, 2004). Recently, raised d-dimer levels at diagnosis strongly predicted CSVT in adults with CSVT (Kosinski *et al.*, 2004), but the significance of this finding in children and neonates remains to be studied.

Despite the reporting of several prothrombotic abnormalities in NCSVT, the persistence and contribution of prothrombotic clotting factors or genetic abnormalities in causing CSVT are not established. The main issue with the thrombophilia laboratory work-up is 'how low' below the accepted normal values (for age) should be considered 'pathologically low'? Another problem is the fact that laboratories across different centres have differing levels of normal ranges and variable methods of testing. Thus it is difficult to pool data from various centres because of these methodological obstacles. There is an urgent need to develop universally acceptable and reproducible methods of testing for prothrombotic risk factors, particularly in neonates.

Overall, the risk of CSVT, and thrombosis in general, is augmented as the number of risk factors increases (Heller *et al.*, 2003). Wu *et al.* (2002) reported multiple risk factors in 18 of 30 neonates with CSVT. In the Toronto study, just over 60 per cent of neonates had acquired postnatal insults that predominantly consisted of head and neck disease, while about 50 per cent had perinatal and intrapartum insults; chief among these was birth asphyxia (unpublished observations). Only about 10 per cent of neonates did not have any identifiable risk factor, while multiple risk factors were identified in nearly one-third of all cases.

Radiographic diagnosis of NCSVT

Various radiographic modes are available to evaluate the cerebral venous system and dural sinuses in the neonate. Each has strengths and limitations. There have been no systematic studies comparing diagnostic methods against a gold standard, especially in neonates. Knowledge of the normal variation in venous anatomy as well as of variations resulting from the use of imaging techniques in neonates is clearly important, as is the correct application of newly available techniques.

Cranial ultrasound

Because of the neonates' open fontanelles, cranial ultrasound is helpful for diagnosing centrally located venous infarcts or haemorrhages in these patients. It is in regular use in most NICUs. As the technique is highly operator-dependent it has some limitations. Its major advantage is that it is a bedside and non-invasive procedure. Doppler ultrasound can define absent or, less reliably, reduced flow in the sinovenous channels in CSVT, mainly in the superior sagittal sinus. Assessment of the transverse sinuses and deep system is more limited (Govaert *et al.*, 1992; Bezinque *et al.*, 1995). Power Doppler, which measures the energy of moving red blood cells instead of the velocity and direction of flow, appears to be better than conventional colour Doppler in the evaluation of CSVT (Tsao *et al.*, 1999). Further research in ultrasound techniques for CSVT diagnosis is desirable. Because of the limitations of ultrasound, it is often difficult to make treatment decisions based only on this technique.

Computed tomography and venography

Computed tomography (CT) is usually the initial imaging mode in neonates after ultrasound for the diagnosis of intracranial abnormalities. This is due to ease of availability, short procedure time, and capacity to detect acute haemorrhage. In the Toronto study, just over 50 per cent of neonates had their CSVT diagnosed by CT or CT venography (CTV) (unpublished observations). In adults and older children, signs indicative of CSVT on a non-contrast CT are the 'filled triangle' or 'dense triangle' sign or the 'cord sign', reflecting the increased density of an intraluminal thrombus in sinovenous channels (Bousser & Russell, 1997) (Fig. 1). On contrast-enhanced CT, the 'empty triangle' or 'empty delta' sign refers to a non-contrast enhancing thrombus surrounded by the dural walls of the sinus, which enhance with contrast. Although the same radiographic signs have been found in neonates, unenhanced CT has significant limitations in the diagnosis of CSVT as it may miss the diagnosis in 20 to 40 per cent of patients, and underestimate both the extent of sinus involvement and the presence and extent of venous infarction (Justich et al., 1984; Barron et al., 1992; Ameri & Bousser, 1992; Davies & Slavotinek, 1994; deVeber et al., 2001). CT can also yield false positive results in neonates (Hamburger et al., 1990), in whom the increased haematocrit, the presence of fetal haemoglobin, and decreased density of unmyelinated brain can combine to produce a high-density triangle in the torcular area on a non-contrast CT which can simulate the dense triangle sign (Ludwig et al., 1980; Davies & Slavotinek, 1994; Kriss, 1998). In addition, unless thinly sliced coronal CT images are obtained it can be difficult to differentiate subdural haemorrhage along the edges of tentorium cerebelli from intraluminal thrombus in the transverse or sigmoid sinus. CT venography using a multislice technique has been reported to be better than routine CT and a good alternative to magnetic resonance venography (MRV) in adults (Casey et al., 1996; Hagen et al., 1996; Ozsvath et al., 1997). However, the radiation dose with multislice CT has been a worry in the neonatal age group (Brenner et al., 2001). With recent advances in CT technology, optimization of the yield of CTV with even lower doses of radiation is expected in the near future. At our centre, techniques of multislice CTV in the coronal and sagittal planes during routine contrast-enhanced CT scanning without resorting to the use of a higher radiation dose have been developed (unpublished observations) (Fig. 2). A comparative study between CTV and MRV in adults has documented the superiority of CTV over the time-of-flight MRV in CSVT (Casey et al., 1996).

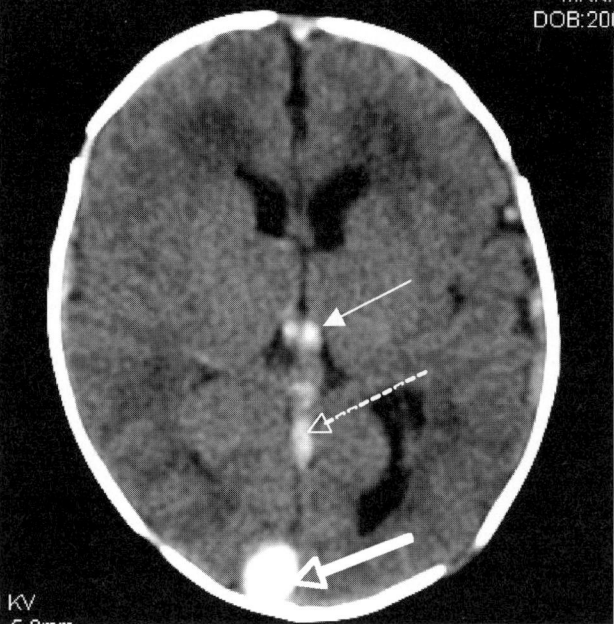

Fig. 1. Axial non-contrast CT scan of 5-days-old male neonate with hyperdense signal in the superior sagittal sinus (thick arrow), the vein of Galen (broken arrow) and both internal cerebral veins (thin arrow) suggestive of acute thrombosis.

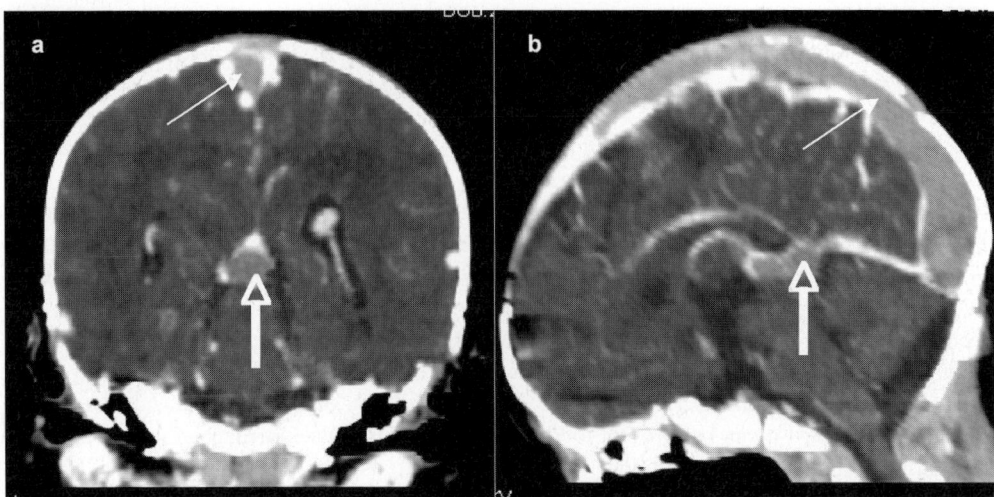

Fig. 2. Coronal (a) and Sagittal (b) contrast-enhanced CT Venogram of the same neonate as in Figure 1 depicting a large filling defect within the superior sagittal sinus (thin arrows) and the vein of Galen (thick arrows) s/o thrombus.

Magnetic resonance imaging and venography

Magnetic resonance imaging (MRI) is at present the preferred diagnostic method in general because of its capacity to demonstrate flow, thrombus, oedema, infarction, and concurrent abnormalities (Macchi *et al.*, 1986; Ameri & Bousser 1992; Medlock *et al.*, 1992; Zimmerman *et al.*, 1992; Dormont *et al.*, 1994). However, only a few studies have addressed the role of MRI in NCSVT (Grossman *et al.*, 1993; Puig *et al.*, 2006). In the Toronto study, just under 50 per cent of neonates had MRI to diagnose CSVT. On conventional MR images, acute thrombus within a cerebral vein or dural sinus is isointense on T1-weighted images (WI) and hypointense on T2-WI. In the subacute stage, thrombus is hyperintense on T1-WI (Fig. 3) as well as on T2-WI images. Slow flow, turbulent flow, angled flow, or flow-related enhancement may cause an increased signal that can imitate intraluminal thrombus. The two dimensional time-of-flight (TOF) MRV has flow gaps in the transverse sinus in up to 30 per cent of normal adults, especially in the non-dominant transverse sinus (Ayanzen *et al.*, 2000). In neonates, moulding of the skull in the occipital region from the dependent position in the MRI head coil often partially compresses the posterior portion of the superior sagittal sinus, resulting in loss of signal on TOF-MRV (Fig. 4). In neonates, subdural blood adjacent to the tentorium and the torcular can be falsely interpreted as transverse sinus thrombosis on MRI or CT. However, subtentorial subdural haemorrhage and thrombosis in the torcular or transverse sinuses may coexist in the same patient and further complicate the issue. To make a distinction between the two conditions, imaging must be done in different planes and with multiple modalities. A recent paper has discussed in detail the pitfalls of two-dimensional TOF-MRV in neonates (Widjaja *et al.*, 2006). Three-dimensional gadolinium-enhanced MRV techniques are being increasingly used in adults (Liang *et al.*, 2001). A more widely used modification of MRI is a dynamic gadolinium bolus injection technique – the three dimensional auto-triggered, elliptic centric ordered (ATECO) gadolinium-enhanced MRV (Farb *et al.*, 2003). This has not been routinely applied in neonates and children owing to technical difficulties but it appears promising (Fig. 5).

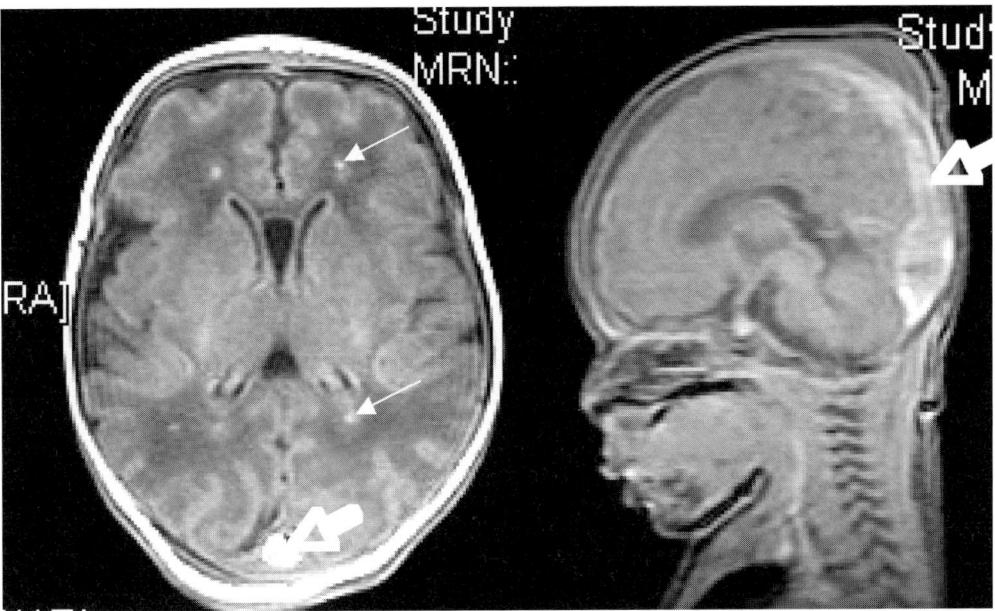

Fig. 3. Axial (on the left) and sagittal (on the right) T1-weighted MRI of a 9-days-old male neonate with E-coli sepsis showing increased signal in superior sagittal sinus and torcular (thick arrows) and bilateral deep white matter small areas of increased signal s/o petechial hemorrhage (thin arrows).

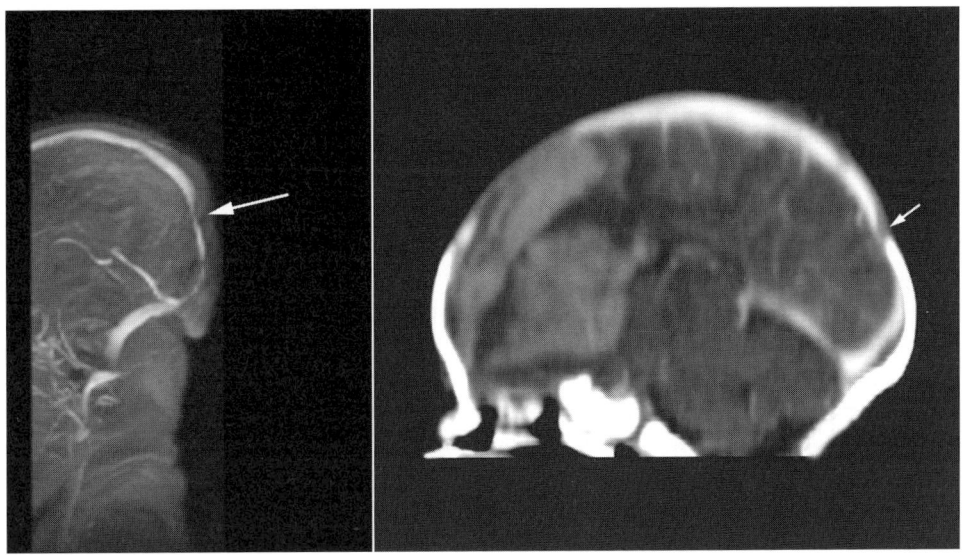

Fig. 4. MR venogram on the left and CT venogram on the right of a 4-days-old male neonate showing compression of the posterior part of superior sagittal sinus in supine position leading to reduced flow in the compressed segment.

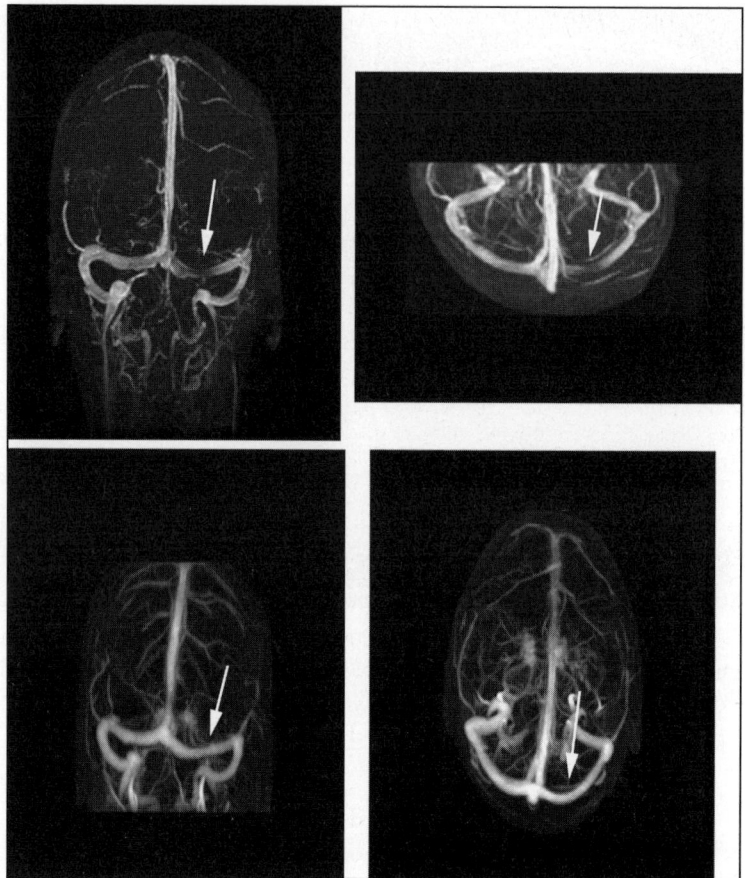

Fig. 5. Time-of-flight (TOF) MR venogram (top two images) and auto-triggered elliptic centric-ordered (ATECO) MR venogram (bottom two images) of a neonate that shows artefactual loss of flow signal in the left transverse sinus on the TOF-MRV that is not evident on the ATECO-MRV.

MRI is the favoured technique for visualizing parenchymal brain changes. In neonates, however, unmyelinated brain presents challenges to T2-WI of venous infarcts. Sedation issues and the availability of urgent time slots for MRI are problematic. For the direct imaging of thrombosis within veins or sinuses, CTV with multislice CT is comparable to gadolinium-enhanced MRV in most stages of the evolution of CSVT, and both these techniques are more accurate than TOF-MRV. There is limited experience with diffusion-weighted imaging (DWI) in neonates with CSVT; however, it has shed light on the presence of cytotoxic and vasogenic oedema during venous infarction in adults with CSVT and the potential reversibility of such changes (Ducreux et al., 2001; Forbes et al., 2001). DWI has recently been reported to be of value in the diagnosis of acute CSVT as well as being a potential predictor of recanalization (Favrole et al., 2004). In acute CSVT, restricted DWI can be seen in the actual clot itself in the affected venous sinus and its presence may predict incomplete recanalization (Moharir et al., 2006a) (Fig. 6). The role of DWI in neonatal CSVT needs further exploration.

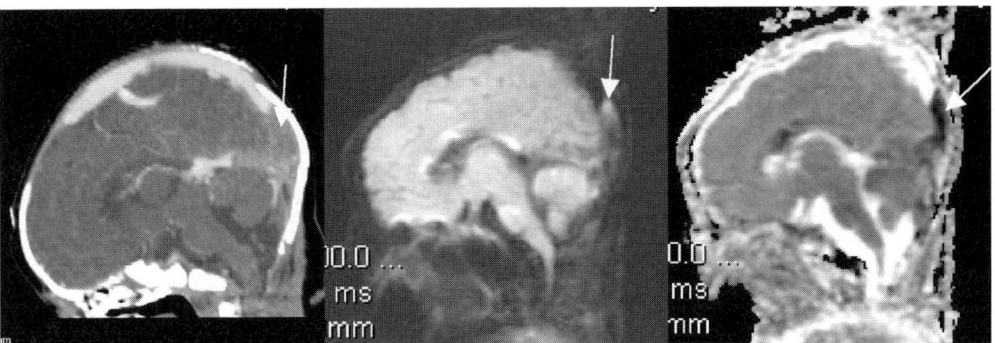

Fig. 6. CT venogram (left panel), sagittal diffusion-weighted MRI (DWI) (centre panel) and sagittal apparent diffusion coefficient (ADC) MRI (right panel) of a 3-days-old male neonate showing thrombus in the posterior part of superior sagittal sinus (SSS), torcular and straight sinus. The thrombus in the SSS is bright on DWI and dark on ADC, suggestive of restricted diffusion within the clot.

Other imaging modes

Conventional cerebral angiography is now rarely used for CSVT diagnosis by itself. Classic angiographic findings are similar to those in adults and include partial or complete lack of filling of cerebral veins or sinuses, enlarged collateral veins, delayed venous emptying, reversal of normal venous flow direction, abnormal cortical veins (broken or corkscrew-like), and regionally or globally delayed venous flow (Ameri & Bousser, 1992).

Neuroimaging findings in NCSVT

Location of thrombosis

NCSVT often involves multiple sites (in about 70 to 80 per cent of neonates in the Toronto study). The superficial sinovenous system, including the superior sagittal sinus and the right transverse sinus, is involved in the majority of neonates (over 50 to 60 per cent), and the deep system and left transverse sinus in the remainder. In severe cases, both systems may be thrombosed. In the Toronto study, over 50 per cent of neonates had involvement of the superior sagittal, torcular, and transverse sinuses (unpublished observations).

Venous infarction

Between 50 and 90 per cent of neonates and children with CSVT have parenchymal lesions, loosely referred to as venous infarcts (deVeber et al., 2001; Fitzgerald et al., 2006). In neonates, the majority of these are haemorrhagic. Diffusion restriction may or may not be seen in venous infarcts, depending on the degree of venous congestion and the reduction of arterial inflow with resultant true ischaemia. With thrombosis of the superficial system, infarcts are usually located in the cortex and white matter and may be bilateral. Typically, superior sagittal sinus thrombosis gives rise to uni- or bilateral high parasagittal venous infarcts. With thrombosis of the deep system, the infarcts are usually located in one or both thalami or the cerebellum. In term neonates with IVH or thalamic haemorrhage, sinovenous thrombosis involving the deep system is the underlying cause in up to one-third of cases and should be looked for (Roland et al., 1990; Wu et al., 2003). In the Toronto study, venous infarction was documented in about 60 per cent of neonates (unpublished observations). Of these about half were frankly haemorrhagic infarcts and the remainder were deep white matter petechial haemorrhagic venous infarcts (Fig. 3).

Recanalization rate

In adults, maximum recanalization occurs by 4 to 6 months after diagnosis, and almost none occurs thereafter (Baumgartner *et al.*, 2003). In the Toronto study, recanalization rates in neonates have been assessed (Moharir *et al.*, 2005; Moharir *et al.*, 2006b). Neonates clearly recanalize faster than older children, with the maximum rate of recanalization in the first 3 months after diagnosis. About 50 per cent of all neonates fully recanalized by 6 weeks to 3 months after diagnosis. The rate fell off to 65 per cent by 6 months and to 75 per cent by 1 year.

Treatment of NCSVT

Currently available treatment for CSVT includes antithrombotic (anticoagulant) therapy, thrombolytic therapy, and supportive therapy. Older children are increasingly treated with anticoagulants on the basis of adult practice. Guidelines for anticoagulant treatment in childhood CSVT have now been published (Monagle *et al.*, 2004), which support the use of anticoagulants (level of evidence grade 2C) for NCSVT fulfilling certain criteria, including a lack of intracranial haemorrhage at diagnosis.

Anticoagulant therapy

The rationale behind anticoagulant therapy is to prevent the propagation of the existing thrombus, and to enable the unopposed dissolution (recanalization) of existing thrombus by the fibrinolytic system. In the Canadian registry study, 37 per cent of 69 neonates with CSVT received anticoagulant therapy without significant haemorrhagic complications. The drugs used were low molecular weight heparin in 29 per cent, unfractionated heparin in nine per cent, and warfarin in one per cent (deVeber *et al.*, 2001). The increasing tendency to treat infants and children with CSVT with anticoagulants is based on the efficacy and safety of anticoagulant treatment in adult clinical trials (Einhaupl *et al.*, 1991; Nagaraja *et al.*, 1995; Preter *et al.*, 1996; Chakrabarti & Maiti, 1997; deBruijn & Stam, 1999), and on emerging evidence of the safety of anticoagulant therapy in children (deVeber *et al.*, 1998b; Dix *et al.*, 2000; deVeber *et al.*, 2001; Barnes *et al.*, 2004; Michaels *et al.*, 2004; Sebire *et al.*, 2005). Unfortunately, case reports and non-consecutive cohort studies cannot establish the efficacy of anticoagulants owing to inherent bias in treatment selection. Consecutive cohort studies in which CSVT is treated using standardized protocols can, however, ascertain the safety of anticoagulants. A large prospective cohort study has analysed the safety of protocol-based anticoagulants for a variety of childhood thrombotic events (Dix *et al.*, 2000). In that study, among 146 children (33 per cent were neonates and 15 per cent had CSVT) who were treated with therapeutic doses of low molecular weight heparin, five per cent had major bleeds. In another cohort study, among 30 children with CSVT (deVeber *et al.*, 1998b) during the acute treatment phase, eight received no anticoagulant therapy because of intracranial haemorrhage, 10 received unfractionated heparin, and 12 received low molecular weight heparin. Eighteen had warfarin for an additional 3 months. Only one child had a clinically silent intracranial haemorrhage, which occurred during treatment with unfractionated heparin. Another recent study documented the safety of low molecular weight heparin in preterm neonates with systemic thrombosis (Michaels *et al.*, 2004). Given the regular occurrence of haemorrhagic venous infarction in CSVT, there has been apprehension about the use of anticoagulants. Data from the available trials in adult patients have shown, however, that even patients with haemorrhagic infarction benefited from heparin therapy (Einhaupl *et al.*, 1991; deBruijn & Stam, 1999). This was also the observation in a recent paediatric study (Sebire *et al.*, 2005). The factors influencing treatment decisions include the extent and location of the thrombus, CSVT propagation (Khurana *et al.*, 1996), the presence of intracranial haemorrhage, the reversibility or irreversibility of risk factors for the CSVT, and the capacity to monitor anticoagulant therapy (Monagle *et al.*, 2006).

In general, neonates with CSVT are not being treated with anticoagulants in most centres because of the lack of safety, efficacy, and outcome data for such treatment in NCSVT. In one study of 42 neonates, only seven per cent received anticoagulants and the outcome was poor in nearly 80 per cent (Fitzgerald *et al.*, 2006). In the Toronto study, the rate of haemorrhagic complications was eight per cent in 37 of 68 treated neonates (Moharir *et al.*, 2006c). Of these, three had major haemorrhagic complications; however, none was fatal. These rates of haemorrhagic complications are comparable to those associated with anticoagulant therapy in adults in general, and in the older children in the Toronto study, suggesting that neonates do not necessarily carry a higher risk of haemorrhage, provided anticoagulant therapy is based on a strict protocol including close clinical and radiographic monitoring for adverse effects. The Toronto study also established that the maximum rate of recanalization occurs by 3 months in neonates and is negligible thereafter, suggesting that the duration of treatment required in neonates is about 3 months (Moharir *et al.*, 2005; Moharir *et al.*, 2006b).

Perhaps the most significant observation in the Toronto study is the risk of propagation of NCSVT. The study has shown for the first time in neonates the effect of untreated CSVT on the acute thrombotic process. Nearly 25 per cent of untreated neonates had progression of thrombosis, compared with only five per cent of treated neonates (Moharir *et al.*, 2006d). Moreover, CSVT propagation resulted in new venous infarction in 10 per cent of all neonates. Importantly, propagation was silent in all cases. This clearly shows that untreated neonatal CSVT is not benign – it can result in worsening of thrombosis, which increases the risk of subclinical parenchymal brain injury. Thus it is essential to monitor untreated neonates radiologically to check for propagation; and if propagation is documented, institution of anticoagulant therapy should be strongly considered.

Thrombolytic therapy

In adults, recanalization with direct catheter thrombolysis of CSVT has been reported (Wasay *et al.*, 2001). Although some investigators have promoted thrombolytic therapy for sinovenous thrombosis as an early intervention, most have recommended limiting its use to patients who have clinical deterioration despite adequate anticoagulant treatment. There are many case reports documenting the successful thrombolytic treatment of CSVT in neonates or children (Wong *et al.*, 1987; Higashida *et al.*, 1989; Griesemer *et al.*, 1994; Tsai *et al.*, 1995). Major haemorrhagic complications have also been reported with this treatment (Horowitz *et al.*, 1995). A consecutive cohort study of seven children with systemic venous thrombosis reported successful lysis in only one, with major complications in three (Monagle *et al.*, 1997). A large population-based study of children with non-cerebral deep vein thrombosis reported a failure of thrombolytic therapy in one-third of the children in whom it was used (Andrew *et al.*, 1994). It must be remembered that the risk/benefit ratio of thrombolytic therapy is not known in neonates with CSVT. Carefully designed cohort studies or randomized controlled trials are needed to support the use of this method of treatment.

Supportive neuroprotective treatment

In acute CSVT, supportive therapy is of paramount importance and is aimed at maintaining adequate perfusion and reducing the metabolic demands of the brain to minimize the extent of cerebral damage. Approaches include maintenance of blood pressure, fluid volume, correction of hyper- or hypoglycaemia, and prevention of seizures. In addition, specific treatment of all reversible underlying risk factors is vital. Neonates with diffuse cerebral swelling at the onset of CSVT may require treatment for persistent intracranial hypertension in the acute and subacute phase.

Clinical outcome

The outcome following neonatal CSVT would be anticipated to be better than in older infants or children owing to theoretically enhanced brain plasticity. In the setting of hypoxic-ischaemic injury, however, evidence from rat models has shown that the neonatal brain is far more vulnerable to harm than that of older animals (Yager & Thornhill, 1997). As with any neurological insult occurring in the neonatal period, detection of the clinical sequelae could understandably be delayed, as the young brain may not be in a position to show many of the neurological deficits that become evident at older ages (Bouza et al., 1994). Studies of outcome of neonates with CSVT are also confounded by the diffuse and subtle nature of the injury, and the high frequency of coexistent CNS insults separate from the CSVT.

Some case series of neonates with CSVT have reported major disability in over 50 per cent of cases (Barron et al., 1992; Fitzgerald et al., 2006), whereas others have reported a normal outcome in over 90 per cent of neonates (Shevell et al., 1989). Two studies have reported the long-term outcome of CSVT in neonates and children (deVeber et al., 2000; deVeber et al., 2001). In the Canadian registry study, nearly 50 per cent of neonates had neurological impairment after a median follow up of 1.6 years. In all age groups, 54 per cent of children were normal, 38 per cent had a neurological deficit, and eight per cent died. The neurological deficits consisted of motor (80 per cent) and cognitive defects (10 per cent), developmental delay (nine per cent), speech deficits (six per cent), visual deficits (six per cent), and other deficits (26 per cent). Six of 12 deaths were attributable to CSVT, with the remainder related to underlying illnesses. Seizures were present in 19 per cent of neonates and 11 per cent of older infants and children. In another consecutive cohort study, 38 infants and children surviving CSVT were evaluated by a standardized neurological examination measure, the Pediatric Stroke Outcome Measure (PSOM) (deVeber et al., 2000) and the modified Euroqual questionnaire for parents (Dorman et al., 1997). Two-thirds had a normal neurological examination, including 14 of 18 neonates and 10 of 20 older infants and children. In the remainder, neurological deficits were mild in seven and moderate or severe in the other seven. In addition to neurological deficits, there were seizures in 16 per cent and headaches in 24 per cent. In the Toronto study, 64 of 68 neonates were followed for a median of 2 years. Neurological outcome was poor in 42 per cent. However, treatment effect could not be studied owing to selection bias for treatment (unpublished observations).

Few studies have looked at the predictors of outcome following childhood or neonatal CSVT (deVeber et al., 2001; Sebire et al., 2005; Fitzgerald et al., 2006). Seizures at presentation, venous infarction, younger age, and lack of anticoagulation therapy have been reported as predictors of poor outcome. However, the influence of anticoagulants on outcome is yet to be thoroughly analysed in neonates and children. In the consecutive cohort study of children with CSVT by deVeber et al. the number of patients treated was small (deVeber et al., 1998b). Three of the eight children who were not treated because of the presence of intracranial haemorrhage expired, and none of the 22 treated children died. After one year of follow up, 67 per cent of treated patients were neurologically normal. In a pooled literature analysis from 1980 to 1996, 150 paediatric patients with CSVT were identified in the same study (deVeber *et al.*, 1998a); 136 were treated supportively without anticoagulants and 14 received anticoagulants. The occurrence of death was similar in treated and untreated patients (14 per cent and 16 per cent, respectively); however, severe neurological morbidity was seen in 22 per cent of untreated patients compared with none of the treated patients. In the Toronto study, younger age, intracranial haemorrhage at diagnosis, associated neurological comorbidity, and longer follow-up duration were independent predictors of poor clinical outcome after paediatric CSVT (unpublished observations).

Recurrent CSVT or other systemic thromboses have been reported in 13 per cent of children with CSVT. This can occur despite initial anticoagulant therapy (deVeber *et al.*, 1998a). In the Canadian study, 19 of 160 patients (13 per cent) had symptomatic recurrence of thrombosis, cerebral in 12 and systemic in seven (deVeber *et al.*, 2001). A recent study reported that four of 42 children with CSVT (9.5 per cent) had recurrent venous thrombosis, one cerebral and three systemic (Sebire *et al.*, 2005). More recently, a multicentre European study has documented a recurrence risk of six per cent for venous thromboembolism in 396 children with CSVT, three per cent (13) of these being cerebral (Kenet *et al.*, 2007). Significantly, none of the recurrences was documented in children under the age of 2 years. In the Toronto study, no neonates had recurrence of CSVT over a median of 2 years of follow-up; however, propagation of the initial thrombus occurred in 25 per cent of cases. Mortality is comparable in children and adults with CSVT. In children, the pooled literature analysis referred to above found a mortality rate of nine per cent (deVeber *et al.*, 1998a). In the Canadian registry study, the mortality was eight per cent (deVeber *et al.*, 2001), but the precise figures for mortality from NCSVT remain unknown.

Conclusions

Neonatal CSVT is increasingly encountered and should be considered in the differential diagnosis of a neonate with seizures and encephalopathy, especially in the setting of difficult birth or neonatal illnesses. Neuroimaging of sinovenous channels must be specifically undertaken or the diagnosis will be missed. Untreated neonates should be closely monitored for propagation of thrombosis. Anticoagulants are strongly recommended in neonates with propagation of CSVT as there are increasing data to suggest that they are safe in this situation. The outcome from neonatal CSVT is poor. There is an urgent need to consider multicentre randomized controlled trials in neonatal CSVT.

References

Abrantes, M., Lacerda, A.F., Abreu, C.R., Levy, A., Azevedo, A. & Da, S.L. (2002): Cerebral venous sinus thrombosis in a neonate due to factor V Leiden deficiency. *Acta Paediatr.* **91**, 243–245.

Ameri, A. & Bousser, M. (1992): Cerebral venous thrombosis. *Neurol. Clin.* **10**, 87–111.

Andrew, M., Paes, B. & Johnston, M. (1990): Development of the hemostatic system in the neonate and young infant. *Am. J. Pediatr. Hematol. Oncol.* **12**, 95–104.

Andrew, M., David, M., Adams, M., Ali, K., Anderson, R., Barnard, D., Bernstein, M., Brisson, L., Cairney, B. & DeSai, D. (1994): Venous thromboembolic complications (VTE) in children: first analyses of the Canadian Registry of VTE. *Blood* **83**, 1251–1257.

Ayanzen, R.H., Bird, C.R., Keller, P.J., McCully, F.J., Theobald, M.R. & Heiserman, J.E. (2000): Cerebral MR venography: normal anatomy and potential diagnostic pitfalls. *Am. J. Neuroradiol.* **21**, 74–78.

Ballem, P. (1998): Acquired thrombophilia in pregnancy. *Semin. Thromb. Hemost.* **24** (Suppl. 1), 41–47.

Barnes, C., Newall, F., Furmedge, J., Mackay, M. & Monagle, P. (2004): Cerebral sinus venous thrombosis in children. *J. Paediatr. Child Health* **40**, 53–55.

Barron, T.F., Gusnard, D.A., Zimmerman, R.A. & Clancy, R.R. (1992): Cerebral venous thrombosis in neonates and children. *Pediatr. Neurol.* **8**, 112–116.

Baud, O., Picard, V., Durand, P., Duchemin, J., Proulle, V., Alhenc-Gelas, M., Devictor, D. & Dreyfus, M. (2001): Intracerebral hemorrhage associated with a novel antithrombin gene mutation in a neonate. *J. Pediatr.* **139**, 741–743.

Baumeister, F.A., Auberger, K. & Schneider, K. (2000): Thrombosis of the deep cerebral veins with excessive bilateral infarction in a premature infant with the thrombogenic 4G/4G genotype of plasminogen activator inhibitor-1. *Eur. J. Pediatr.* **159**, 239–242.

Baumgartner, R.W., Studer, A., Arnold, M. & Georgiadis, D. (2003): Recanalization of cerebral venous thrombosis. *J. Neurol. Neurosurg. Psychiatry* **74**, 459–461.

Bezinque, S.L., Slovis, T.L. & Touchette, A.S. (1995): Characterization of superior sagittal sinus blood flow velocity using colour flow Doppler in neonates and infants. *Pediatr. Radiol.* **25**, 175–179.

Bonduel, M., Sciuccati, G., Hepner, M., Torres, A.F., Pieroni, G. & Frontroth, J.P. (1999): Prothrombotic disorders in children with arterial ischemic stroke and sinovenous thrombosis. *Arch. Neurol.* **56**, 967–971.

Bousser, M.G. & Russell, R.R. (1997): Cerebral venous thrombosis. In: *Major problems in neurology*, eds. C.P. Warlow & J. Van Gijn, p. 104. London: W.B. Saunders.

Bouza, H., Rutherford, M., Acolet, D., Pennock, J.M. & Dubowitz, L.M.S. (1994): Evolution of early hemiplegic signs in full term infants with unilateral brain lesions in the neonatal period: a prospective study. *Neuropediatrics* **25**, 201–207.

Brenner, D., Elliston, C. & Hall, E. (2001): Estimated risks of radiation-induced fatal cancer from pediatric CT. *Am. J. Roentgenol.* **176**, 289–296.

Burneo, J.G., Elias, S.B. & Barkley, G.L. (2002): Cerebral venous thrombosis due to protein S deficiency in pregnancy. *Lancet* **359**, 892.

Capra, N. & Anderson, K. (1984): Anatomy of the cerebral venous system. In: *The cerebral venous system and its disorders*, eds. J.P. Knapp & H.H. Schmidek, pp. 1–36. Orlando, Florida: Grune & Stratton.

Carvalho, K.S., Bodensteiner, J.B., Connolly, P.J. & Garg, B.P. (2001): Cerebral venous thrombosis in children. *J. Child Neurol.* **16**, 574–580.

Casey, S.O., Alberico, R.A., Patel, M., Jimenez, J.M., Ozsvath, R.R., Maguire, W.M. & Taylor, M.L. (1996): Cerebral CT venography. *Radiology* **198**, 163–170.

Chakrabarti, I. & Maiti, B. (1997): Study on cerebral venous thrombosis with special reference to efficacy of heparin [abstract]. *J. Neurol. Sci.* **150**, S147.

Cowan, F. & Thoresen, M. (1985): Changes in superior sagittal sinus blood velocities due to postural alterations and pressure on the head of the newborn infant. *Pediatrics* **75**, 103–1047.

Davies, R.P. & Slavotinek, J.P. (1994): Incidence of the empty delta sign in computed tomography in the paediatric age group. *Aust. Radiol.* **38**, 17–19.

Delorme, M.A., Burrows, R.F., Ofosu, F.A. & Andrew, M. (1992): Thrombin regulation in mother and fetus during pregnancy. *Semin. Thromb. Hemost.* **18**, 81–90.

de Bruijn, S.F. & Stam, J. (1999): Randomized, placebo-controlled trial of anticoagulant treatment with low molecular weight heparin for cerebral sinus thrombosis. *Stroke* **30**, 484–488.

deVeber, G. & Adams, M. on behalf of the Canadian Pediatric Ischemic Stroke Study Group (1996): Neonatal sinovenous thrombosis and arterial ischemic stroke: prospective study of clinical and radiographic features [abstract]. *Can. J. Neurosci.* **23** (Suppl. 1), S16.

deVeber, G., Monagle, P., Chan, A., MacGregor, D., Curtis, R., Lee, S., Vegh, P., Adams, M., Marzinotto, V., Leaker, M., Massicotte, M.P., Lillicrap, D. & Andrew, M. (1998a): Prothrombotic disorders in infants and children with cerebral thromboembolism. *Arch. Neurol.* **55**, 1539–1543.

deVeber, G., Chan, A., Monagle, P., Marzinotto, V., Armstrong, D., Massicotte, P., Leaker, M. & Andrew, M. (1998b): Anticoagulation therapy in pediatric patients with sinovenous thrombosis: a cohort study. *Arch. Neurol.* **55**, 1533–1537.

deVeber, G., MacGregor, D., Curtis, R. & Mayank, S. (2000): Neurologic outcome in survivors of childhood arterial ischemic stroke and sinovenous thrombosis. *J. Child Neurol.* **15**, 316–324.

deVeber, G., Andrew, M., Adams, C., Bjornson, B., Booth, F., Buckley, D.J., Camfield, C.S., David, M., Humphreys, P., Langevin, P., MacDonald, E.A., Gillett, J., Meaney, B., Shevell, M., Sinclair, D.B. & Yager, J. for Canadian

Pediatric Ischemic Stroke Study Group (2001): Cerebral sinovenous thrombosis in children. *N. Engl. J. Med.* **345**, 417–423.

Dix, D., Andrew, M., Marzinotto, V., Charpentier, K., Bridge, S., Monagle, P., deVeber, G., Leaker, M., Chan, A. & Massicotte, P. (2000): The use of low molecular weight heparin in pediatric patients: a prospective cohort study. *J. Pediatr.* **136**, 439–445.

Dorman, P., Waddell, F., Slattery, J., Dennis, M. & Sandercock, P. (1997): Is the EuroQol a valid measure of health related quality of life after stroke? *Stroke* **28**, 1876–1882.

Dormont, D., Anxionnat, R., Everard, S., Louaille, C., Chiras, J. & Marsault, C. (1994): MRI in cerebral venous thrombosis. *J. Neuroradiol.* **21**, 81–99.

Ducreux, D., Oppenheim, C., Vandamme, X., Dormont, D., Samson, Y., Rancurel, G., Cosnard, G. & Marsault, C. (2001): Diffusion-weighted imaging patterns of brain damage associated with cerebral venous thrombosis. *Am. J. Neuroradiol.* **22**, 261–268.

Einhaupl, K.M., Villringer, A., Meister, W., Mehraein, S., Garner, C., Pellkofer, M., Haberl, R.L., Pfister, H.W. & Schmiedek, P. (1991): Heparin treatment in sinus venous thrombosis. *Lancet* **338**, 597–600.

Ergenekon, E., Gucuyener, K., Atalay, Y., Serdarolu, A., Tali, T., Koc, E. & Turkyilmaz, C. (2000): Neonatal cerebral venous thrombosis coexisting with bilateral adrenal hemorrhage. *Ind. J. Pediatr.* **67**, 591–594.

Ezgu, F.S., Atalay, Y., Hasanolu, A., Gucuyener, K., Koc, E. & Ergenekon, E. (2004): Intracranial venous thrombosis after hypoxic-ischemic brain insult in two newborns: could low serum carnitine levels have contributed? *Nutr. Neurosci.* **7**, 63–65.

Farb, R., Scott, J., Willinsky, R., Montanera, W., Wright, G. & ter Brugge, K. (2003): Intracranial venous system: gadolinium-enhanced three-dimensional MR venography with auto-triggered elliptic centric-ordered sequence-initial experience. *Radiology* **206**, 203–209.

Farstad, H., Gaustad, P., Kristiansen, P., Perminov, G. & Abrahamsen, T.G. (2003): Cerebral venous thrombosis and Escherichia coli infection in neonates. *Acta Paediatr.* **92**, 254–257.

Favrole, P., Guichard, J.-P., Crassard, I., Bousser, M.-G. & Chabriat, H. (2004): Diffusion-weighted imaging of intra-vascular clots in cerebral venous thrombosis. *Stroke* **35**, 99–105.

Ferro, J.M., Correia, M., Pontes, C., Baptista, M.V. & Pita, F., for the Cerebral Venous Thrombosis Portuguese Collaborative Study Group (2001): Cerebral vein and dural sinus thrombosis in Portugal: 1980–1998. *Cerebrovasc. Dis.* **11**, 177–182.

Fitzgerald, K.C., Williams, L.S., Garg, B.P., Carvalho, K.S. & Golomb, M.R. (2006): Cerebral sinovenous thrombosis in the neonate. *Arch. Neurol.* **63**, 405–409.

Fofah, O. & Roth, P. (1997): Congenital nephrotic syndrome presenting with cerebral venous thrombosis, hypocalcemia, and seizures in the neonatal period. *J. Perinatol.* **17**, 492–494.

Forbes, K.P., Pipe, J.G. & Heiserman, J.E. (2001): Evidence for cytotoxic edema in the pathogenesis of cerebral venous infarction. *Am. J. Neuroradiol.* **22**, 450–455.

Friese, S., Muller-Hansen, I., Schoning, M., Nowak-Gottl, U. & Kuker, W. (2003): Isolated internal cerebral venous thrombosis in a neonate with increased lipoprotein (a) level: diagnostic and therapeutic considerations. *Neuropediatrics* **34**, 36–39.

Fumagalli, M., Ramenghi, L.A. & Mosca, F. (2004): Palpebral ecchymosis and cerebral venous thrombosis in a near term infant. *Arch. Dis. Child. Fetal Neonat. Ed.* **89**, F530.

Gebara, B.M. & Everett, K.O. (2001): Dural sinus thrombosis complicating hypernatremic dehydration in a breastfed neonate. *Clin. Pediatr.* **40**, 45–48.

Golomb, M.R., Dick, P.T., MacGregor, D.L., Curtis, R., Sofronas, M. & deVeber, G.A. (2004): Neonatal arterial ischemic stroke and cerebral sinovenous thrombosis are more commonly diagnosed in boys. *J. Child Neurol.* **19**, 493–497.

Govaert, P., Achten, E., Vanhaesebrouck, P., De Praeter, C. & Van Damme, J. (1992): Deep cerebral venous thrombosis in thalamo-ventricular hemorrhage of the term newborn. *Pediatr. Radiol.* **22**, 123–127.

Govaert, P., Voet, D., Achten, E., Vanhaesebrouck, P., van Rostenberghe, H., van Gysel, D. & Afschrift, M. (1992): Noninvasive diagnosis of superior sagittal sinus thrombosis in a neonate. *Am. J. Perinatol.* **9**, 201–204.

Griesemer, D.A., Theodorou, A,A.. Berg, R,A. & Spera, T.D. (1994): Local fibrinolysis in cerebral venous thrombosis. *Pediatr. Neurol.* **10**, 78–80.

Grossman, R., Novak, G., Patel, M., Maytal, J., Ferreira, J. & Eviatar, L. (1993): MRI in neonatal dural sinus thrombosis. *Pediatr. Neurol.* **9**, 235–238.

Grow, J.L., Fliman, P.J. & Pipe, S.W. (2002): Neonatal sinovenous thrombosis associated with homozygous thermolabile methylenetetrahydrofolate reductase in both mother and infant. *J. Perinatol.* **22**, 175–178.

Hagen, T., Bartylla, K., Waziri, A., Schmitz, B. & Piepgras, U. (1996): Value of CT angiography in the diagnosis of cerebral sinus and venous thromboses. *Radiology* **36,** 859–866.

Hamburger, C., Villringer, A. & Bauer, M. (1990): Delta (empty triangle) sign in patients without thrombosis of the superior sagittal sinus. In: *Cerebral sinus thrombosis: experimental and clinical aspects,* eds. K. Einhaupl, O. Kempski & A. Baethmann, pp. 211–217. New York: Plenum Press.

Hanigan, W.C., Tracy, P.T., Tadros, W.S. & Wright, R.M. (1988): Neonatal cerebral venous thrombosis. *Pediatr. Neurosci.* **14,** 177–183.

Hanigan, W.C., Fraser, K., Tarantino, M. & Wang, H. (2005): Tumefaction of the dural sinuses associated with a coagulopathy following treatment of hydrocephalus in a perinate: case report. *J. Neurosurg.* **102 (Suppl. 4),** 426–430.

Hartmann, A., Wappenschmidt, J. & Solymosi, L. (1987): Clinical findings and differential diagnosis of cerebral vein thrombosis. In: *Cerebral sinus thrombosis: experimental and clinical aspects,* eds. K. Einhaupl, O. Kempski & A. Baethmann, pp. 171–186. New York: Plenum Press.

Heller, C., Heinecke, A., Junker, R., Knofler, R., Kosch, A., Kurnik, K., Schobess, R., von Eckardstein, A., Strater, R., Zieger, B. & Nowak-Gottl, U. (2003): Childhood Stroke Study Group. Cerebral venous thrombosis in children: a multifactorial origin. *Circulation* **108,** 1362–1367.

Herman, T.E. & Siegel, M.J. (1995): Special imaging casebook. Neonatal dural sinus thrombosis. *J. Perinatol.* **15,** 507–509.

Higashida, R.T., Helmer, E., Halbach, V.V. & Hieshima, G.B. (1989): Direct thrombolytic therapy for superior sagittal sinus thrombosis. *Am. J. Neuroradiol.* **10,** S4–S6.

Horowitz, M., Purdy, P., Unwin, H., Carstens, G., Greenlee, R., Hise, J., Kopitnik, T., Batjer, H., Rollins, N. & Samson, D. (1995): Treatment of dural sinus thrombosis using selective catheterization and urokinase. *Ann. Neurol.* **38,** 58–67.

Ibrahim, A., Damon, G., Teyssier, G., Billiemaz, K., Rayet, I. & Tardy, B. (2000): Heterozygous protein C deficiency: apropos of 2 cases with cerebral venous thrombosis in the neonatal period. *Arch. Pediatr.* **7,** 158–162.

Justich, E., Lammer, J., Fritsch, G., Beitzke, A. & Walter, G.F. (1984): CT diagnosis of thrombosis of dural sinuses in childhood. *Eur. J. Radiol.* **4,** 294–295.

Kenet, G., Kirkham, F., Neiderstadt, T., Heinecke, A., Saunders, D., Stoll, M., Brenner, B., Bidlingmaier, C., Heller, C., Knofler, R., Schobess, R., Zeiger, B., Sebire, G., Nowak-Gottl, U., and the European Thromboses Study Group (2007): Risk factors for recurrent venous thromboembolism in the European collaborative database on cerebral venous thrombosis: a multicentre cohort study. *Lancet Neurol.* **6,** 595–603.

Khurana, D.S., Buonanno, F., Ebb, D. & Krishnamoorthy, K.S. (1996): The role of anticoagulation in idiopathic cerebral venous thrombosis. *J. Child Neurol.* **11,** 248–250.

Klein, L., Bhardwaj, V. & Gebara, B. (2004): Cerebral venous sinus thrombosis in a neonate with homozygous prothrombin G20210A genotype. *J. Perinatol.* **24,** 797–799.

Kosinski, C.M., Mull, M., Schwarz, M., Schläfer, J., Milkereit, E., Willmes, K., Schiefer, J., Koch, B. & Biniek, R. (2004): Do normal D-dimer levels reliably exclude cerebral sinus thrombosis? *Stroke* **35,** 2820–2825.

Kriss, V.M. (1998): Hyperdense posterior falx in the neonate. *Pediatr. Radiol.* **28,** 817–819.

Kudo, L., Terae, S., Ishii, A., Omatsu, T., Asano, T., Tha, K. & Miyasaka, K. (2004): Physiologic change in flow velocity and direction of dural venous sinuses with respiration: MR venography and flow analysis. *Am. J. Neuroradiol.* **25,** 551–557.

Liang, L., Korogi, Y., Sugahara, T., Onomichi, M., Shigematsu, Y., Yang, D., Kitajima, M., Hiai, Y. & Takahashi, M. (2001): Evaluation of the intracranial dural sinuses with a 3D contrast-enhanced MP-RAGE sequence: prospective comparison with 2D-TOF MR venography and digital subtraction angiography. *Am. J. Neuroradiol.* **22,** 481–492.

Ludwig, B., Brand, M. & Brockerhoff, P. (1980): Postpartum CT examination of the heads of full term infants. *Neuroradiology* **20,** 145–154.

Macchi, P.J., Grossman, R.I., Gomori, J.M., Goldberg, H.I., Zimmerman, R.A. & Bilaniuk, L.T. (1986): High field MR imaging of cerebral venous thrombosis. *J. Comput. Assist. Tomogr.* **10,** 10–15.

Martinez-Menendez, B., Perez Sempere, A., Simon, R. & Mateos, F. (1992): Cerebral venous thrombosis as a cause of neonatal focal clonic seizures. *J. Neurol.* **239,** 294.

Medlock, M.D., Olivero, W.C., Hanigan, W.C., Wright, R.M. & Winek, S.J. (1992): Children with cerebral venous thrombosis diagnosed with magnetic resonance imaging and magnetic resonance angiography. *Neurosurgery* **31,** 870–876.

Mehta, N., Jones, L., Kraut, M.A. & Melhem, E.R. (2000): Physiologic variations in dural venous sinus flow on phase contrast MR imaging. *Am. J. Roentgenol.* **175,** 221–225.

Michaels, L.A., Gurian M., Hegyi, T. & Drachtman, R.A. (2004): Low molecular weight heparin in the treatment of venous and arterial thromboses in the premature infant. *Pediatrics* **114,** 703–707.

Moharir, M., Shroff, M., Adams, M., Chan, A., Bharucha, P. & deVeber, G. (2005): Childhood cerebral sinovenous thrombosis: a study of recanalisation rates [abstract]. *Ann. Neurol.* **58 (Suppl. 9)**, S110.

Moharir, M., Shroff, M. & deVeber, G. (2006a): Diffusion-weighted imaging of venous clots in childhood cerebral sinovenous thrombosis: an aid to diagnosis and a potential predictor of recanalization outcome [abstract]. *Ann. Neurol.* **60**, S157.

Moharir, M., Shroff, M., Adams, M., Chan, A., Bharucha, P. & deVeber, G. (2006b): Childhood cerebral sinovenous thrombosis: a study of clinical and radiographic outcomes [abstract]. *Stroke* **37**, 640.

Moharir, M., Shroff, M., Adams, M., Chan, A., Bharucha, P. & deVeber, G. (2006c): Cerebral sinovenous thrombosis in children: a study of safety of anticoagulant therapy [abstract]. *Neuropediatrics* **37**, S1.

Moharir, M., Shroff, M., MacGregor, D., Adams, M., Chan, A., Bharucha, P. & deVeber, G. (2006d): Clinical and radiographic features of thrombosis propagation in childhood cerebral sinovenous thrombosis [abstract]. *Ann. Neurol.* **60**, S141–S142.

Moliner, C.E., Lopez, B.E., Ginovart, G.G., Nadal, A.J. & Cubells, R.J. (2000): Neonatal cerebral thrombosis and deficit of factor V Leiden. *Ann. Espanol Pediatr.* **52**, 52–55.

Monagle, P., Phelan, E., Downie, P. & Andrew, M. (1997): Local thrombolytic therapy in children [abstract]. *Thromb. Haemost.* **77 (Suppl.)**, 504.

Monagle, P., Chan, A., Massicotte, P., Chalmers, E. & Michelson, A.D. (2004): Antithrombotic therapy in children: the seventh accp conference on antithrombotic and thrombolytic therapy. *Chest* **126**, 645S–687S.

Monagle, P., Chan, A., deVeber, G. & Massicotte, P. (2006): *Andrew's Pediatric thromboembolism and stroke*, 3rd edition, pp. 196, 198. Hamilton: BC Decker.

Nagaraja, D., Rao, B.S.S. & Taly, A.B. (1995): Randomized controlled trial of heparin in puerperal venous sinus thrombosis. *NIMHANS J.* **13**, 111–115.

Nakase, H., Heimann, A. & Kempski, O. (1996): Alterations of regional cerebral blood flow and oxygen saturation in a rat sinus-vein thrombosis model. *Stroke* **27**, 720–728.

Newton, T.H. & Gooding, C.A. (1975): Compression of superior sagittal sinus by neonatal calvarial molding. *Neuroradiology* **115**, 635–639.

Ozsvath, R.R., Casey, S.O., Lustrin, E.S., Alberico, R.A., Hassankhani, H. & Patel, M. (1997): Cerebral venography: comparison of CT and MR projection venography. *Am. J. Roentgenol.* **169**, 1699–1707.

Porto, L., Kieslich, M., Yan, B., Zanella, F.E. & Lanfermann, H. (2006): Accelerated myelination associated with venous congestion. *Eur. Radiol.* **16**, 922–926.

Preter, M., Tzourio, C., Amen, A. & Bousser, M.G. (1996): Long term prognosis in cerebral venous thrombosis: follow-up of 77 patients. *Stroke* **27**, 243–246.

Puig, J., Pedraza, S., Mendez, J. & Trujillo, A. (2006): Neonatal cerebral venous thrombosis: diagnosis by magnetic resonance angiography. *Radiologia* **48**, 169–171.

Ramenghi, L.A., Gill, B.J., Tanner, S.F., Martinez, D., Arthur, R. & Levene, M.I. (2002): Cerebral venous thrombosis, intraventricular haemorrhage and white matter lesions in a preterm newborn with factor V (Leiden) mutation. *Neuropediatrics* **33**, 97–99.

Ridley, P.D., Ledingham, S.J., Lennox, S.C., Burman, J.F., Chung, H.I., Sheffield, E.A., Talbot, S. & Bevan, D. (1990): Protein C deficiency associated with massive cerebral thrombosis following open heart surgery. *J. Cardiovasc. Surg.* **31**, 249–251.

Rivkin, M.J., Anderson, M.L. & Kaye, E.M. (1992): Neonatal idiopathic cerebral venous thrombosis: an unrecognized cause of transient seizures or lethargy. *Ann. Neurol.* **32**, 51–56.

Roland, E.H., Flodmark, O. & Hill, A. (1990): Thalamic hemorrhage with intraventricular hemorrhage in the full-term newborn. *Pediatrics* **85**, 737–742.

Röther, J., Waggie, K., van Bruggen, N., de Crespigny, A.J. & Moseley, M.E. (1996): Experimental cerebral venous thrombosis: evaluation using MR imaging. *J. Cerebral Blood Flow Metab.* **16**, 1353–1361.

Rottger, C., Madlener, K., Heil, M., Gerriets, T., Walberer, M., Wessels, T., Bachmann, G., Kaps, M. & Stoltz, E. (2005): Is heparin treatment the optimal treatment for cerebral venous thrombosis? *Stroke* **36**, 841–846.

Sagrera, F.X., Raspall, T.F., Sala, C.P., Vila, C.C. & Campistol, P.J. (1996): Cephalic trembling as a result of neonatal cerebral venous thrombosis. *Ann. Espanol Pediatr.* **45**, 431–433.

Schreiber, S.J., Lurtzing, F., Gotze, R., Doepp, F., Klingebiel, R. & Valdueza, J.M. (2003): Extrajugular pathways of human cerebral venous drainage assessed by duplex ultrasound. *J. Appl. Physiol.* **94**, 1802–1805.

Sebire, G., Tabarki, B., Saunders, D.E., Leroy, I., Liesner, R., Saint-Martin, C., Husson, B., Williams, A.N., Wade, A. & Kirkham, F.J. (2005): Cerebral venous sinus thrombosis in children: risk factors, presentation, diagnosis and outcome. *Brain* **128**, 477–489.

Shevell, M.I., Silver, K., O'Gorman, A.M., Watters, G.V. & Montes, J.L. (1989): Neonatal dural sinus thrombosis. *Pediatr. Neurol.* **5,** 161–165.

Shroff, M. & deVeber, G. (2003): Sinovenous thrombosis in children. *Neuroimaging Clin. North Am.* **13,** 115–138.

Soman, T.B., Moharir, M., DeVeber, G. & Weiss, S. (2006): Infantile spasms as an adverse outcome of neonatal cortical sinovenous thrombosis. *J. Child Neurol.* **21,** 126–131.

Tardy-Poncet, B., Rayet, I., Damon, G., Alhenc-Gelas, M., Dutour, N. & Lavocat, M.P. (2001): Protein C concentrates in a neonate with a cerebral venous thrombosis due to heterozygous type 1 protein C deficiency. *Thromb. Haemost.* **85,** 1118–1119.

Tarras, S., Gadia, C., Meister, L., Roldan, E. & Gregorios, J.B. (1988): Homozygous protein C deficiency in a newborn. Clinicopathologic correlation. *Arch. Neurol.* **45,** 214–216.

Tsai, F.Y., Wang, A.M., Matovich, V.B., Lavin, M., Berberian, B., Simonson, T.M., Yuh & W.T. (1995): MR staging of acute dural sinus thrombosis: correlation with venous pressure measurements and implications for treatment and prognosis. *Am. J. Neuroradiol.* **16,** 1021–1029.

Tsao, P.N., Lee, W.T., Peng, S.F., Lin, J.H. & Yau, K.I. (1999): Power Doppler ultrasound imaging in neonatal cerebral venous sinus thrombosis. *Pediatr. Neurol.* **21,** 652–655.

Ungersbock, K., Heimann, A. & Kempski, O. (1993): Cerebral blood flow alterations in a rat model of cerebral sinus thrombosis. *Stroke* **24,** 563–569.

Valdueza, J.M., von Munster, T., Hoffman, O., Schreiber, S. & Einhäupl, K.M. (2000): Postural dependency of cerebral venous outflow. *Lancet* **355,** 200–201.

van Amerongen, R.H., Moretta, A.C. & Gaeta, T.J. (2001): Severe hypernatremic dehydration and death in a breast-fed infant. *Pediatr. Emerg. Care.* **17,** 175–180.

Wasay, M., Bakshi, R., Kojan, S., Bobustuc, G., Dubey N. & Unwin, H. (2001): Nonrandomized comparison of local urokinase thrombolysis versus systemic heparin anticoagulation for superior sagittal sinus thrombosis. *Stroke* **32,** 2310–2317.

Widjaja, E., Shroff, M., Blaser, S., Laughlin, S. & Raybaud, C. (2006): 2D Time-of-flight MR venography in neonates: anatomy and pitfalls. *Am. J. Neuroradiol.* **27,** 1913–1918.

Woodhall, B. (1936): Variations of the cranial venous sinuses in the region of the torcular herophili. *Arch. Surg.* **33,** 297–314.

Wong, V.K., LeMesurier, J., Franceschini, R., Heikali, M. & Hanson, R. (1987): Cerebral venous thrombosis as a cause of neonatal seizures. *Pediatr. Neurol.* **3,** 235–237.

Wu, Y.W., Miller, S.P., Chin, K., Collins, A.E., Lomeli, S.C., Chuang, N.A., Barkovich, A.J. & Ferriero, D.M. (2002): Multiple risk factors in neonatal sinovenous thrombosis. *Neurology* **59,** 438–440.

Wu, Y.W., Hamrick, S.E., Miller, S.P., Haward, M.F., Lai, M.C., Callen, P.W., Barkovich, A.J. & Ferriero, D.M. (2003): Intraventricular hemorrhage in term neonates caused by sinovenous thrombosis. *Ann. Neurol.* **54,** 123–126.

Yager, J.Y. & Thornhill, J.A. (1997): The effect of age on susceptibility to hypoxic-ischemic brain damage. *Neurosci. Biobehav. Rev.* **21,** 167–174.

Zimmerman, R.A., Bogdan, A.R. & Gusnard, D.A. (1992): Pediatric magnetic resonance angiography: assessment of stroke. *Cardiovasc. Intervent. Radiol.* **15,** 60–64.

Chapter 17

The spectrum of visual disorders in children with perinatal brain lesions: long-term effects

Giovanni Cioni [*][°], Francesca Tinelli [*][°] and Andrea Guzzetta [*]

[*] Department of Developmental Neuroscience, Stella Maris Scientific Institute, via dei Giacinti 2, 56128 Pisa, Italy;
[°] Division of Child Neurology and Psychiatry, University of Pisa, Italy
g.cioni@inpe.unipi.it

Summary

Improved survival in high-risk infants has broadened our interest in their cognitive and neuropsychological outcome, and particularly in their visual and visuo-perceptual development. Normal visual function depends largely on the integrity of a network which includes the optic radiations and the primary visual cortex, but also other cortical and subcortical areas, such as the frontal or temporal lobes and even the basal ganglia, which are known to be associated with visual attention and with other aspects of visual function. All these areas are highly vulnerable to brain lesions. Conversely, in newborns with congenital lesions or lesions acquired in the perinatal period the damage caused by the cerebral insult can be compensated by mechanisms of brain plasticity. It is necessary to evaluate not only basic visual functions but also 'higher' modes of visual processing, such as object recognition and motion perception, for which the plasticity cannot be sufficient to compensate the damage caused by the lesion. In this chapter we will report briefly on the methods used for the assessment of basic and higher visual functions and describe the principal patterns of visual function observed in infants with neonatal brain lesions. Finally we will describe the possibility of utilizing, in the first months of life, tests based on visual information processing that may be better predictors of intelligence quotient at a later age than traditional developmental scales.

Introduction

Recent advances in neonatal intensive care have led to dramatic improvements in the survival of high-risk neonates paralleling an increase in preterm live births. This improvement has been particularly striking in very low birth weight infants. Improved survival of preterm infants has broadened our interest in their cognitive and neuropsychological outcomes. The incidence of major disabilities (moderate to severe mental retardation, neurosensory disorders, epilepsy, cerebral palsy) has remained constant, but high prevalence/low severity dysfunction (learning disabilities, attention deficit hyperactivity disorder (ADHD), borderline mental retardation, specific neuropsychological deficits, and behavioural disorders) has increased (Aylward, 2002).

In this context an important role has been played by the investigation of visual and visuo-perceptual disorders. The normal development of visual function depends on the integrity of a network which includes the optic radiations and the primary visual cortex, but also other cortical and subcortical areas such as the frontal and temporal lobes and the basal ganglia, which are known to be associated with visual attention and with other aspects of visual function. While most of the early studies reported only on the prevalence of abnormal visual function in retrospective studies in children with cerebral palsy, increasing attention has been devoted in the past few years to the development of visual function in infants with brain lesions, thanks to major improvements in neonatal imaging and to the possibility of assessing visual function very early in life.

In this chapter we describe the main tests used to assess basic visual functions and the patterns of visual function observed in the first years of life in infants with neonatal brain lesions; we describe higher visual functions and their possible impairment in children with brain lesions; and we report on the possibility of using tests based on visual information processing as predictors of intelligence quotient.

Assessment of basic visual functions in the first years of life

The assessment of visual function in young infants includes behavioural and electrophysiological techniques to evaluate oculomotor behaviour, acuity, visual fields, and optokinetic nystagmus. These functions undergo rapid maturation in the first year after term delivery (Fig. 1).

The application of these tests should be preceded by a standard ophthalmological examination to exclude the presence of eye abnormalities such as retinopathy, cataract, or optic atrophy.

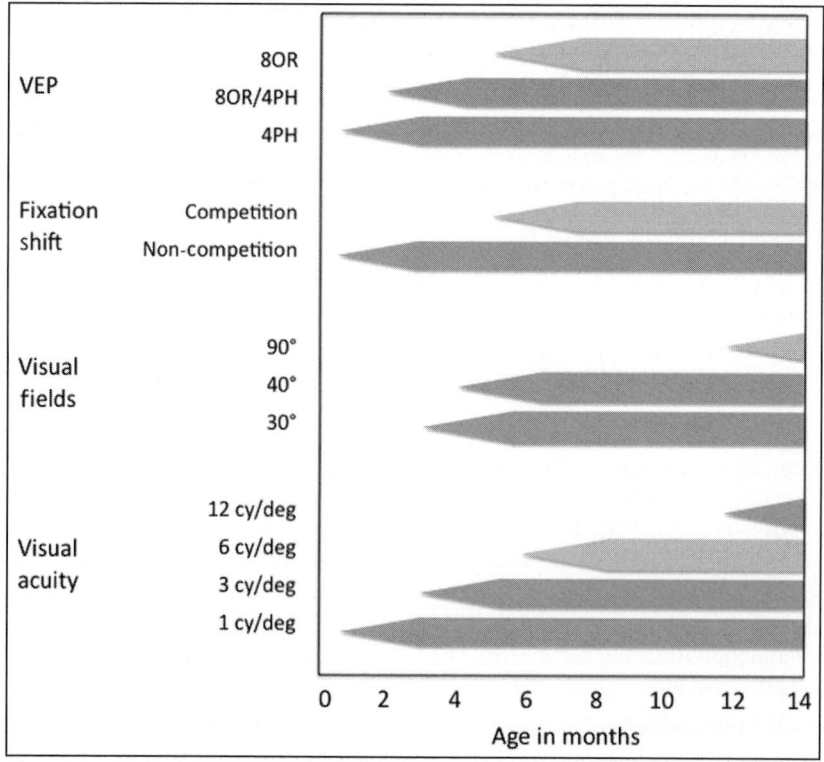

Fig. 1. Maturation of different aspects of visual function during the first year of life. Cy, cycles.

Behavioural techniques

Oculomotor behaviour

Oculomotor behaviour can be assessed by observing fixation, following, and the presence of abnormal eye movements such as spontaneous nystagmus. Strabismus is tested by examining the symmetry of the corneal light reflex and by the cover test.

Visual acuity

Visual acuity can be tested by using forced choice preferential looking (FCPL). The infant is presented at eye level on one side of the midline with a target consisting of black and white stripes paired with a uniform grey background on the other side. The level of acuity is measured as the finest grating (that is, the width of the black and white stripes) for which the infant shows a consistent preference (in cycles/degree), and compared with age-specific normative data (Teller *et al.*, 1986).

Visual field size

Visual field size can be assessed using kinetic perimetry (Mohn & Van Hof-van Duin, 1986). During central fixation of a centrally positioned white ball, an identical target is moved from the periphery towards the fixation point along one arc of the perimeter. Eye and head movements towards the peripheral ball are used to estimate the outline of the visual field. Normative data for full term and preterm infants are available (van Hof-van Duin *et al.*, 1992).

Optokinetic nystagmus

Optokinetic nystagmus (OKN) can be elicited using a large piece of paper or a computer-generated random dot pattern in front of the infant's face. The examiner observes the infant's eye movements, recording the presence and symmetry of any OKN generated in response to the movement of the pattern in either direction. Normally, binocular OKN is symmetrical from birth onwards, whereas monocular OKN shows a better response to stimulation in a temporo-nasal direction up to about 3 to 6 months of corrected age (Atkinson & Braddick, 1981).

Fixation shift

Fixation shift is a test of visual attention evaluating the direction and the latency of saccadic eye movements in response to a peripheral target in the lateral field. A central target is used as a fixation stimulus before the appearance of the peripheral target. While in some trials the central target disappears simultaneously with the appearance of the peripheral target (non-competition), in others the central target remains visible, generating a situation of competition between the two stimuli. Normal children can reliably shift their attention in a situation of non-competition during the first weeks after birth, but brisk refixation in a situation of competition is only found after 6 to 8 weeks post-term, and reliably by 12 to 18 weeks post-term. Absent or delayed (with a latency of more than 1.2 seconds) refixation at 5 months of age is considered abnormal (Atkinson *et al.*, 1992).

Electrophysiological techniques

Visual evoked potentials

Visual evoked potentials (VEPs) can be recorded using flash or orientation-reversal and phase-reversal stimuli. Using flash stimuli it is possible to follow the normal or abnormal maturation of the visual pathway. Steady state flash VEPs have also been used to assess the maturation of cortical and subcortical processing of the visual pathway (Mercuri et al., 1998). For phase-reversal VEPs the orientation of the black and white stripes is fixed but the contrast is reversed periodically. For orientation-reversal VEPs, stimuli periodically change orientation between 45 and 135 degrees. The phase-reversal response is already present at term, while the orientation-reversal response is only consistently elicited at 10 weeks post-term for slow changes (four reversals per second) and after 12 weeks for faster changes (eight reversals per second) (Braddick et al., 1986).

Pattern of visual function in infants with neonatal brain lesions

Neonatal focal lesions

The most common type of stroke in infants is an arterial infarct. This typically occurs in full-term infants and in the great majority of cases involves the left middle cerebral artery. Adults who suffer an ischaemic brain stroke with lesions affecting the striate occipital cortex and the optic radiations always have associated contralateral hemianopia, but infants with congenital lesions behave differently. In 1996 Mercuri et al. reported that, in a cohort of 12 infants with neonatal infarction, only 50 per cent of those with unilateral involvement of the optic radiations or the visual areas in the occipital cortex had contralateral visual field abnormalities in the first year of life. Similarly, although in all 12 patients the infarcted area involved the parietal lobe, only a few had an abnormal fixation shift in the first year of life. When the same infants were tested at school age, the proportion of children with visual abnormalities was even lower than on the assessment carried out in the neonatal period (Mercuri et al., 2003).

These findings suggest that early lesions affecting the visual pathway are, to some extent, compensated for by the immature brain but we were unable to identify any other marker which could help to discriminate infants with normal visual function from those with visual abnormalities.

In our experience the risk of developing visual abnormalities is greater in children who develop hemiplegia (33 per cent) than in those with a normal outcome. This is probably linked to the extent of the lesion.

Hypoxic-ischaemic encephalopathy

A few studies in the early 1990s, including both preterm and full term infants with hypoxic-ischaemic lesions, reported that visual abnormalities were very common in such infants (Groenendaal et al., 1989; Groenendaal & van Hof-van Duin, 1992; Cioni et al., 1996). The severity of hypoxic-ischaemic encephalopathy at birth, graded according to Sarnat & Sarnat (1976), cannot always predict the severity of visual impairment (Mercuri et al., 1997a); however, involvement of the basal ganglia and thalami appears to be very important for the presence and severity of visual impairment. When the basal ganglia and thalami are not involved, not all lesions involving the occipital lobes are associated with impaired visual function, suggesting possible plasticity of the brain. However, involvement of the basal ganglia and thalami is most often associated with visual impairment. More specifically, children with severe basal ganglia lesions have very severe visual impairment from the early months and show no improvement with age, generally having only a response to light. Children with moderate basal ganglia lesions also have abnormal results on various tests of visual function – such as acuity, fields, and fixation shift – but they have much better residual vision that can be used in everyday life. When tested at school age these infants show a similar degree of persisting impairment even when more mature aspects of visual function, such as crowding acuity or stereopsis, are tested (Mercuri *et al.*, 2004). The only infants who show different results on assessments carried out during the first year and at school age are those with minimal basal ganglia lesions. Though some infants with minimal lesions may also have visual abnormalities in the first months after birth, these tend to recover by the end of the first year (Mercuri *et al.*, 1997b). These infants are described as having 'delayed visual maturation', a term used to describe infants with reduced vision at birth which improves by the end of the first year of life (Tresidder *et al.*, 1990). The role played by the basal ganglia and the thalami in visual maturation is still not fully understood but several studies have reported extensive reciprocal connections between visual cortical areas and the basal ganglia (Ungerleider *et al.*, 1984; Updyke, 1993; Serizawa *et al.*, 1994). One hypothesis is that the integrity of these connections is essential not only for the normal development of visual function but also for an exchange of information within the brain when damage to the developing brain occurs. An interruption to these connections may preclude the possibility of functional reorganization, reducing the possibility that other cortical areas may take over the function of a damaged occipital region.

Periventricular leucomalacia

The term 'periventricular leucomalacia' (PVL) was coined in 1962. In the original description of the pathology of PVL, Banker and Larroche already highlighted that the lesion often involves the axons in the optic radiations and is therefore likely to lead to abnormal visual function (Banker & Larroche, 1962).

Several studies using a combined clinical and imaging approach have shown that the presence and severity of visual abnormalities is related to the severity and extent of the lesion. Infants with 'prolonged flares', persisting for more than 7 days (PVL type 1 according to the classification proposed by de Vries & Dubowitz, 1985) or evolving into small localized frontoparietal cysts (PVL type 2), generally had normal acuity (Eken *et al.*, 1995; Cioni *et al.*, 1997). Isolated abnormalities of ocular movements, usually squint (50 per cent), or of other aspects of visual function such as visual fields (22 per cent) or OKN (35 per cent), could, however, occasionally be found in infants with such lesions (Eken *et al.*, 1995; Uggetti *et al.*, 1996; Cioni *et al.*, 1997).

In contrast, severe visual abnormalities with impairment of various aspects of visual function are much more frequent in infants with PVL grades 3 and 4 (Cioni *et al.*, 1997; Lanzi *et al.*, 1998) – in particular squint, impaired visual acuity, and impaired visual fields.

The presence of abnormal acuity, and more generally of abnormal visual function, has been related to lesions in the peritrigonal white matter and the optic radiations as well as to the extent of occipital cortex involvement (Eken *et al.*, 1995; Uggetti *et al.*, 1996; Cioni *et al.*, 1997).

Although the association between the involvement of optic radiations/occipital cortex and abnormal visual findings was statistically significant, the correlation did not hold true in all cases, suggesting that other factors may play a role in determining visual impairment.

Ricci *et al.* (2006) recently reviewed magnetic resonance imaging (MRI) scans done after 6 months in a cohort of 12 infants with severe PVL (type 3 according to de Vries), in whom a more detailed assessment of visual function – including ocular movements, acuity, and visual fields but also fixation shift and pattern VEP – had been undertaken. In agreement with previous studies these investigators found that visual abnormalities were more frequent in infants with abnormal optic radiations and an abnormal occipital cortex, but they were able to demonstrate that the severity of visual impairment was also correlated with involvement of other cortical and subcortical areas. More specifically, infants with abnormal optic radiations but with lesions located more posteriorly, with no or little involvement of the middle and anterior parietal and frontal lobes and with normal basal ganglia on MRI, had better visual function overall, with normal acuity and fixation shift. In contrast, infants with anterior and posterior periventricular involvement and atrophy of the thalamus had more severe involvement of visual function with abnormalities on all the aspects assessed.

The early diagnosis of visual impairment in infants with PVL is important because of the relation between visual function and neurodevelopment in these children. Our group (Cioni et al., 1997) and others (Eken et al., 1995) have previously reported that infants with more severe and diffuse abnormalities of visual function also had a low developmental quotient (DQ). Multivariate analysis showed that visual impairment was the most important variable in determining the neurodevelopmental scores in these infants – more than the severity of motor disability or the extent of lesions on MRI.

Intraventricular haemorrhage

Abnormalities of visual function are frequent among preterm infants with intraventricular haemorrhages (IVH) but they are less common and generally less severe than in infants with periventricular leucomalacia. A recent study investigated visual function in a large cohort of 171 infants with different degrees of IVH, reporting a deficit of visual acuity and visual fields. While the visual field defects were usually transient and only persisted until 1 year of age, the reduction of visual acuity did persist over the fourth year. In this study visual impairment did not correlate with the severity of the haemorrhage (Papile et al., 1983) but was more often observed in infants who subsequently developed cerebral palsy. These results are in partial agreement with previous studies that showed a reduction of visual acuity in infants with IVH during the neonatal period (Morante et al., 1982; Dubowitz et al., 1983), though this tended to recover during the first months of life (Eken et al., 1994). In the latter study, a correlation with the degree of IVH was also found.

Transient anomalies of visual function may be caused by the effect of an intraventricular haemorrhage on the thalamus or the inferior colliculi, or by bleeding in the germinal matrix at the origin of the optic radiations and the posterior thalami. On the other hand, permanent effects may be present where there is deeper tissue involvement, as demonstrated by the positive association between visual deficit and neuromotor impairment. It should be noted, however, that not all infants with parenchymal involvement (grade IV lesions) show a deficit of visual function, as the lesion is more often located in the mid-anterior parietal lobe and is not therefore in sites affecting the primary visual pathway – that is, the posterior parietal and occipital lobes.

Visual-perceptual deficits: high level visual processing

From the early 1990s there has been renewed interest in visual-perceptual problems in children with early brain damage, particularly in attempting to link reduced perceptual ability to abnormalities on MRI. These studies reported visual-perceptual impairments in 55 to 60 per cent of children born prematurely with spastic diplegic cerebral palsy (Koeda & Takeshita, 1992). Stiers and colleagues (Stiers et al., 1998; Stiers et al., 1999; Stiers et al., 2002) defined visual-perceptual impairment as a specific impairment comparable with performance level on non-verbal intelligence subtests. Stiers et al. studied visual perceptual disorders by means of a test called L-94 and found that in the cerebral palsy group 40 per cent of the children were impaired on at least one visual-perceptual task, most severely in children with diplegia and quadriplegia and least severely in those with hemiplegia.

These data were confirmed in a study by Fazzi *et al.* (2004), who administered the Developmental Test of Visual Disorder in 20 children with PVL and spastic diplegia. They found a specific deficit in eye-hand coordination and in praxic-constructional abilities, suggesting that this could be an expression of malfunctioning of the occipital-parietal pathway of visual integration, the so-called 'dorsal stream'.

Ventral and dorsal stream

It is now widely recognized that a major role in processing visual information is played by the extrastriatal visual pathways, consisting of two specialized processing streams that originate beyond the primary visual cortex: the 'ventral stream' projecting to the temporal lobe, mainly devoted to object and face recognition, and the 'dorsal stream' projecting to the parietal lobe, involved in processing spatial information and visuomotor planning. Adult functional magnetic resonance imaging (fMRI) studies have confirmed the existence of two independent parallel networks specifically activated by form and motion coherence, which include specific areas within the occipital, parietal, and temporal lobes (Braddick *et al.*, 2000).

To specifically assess and compare dorsal and ventral stream functions, two different psychophysical measures have recently been proposed. The measurement of motion coherence thresholds (detecting signal dots moving coherently in a field of randomly moving noise dots) has been used to test dorsal stream function, while form coherence tasks (detecting a region of concentrically aligned segments in a field of randomly oriented line segments) have been used to test ventral stream function. These tests have been applied to various developmental disabilities – including William's syndrome, fragile-X syndrome, dyslexia, autism, and dyspraxia – and different degrees of functional impairment for the dorsal and ventral streams have been demonstrated. In a recent study (Gunn *et al.*, 2002) we have investigated dorsal and ventral stream function in a group of children with congenital hemiplegia caused by prenatal and perinatal brain damage, and a greater vulnerability of the dorsal pathway was shown in these children, though there was no apparent correlation with cerebral aetiology and the location of the damage.

We also have investigated the potential independent role of dorsal and ventral stream impairment in relation to different categories of neuropsychological visuo-perceptual tests. A positive correlation was found between form coherence thresholds and the VMI test, a pen-and-paper task assessing the ability to copy geometric figures. This would suggest that form coherence processing may be heavily involved in visuomotor tasks. The ability to copy complex figures, as required in the VMI test, may need a degree of form perception for detail memorization, particularly with older children able to develop more mature working strategies.

The assessment of dorsal and ventral stream sensitivity can provide important cues for the interpretation of visuoperceptual and visuospatial deficits, as extrastriatal visual functions are heavily involved in visual processing. However, although selective correlations can be identified between the single tests and ventral/dorsal stream functions, both systems seem generally to be involved in visual processing with different degrees of contribution, supported by extensive interconnections that may provide the structural basis for recruitment in response to injury.

Motion perception

In humans, motion is analysed at various cortical levels, including the primary and secondary visual cortex. The main area that is specialized for motion analysis in the human is the middle temporal (MT) area or V5, the homologue of the MT monkey cortex (Zeki, 1980; Tootell *et al.*, 1995). Neural activity in this region (in humans) shows strong motion opponency, increases linearly with motion coherence (Rees *et al.*, 2000), and has been found (in monkeys and humans) to correlate closely with motion perception (Britten *et al.*, 1996; Rees *et al.*, 2000). In addition, area MT responds well with coherent *vs* random motion, suggesting that it is implicated in the perception of global rather than local motion (Van Oostende *et al.*, 1997; Morrone *et al.*, 2000; Smith *et al.*, 2006).

In adults, acquired bilateral damage of the lateral temporo-occipital cortex and the underlying white matter (bilaterally involving MT) was found to be strongly associated with abnormalities of motion perception (Zihl *et al.*, 1983; Vaina *et al.*, 1990; Beardsley & Vaina, 2006). Impairment of motion perception in these conditions appears to be almost irreversible (Zihl *et al.*, 1991), possibly as a result of the limited potential for functional reorganization associated with the late acquisition of bilateral damage. Conversely, very little is known about the possible effects of lesions occurring prenatally or around the time of birth, when the nervous system is still largely immature and different pathways of functional reorganization might be expected to be activated.

Our group (Guzzetta, A. *et al.*, unpublished data) has recently measured coherence sensitivity for global motion along a translational or circular trajectory in 13 children with PVL. Subjects were required to discriminate the direction of motion, either rightwards from the left (translational motion) or clockwise from counter-clockwise (circular motion).

The main result of the study indicates that in children with PVL, sensitivity both to translational and rotational motion is on average significantly reduced compared with age-matched controls (Fig. 2). Deficits of motion processing were not related to the number of other visual abnormalities or to the results on any single visual test, suggesting a different mechanism for these disorders.

Of particular note, our group (Morrone *et al.*, 2007) found that two children with PVL perceived translational motion of a random dot display to move in the opposite direction, consistently and with high sensitivity. The apparent inversion was specific for translation motion (Fig. 3).

The perceptual deficit for translational motion was reinforced by fMRI studies. Translational motion elicited no response in the MT complex, although it did produce a strong response in many visual areas when contrasted with blank stimuli. However, rotational motion produced a normal pattern of activation in a subregion of the MT complex (Fig. 4). The severe deficit for motion perception was also evident in the semi-natural situation of a driving simulation videogame.

The bizarre inversion of motion direction suggests that the system is somehow 'aliasing' the motion signal, in a form of a 'wagon wheel effect' (where the spoked wheels in a Western movie seem to move backwards when they reach a certain speed). This results from the periodic nature of the spokes of the rotating wheels, so if one spoke moves more than halfway towards the position of the next spoke in the time of one frame, it will be paired with the successive spoke, causing the direction of motion to invert (Roget, 1825). Technically the inversion is known as *aliasing*, resulting from the fact that the rate of sampling by the filming technique is less than twice that of the repetition rate of the spokes, which is the minimum frequency necessary for vertical sampling.

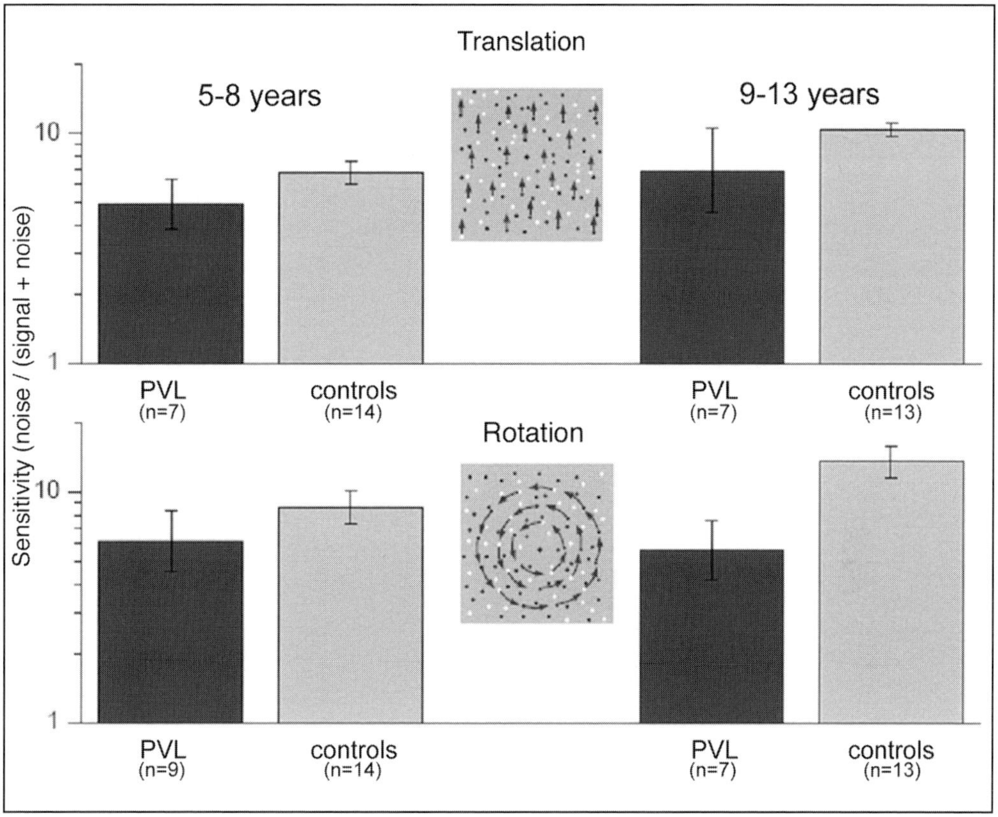

Chapter 17 The spectrum of visual disorders in children with perinatal brain lesions: long-term effects

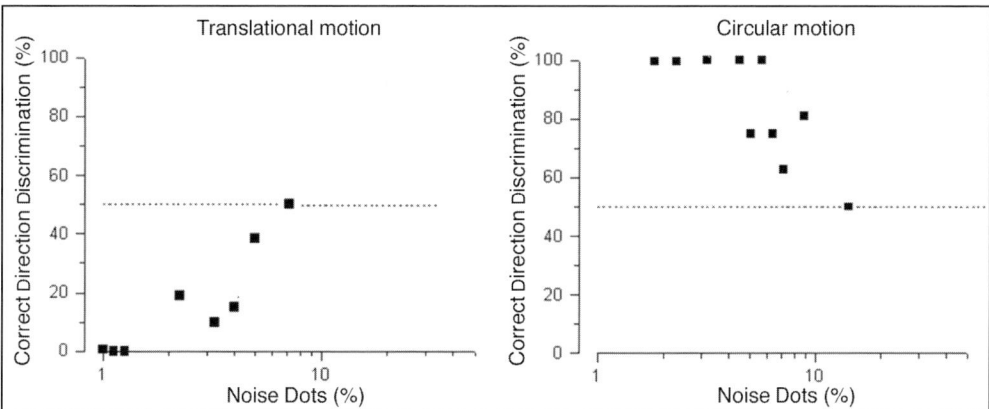

Fig. 2. Average sensitivity for two types of coherent motion, translation (upper graphs) and rotation (lower graphs), divided into two age groups. Error bars indicate the standard error of the mean.

Fig. 3. The subject reported in figure (black squares) always perceived the opposite direction of motion for translation, performing at 0 per cent correct for the maximum signal. Motion discrimination for circular motion was normal.

189

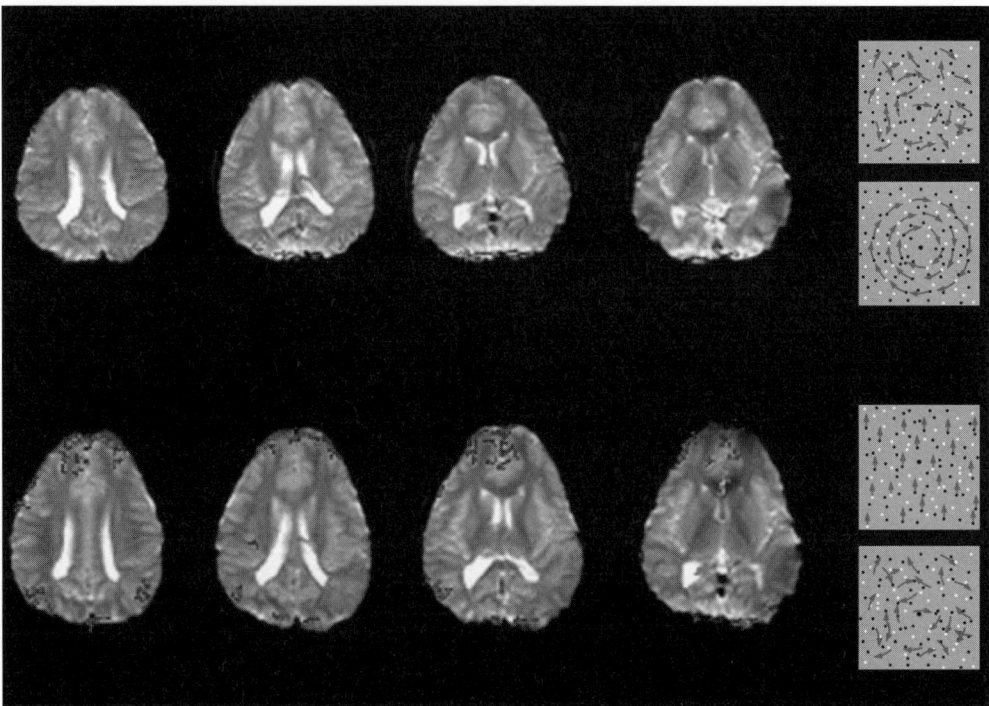

Fig. 4. fMRI BOLD response. Upper row: strong activation elicited by alternation of circular motion with random noise in the low hMT+ area. Lower row: no activation elicited by alternation of translational motion with random noise in the low or high hMT+ area.

Why the reversed motion should occur only for translational motion and not for circular motion is far from obvious. However, as there is evidence that translational motion is processed in different neural centres with respect to rotational motion (Morrone et al., 2000), it is conceivable that one of these areas, with smaller receptive fields, is more vulnerable and less plastic to the prenatal damage.

Although the full details of the purported aliasing mechanisms are obscure at present, lesion-created spatial undersampling seems to be the most promising hypothesis to explain the curious inversion of apparent direction of drifting random-dot kinematograms in the two PVL subjects.

A more specific correlation with the site and extent of periventricular brain damage in children with PVL was reported for the impairment of visual processing of biological motion – that is, the capacity to recognize the movement of an invisible human actor by means of a 'light-point' attached to the head and the major limb joints of a man (Pavlova et al., 2003; Pavlova et al., 2006a; Pavlova et al., 2006b). In these studies, the investigators were able to demonstrate how the severity of visual impairment was not related to the degree of prematurity or to motor ability but rather to the extent of PVL over the parieto-occipital complex, suggesting a specific lesion-related restriction of the brain's spontaneous compensatory plasticity in the development of this type of visuo-perceptual competence.

In the light of our results on flow motion perception (translational and rotational) in PVL, the visual streams underlying biological and flow motion can be more globally impaired in children with PVL or with mechanisms that to some extent overlap. The finding in separate studies and cohorts of an impairment of biological motion and flow motion in children with PVL may support this hypothesis, while the different measures used to assess periventricular brain damage in these studies may account for the lack of accordance. This, however, is not sufficient to exclude different underlying mechanisms for the two disorders.

On the whole the data presented here extend previous findings by other groups on the impairment of motion sensitivity in children with PVL, showing how they might be vulnerable to a more basic impairment of the motion processing stream. Nevertheless, very little is known about the neurophysiological bases of these disorders or about their functional consequences in everyday life. It is conceivable that an impairment of motion sensitivity may play a role in the functional abilities of these children, including locomotion and goal-directed motor function (Schenk *et al.*, 2000).

Early visual information processing as predictor of intelligence quotient

New instruments for the assessment of infants' intelligence based on information processing (IP) abilities have been introduced recently, mainly in experimental settings, showing a greater predictive power. These measures refer to the ability of the infant to encode a familiar stimulus, remember it, and discriminate it from a newly presented one, and are thought to reflect more stable cognitive processes during development, therefore allowing a better prediction of later IQ. One of the instruments, based on visual information processing, is the Fagan test (FTII), which consists of 10 trials in which a familiarization phase precedes the novelty problem. In the familiarization phase, a pair of identical stimuli (human faces) or a single stimulus are presented on a screen for a variable time, according to the age of the subjects. Following this phase, the familiar stimulus and a novel stimulus are presented simultaneously for two successive trials, with the left-right positions reversed in the second trial. The experimenter, sitting behind the screen, records the time the infant spends looking at the novel and the familiar stimulus (Fig. 5). The dependent variable, which reflects the magnitude of the novelty effect, is the percentage of time spent looking at the novel stimulus divided by the total looking time for both familiar and novel stimuli. The FTII has been standardized for four precise time windows: 67, 69, 79, and 92 weeks postmenstrual age, corresponding respectively to about 6 months, $6^{1/2}$ months, 9 months, and 1 year of post-term age.

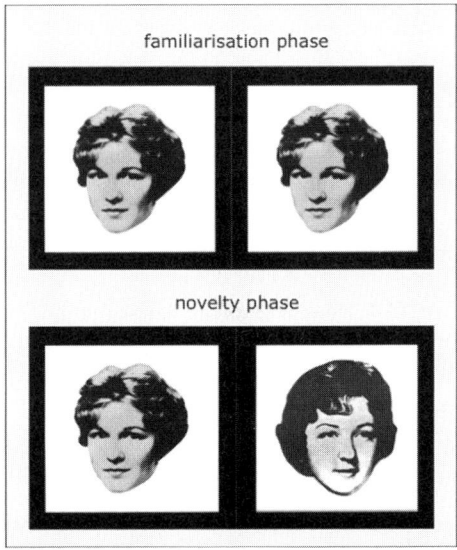

Fig. 5. Fagan test of infant intelligence: pictures showing familiarization and novelty phases.

Recently, our group (Guzzetta et al., 2006) has investigated the role of the FTII for the early prediction of the psychological short-term outcome in a population of high-risk preterm infants consecutively enrolled in a follow-up programme, and we found that the assessment done at 9 months appeared to be the most predictive of later general quotient (GQ) evaluated by means of Griffiths developmental scale at 2 years. In particular, the group of infants at low risk on the FTII showed later GQs that were higher (mean value of 89) than those who were suspect or at high risk (mean values of 82 and 79, respectively). The FTII was found to have high sensitivity (100 per cent). In particular, the two infants who showed an abnormal GQ at two years presented an abnormal result on the FTII, one in the suspect and one in the high risk category. Conversely, the presence of five false negative results reduced the specificity to 68 per cent. It is of interest that two of the three children with cerebral palsy and GQs within the normal range had normal results on the FTII, which therefore proved effective in the early detection of a good short-term cognitive outcome even in cases of severe neuromotor abnormalities. Of the two infants with late abnormal GQs only one developed cerebral palsy, but both showed abnormal results on the FTII.

In summary, the time for the assessment that was most effective in predicting short-term developmental outcome in our infants corresponded to 79 weeks' postmenstrual age. At this age, the overall maturation of the attentional and visual systems resulted in a less laborious and more reliable assessment using the FTII than if carried out earlier. Moreover, as the test was only weakly influenced by motor behaviour because of the limited motor skills required, good predictive power was assured even among those infants with specific neuromotor disorders.

Conclusions

Early detailed neuroimaging provides important information on the specific risk of visual problems of central origin, and new reliable methods can be applied in early infancy for the assessment and monitoring of visual disorders in neonates at risk. These findings are particularly relevant because of the essential role of early visual function in cognitive development (Mercuri et al., 1998; Cioni et al., 2000), and for the early planning of specific rehabilitation. Infants in whom visual impairment is detected should be enrolled in early intervention programmes, which have been shown to have a favourable influence on the visual outcome of these infants (Sonksen et al., 1991).

Acknowledgments: This work was supported by grant of the Italian Ministry of Research and Universities (MIUR: Cofin 2005) and the Mariani Foundation from Milan.

References

Atkinson, J. & Braddick, O.J. (1981): Development of optokinetic nystagmus in infants: an indicator of cortical binocularity. In: *Eye movements: cognition and visual perception*, eds. D.F. Fisher, R.A. Monty & J.W. Sender, pp. 53–64. Hillsdale, N.J.: Lawrence Erlbaum Associates.

Atkinson, J., Hood, B., Wattam-Bell, J. & Braddick, O. (1992): Changes in infants' ability to switch visual attention in the first three months of life. *Perception* **21,** 643–653.

Aylward, G.P. (2002): Cognitive and neuropsychological outcomes: more than IQ scores. *Ment. Retard. Dev. Disabil. Res. Rev.* **8,** 234–240.

Banker, B. & Larroche, J. (1962): Periventricular leucomalacia of infancy. *Arch. Neurol.* **7,** 386–410.

Beardsley, S.A. & Vaina, L.M. (2006): Global motion mechanisms compensate local motion deficits in a patient with a bilateral occipital lobe lesion. *Exp. Brain Res.* **173,** 724–732.

Braddick, O.J., Wattam-Bell. J. & Atkinson, J. (1986): Orientation-specific cortical responses develop in early infancy. *Nature* **320,** 617–619.

Braddick, O.J., O'Brien, J.M., Wattam-Bell, J., Atkinson, J. & Turner, R. (2000): Form and motion coherence activate independent, but not dorsal/ventral segregated, networks in the human brain. *Curr. Biol.* **10,** 731–734.

Britten, K.H., Newsome, W.T., Shadlen, M.N., Celebrini, S. & Movshon, J.A. (1996): A relationship between behavioral choice and the visual responses of neurons in macaque MT. *Vis. Neurosci.* **13,** 87–100.

Cioni, G., Fazzi, B., Ipata, A.E., Canapicchi, R. & van Hof-van Duin, J. (1996): Correlation between cerebral visual impairment and magnetic resonance imaging in children with neonatal encephalopathy. *Dev. Med. Child Neurol.* **38,** 120–132.

Cioni, G., Fazzi, B., Coluccini, M., Bartalena, L., Boldrini, A. & van Hof-van Duin, J. (1997): Cerebral visual impairment in preterm infants with periventricular leucomalacia. *Pediatr. Neurol.* **17,** 331–338.

Cioni, G., Bertuccelli, B., Boldrini, A., Canapicchi, R., Fazzi, B., Guzzetta, A. & Mercuri, E. (2000): Correlation between visual function, neurodevelopmental outcome, and magnetic resonance imaging findings in infants with periventricular leucomalacia. *Arch. Dis. Child. Fetal Neonat. Ed.* **82,** F134–F140.

de Vries, L.S. & Dubowitz, L.M.S. (1985): Cystic leucomalacia in the preterm infant: site of lesion in relation to prognosis. *Lancet* ii, 1075–1076.

Dubowitz, L.M.S., Mushin, J., Morante, A. & Placzek, M. (1983): The maturation of visual acuity in neurologically normal and abnormal newborn infants. *Behav. Brain. Res.* **10,** 39–45.

Eken, P., van Nieuwenhuizen, O., van der Graaf, Y., Schalij-Delfos, N.E. & de Vries, L. (1994): Relation between neonatal cranial ultrasound abnormalities and cerebral visual impairment in infancy. *Dev. Med. Child Neurol.* **36,** 3–15.

Eken, P., de Vries, L., van der Graaf, Y., Meiners, L.C. & van Nieuwenhuizen, O. (1995): Haemorrhagic-ischaemic lesions of the neonatal brain: correlation between cerebral visual impairment, neurodevelopmental outcome and MRI in infancy. *Dev. Med. Child Neurol.* **37,** 41–55.

Fazzi, E., Bova, S.M., Uggetti, C., Signorini, S.G., Bianchi, P.E., Maraucci, I., Coppello, M. & Lanzi, G. (2004): Visual-perceptual impairment in children with periventricular leucomalacia. *Brain Dev.* **26,** 506–512.

Groenendaal, F. & van Hof-van Duin, J. (1992): Visual deficits and improvements in children after perinatal hypoxia. *J. Vis. Impair. Blind.* **86,** 215–218.

Groenendaal, F., van Hof-van Duin, J., Baerts, W. & Fetter, W.P. (1989): Effects of perinatal hypoxia on visual development during the first year of (corrected) age. *Early Hum. Dev.* **20,** 267–279.

Gunn, A., Cory, E., Atkinson, J., Braddick, O., Wattam-Bell, J., Guzzetta, A. & Cioni, G. (2002): Dorsal and ventral stream sensitivity in normal development and hemiplegia. *Neuroreport* **13,** 843–847.

Guzzetta, A., Mazzotti, S., Tinelli, F., Bancale, A., Ferretti, G., Battini, R., Bartalena, L., Boldrini, A. & Cioni, G. (2006): Early assessment of visual information processing and neurological outcome in preterm infants. *Neuropediatrics* **37,** 278–285.

Koeda, T. & Takeshita, K. (1992): Visuo-perceptual impairment and cerebral lesions in spastic diplegia with preterm birth. *Brain Dev.* **14,** 239–244.

Lanzi, G., Fazzi, E., Uggetti, C., Cavallini, A., Danova, S., Egitto, M.G., Ginevra, O.F., Salati, R. & Bianchi, P.E. (1998): Cerebral visual impairment in periventricular leucomalacia. *Neuropediatrics* **29,** 145–150.

Mercuri, E., Atkinson, J., Braddick, O., Anker S., Nokes, L., Cowan, F., Rutherford, M., Pennock, J. & Dubowitz, L. (1996): Visual function and perinatal focal cerebral infarction. *Arch. Dis. Child. Fetal Neonat. Ed.* **75,** F76–F81.

Mercuri, E., Atkinson, J., Braddick, O., Anker, S., Cowan, F., Rutherford, M., Pennock, J. & Dubowitz, L. (1997a): Basal ganglia damage and impaired visual function in the newborn infant. *Arch. Dis. Child. Fetal Neonat. Ed.* **77,** F111–F114.

Mercuri, E., Atkinson, J., Braddick, O., Anker, S., Cowan, F., Pennock, J., Rutherford, M.A., & Dubowitz, L.M. (1997b): The aetiology of delayed visual maturation: short review and personal findings in relation to magnetic resonance imaging. *Eur. J. Paediatr. Neurol.* **1,** 31–34.

Mercuri, E., Braddick. O., Atkinson. J., Cowan, F., Anker, S., Andrew, R., Wattam-Bell, J., Rutherford M., Counsell S. & Dubowitz L. (1998): Orientation-reversal and phase-reversal visual evoked potentials in full-term infants with brain lesions: a longitudinal study. *Neuropediatrics* **29,** 169–174.

Mercuri, E., Anker, S., Guzzetta, A., Barnett, A.L., Haataja, L., Rutherford, M., Cowan, F., Dubowitz, L., Braddick, O. & Atkinson, J. (2004): Visual function at school age in children with neonatal encephalopathy and low Apgar scores. *Arch. Dis. Child. Fetal Neonat. Ed.* **89,** F258–F262.

Mercuri, E., Anker, S., Guzzetta, A., Barnett, A., Haataja, L., Rutherford, M., Cowan, F., Dubowitz, L., Braddick, O. & Atkinson, J. (2003): Neonatal cerebral infarction and visual function at school age. *Arch. Dis. Child. Fetal Neonat. Ed.* **88,** F487-F491. Erratum: 2004, **89,** F187.

Mohn, G. & van Hof-van Duin, J. (1986): Development of the binocular and monocular visual field during the first year of life. *Clin. Vis. Sci.* **1**, 51–64.

Morante, A., Dubowitz, L.M.S., Levene, M.I. & Dubowitz, V. (1982): The development of visual function in normal and neurologically abnormal preterm and full term infants. *Dev. Med. Child. Neurol.* **24**, 771–784.

Morrone, M.C., Tosetti, M., Montanaro, D., Fiorentini, A., Cioni, G. & Burr, D.C. (2000): A cortical area that responds specifically to optic flow, revealed by fMRI. *Nat. Neurosci.* **3**, 1322–1328.

Morrone, M.C., Guzzetta, A., Tinelli, F., Tosetti, M., Del Viva, M., Montanaro, D., Burr, D. & Cioni, G. (2008): Inversion of perceived direction of motion caused by spatial under-sampling in two children with periventricular leucomalacia. *J. Cogn. Neurosci.* Jan 22 (Epub ahead of print).

Papile, L.A., Munsick-Bruno, G. & Schaefer, A., (1983): Relationship of cerebral intraventricular hemorrhage and early childhood neurologic handicaps. *J. Pediatr.* **103**, 273–277.

Pavlova, M., Staudt, M., Sokolov, A., Birbaumer, N. & Krageloh-Mann, I. (2003): Perception and production of biological movement in patients with early periventricular brain lesions. *Brain* **126**, 692–701.

Pavlova, M., Marconato, F., Sokolov, A., Braun, C., Birbaumer, N. & Krageloh Mann, I. (2006a): Periventricular leucomalacia specifically affects cortical MEG response to biological motion. *Ann. Neurol.* **59**, 415–419.

Pavlova, M., Sokolov, A., Birbaumer, N. & Krageloh-Mann, I. (2006b): Biological motion processing in adolescents with early periventricular brain damage. *Neuropsychologia* **44**, 586–593.

Rees, G., Friston, K. & Koch, C. (2000): A direct quantitative relationship between the functional properties of human and macaque V5. *Nat. Neurosci.* **3**, 716–723.

Ricci, D., Anker, S., Cowan, F., Pane, M., Gallini, F., Luciano, R., Convito, V., Baranello, G., Cesarini, L., Bianco, F., Rutherford, M., Romagnoli, C., Atkinson, J., Braddick, O., Guzzetta, F. & Mercuri, E. (2006): Thalamic atrophy in infants with PVL and cerebral visual impairment. *Early Hum. Dev.* **82**, 591–595.

Roget, P.M. (1825): Explanation of an optical deception in the appearance of the spokes of a wheel seen through vertical apertures. *Phil. Trans. R. Soc.* **115**, 131–140.

Sarnat, H.B. & Sarnat, M.S. (1976): Neonatal encephalopathy following neonatal distress. A clinical and electroencephalographic study. *Arch. Neurol.* **33**, 696–705.

Schenk, T., Mai, N., Ditterich, J. & Zihl, J. (2000): Can a motion-blind patient reach for moving objects? *Eur. J. Neurosci.* **12**, 3351–3360.

Serizawa, M., McHaffie, J.G., Hoshino, K. & Norita, M. (1994): Corticostriatal and corticotectal projections from visual cortical areas 17, 18 and 18a in the pigmented rat. *Arch. Histol. Cytol.* **57**, 493–507.

Smith, A.T., Wall, M.B., Williams, A.L. & Singh, K.D. (2006): Sensitivity to optic flow in human cortical areas MT and MST. *Eur. J. Neurosci.* **23**, 561–569.

Sonksen, P.M., Petrie, A. & Drew, K.J. (1991): Promotion of visual development of severally visual impaired babies: evaluation of a developmentally based program. *Dev. Med. Child Neurol.* **22**, 320–335.

Stiers, P., De Cock, P. & Vandebussche, E. (1998): Impaired visual perceptual performance on an object recognition task in children with cerebral visual impairment. *Neuropediatrics* **29**, 80–88.

Stiers, P., De Cock, P. & Vandebussche, E. (1999): Separating visual perception and non-verbal intelligence in children with early brain injury. *Brain Dev.* **21**, 397–406.

Stiers, P., Vanderkelen, R., Vanneste, G., Coene, S., De Rammelaere, M. & Vandenbussche, E. (2002): Visual-perceptual impairment in a random sample of children with cerebral palsy. *Dev. Med. Child Neurol.* **44**, 370–382.

Teller, D.Y., McDonald, M.A., Preston, K., Sebris, S.L. & Dobson, V.(1986): Assessment of visual acuity in infants and children: the acuity card procedure. *Dev. Med. Child Neurol.* **26**, 779–789.

Tootell, R.B.H., Reppas, J.B, Kwong, K.K., Malach, R., Born, R.T., Brady, T.J., Rosen, B.R. & Belliveau, J.W. (1995): Functional analysis of human MT and related visual cortical areas using magnetic resonance imaging. *J. Neurosci.* **15**, 3215–3230.

Tresidder, J., Fielder, A.R. & Nicholson, J., (1990): Delayed visual maturation: ophthalmic and neurodevelopmental aspects. *Dev. Med. Child Neurol.* **32**, 872–881.

Uggetti, C., Egitto, M.G., Fazzi, E., Bianchi, P.E., Bergamaschi, R., Zappoli, F., Sibilla, L., Martelli A. & Lanzi G., (1996): Cerebral visual impairment in periventricular leucomalacia: MR correlation. *Am. J. Neuroradiol.* **17**, 979–985.

Ungerleider, L.G., Desimone, R., Galwin, T.W. & Mishkin, M. (1984): Subcortical projections of area MT in the macaque. *J. Comp. Neurol.* **223**, 368–386.

Updyke, B.V. (1993): Organisation of visual corticostriatal projections in the cat, with observations on visual projections to claustrum and amygdala. *J. Comp. Neurol.* **327**, 159–193.

Vaina, L.M., Lemay, M., Bienfang, D.C., Choi, A.Y. & Nakayama, K. (1990): Intact 'biological motion' and 'structure from motion' perception in a patient with impaired motion mechanisms: a case study. *Vis. Neurosci.* **5**, 353–369.

van Hof-van Duin, J., Heersema, D.J., Groenendaal, F., Baerts, W. & Fetter, W.P.F. (1992): Visual field and grating acuity development in low-risk preterm infants during the first 2 1/2 years after term. *Behav. Brain Res.* **49,** 115–122.

Van Oostende, S., Sunaert, S., Van Hecke, P., Marchal, G. & Orban, G.A. (1997): The kinetic occipital (KO) region in man: an fMRI study. *Cereb. Cortex* **7,** 690–701.

Zeki, S.M. (1980): The response properties of cells in the middle temporal area (area MT) of owl monkey visual cortex. *Proc. R. Soc. Lond. B* **207,** 239–248.

Zihl, J., von Cramon, D. & Mai, N. (1983): Selective disturbance of movement vision after bilateral brain damage. *Brain* **106,** 313–340.

Zihl, J., von Cramon, D., Mai, N. & Schmid, C. (1991): Disturbance of movement vision after bilateral posterior brain damage. Further evidence and follow up observations. *Brain* **114,** 2235–2252.

Chapter 18

Early predictors of cognitive development in very low birth weight children

Roberto Militerni *, Bianca Adinolfi °, Luigi Falco ^, Alessandro Frolli *
and Guido Militerni *

* II Policlinico, Cattedra di Neuropsichiatria Infantile, via Pansini 5, 80121 Naples, Italy;
° UOC Pediatria, Azienda Ospedaliera 'San Sebastiano' di Caserta, Caserta, Italy;
^ UOC Terapia Intensiva Neonatale, Azienda Ospedaliera 'San Sebastiano' di Caserta
roberto.militerni@unina2.it

Summary

Survival of very preterm and very low birth weight (VLBW) live-born infants has increased substantially in recent years. Follow-up during the first 2 years of life showed the presence of neurodevelopmental disabilities such as cerebral palsy and mental retardation in 10 to 20 per cent. Long-term follow-up to school age revealed an even higher frequency of developmental impairments. These include problems in cognitive and behavioural development, and school failure. To examine the predictive power of measures taken in the first 2 years of life, 18 very low birth weight children were tested at ages of 18 and 60 months. Among the variables used, the early social communication skills, with special regard to the 'joint attention', were included. The results suggest that early joint attention skills are significantly associated with cognitive measures at age 5 years. The nature and meaning of joint attention are considered.

Introduction

Survival of very preterm and very low birth weight (VLBW) live-born infants has increased substantially in recent years, with some variation depending on the population investigated and the mortality definition used. Developmental sequelae, however, are still a major problem, mostly because babies who would previously have been expected to die are now surviving neonatal intensive care. Developmental outcome varies even more depending on the age of the child at assessment, the population studied, and the definition of handicap used. Follow-up studies have shown that developmental problems increase with age, and seemingly healthy toddlers may still have developmental problems and school failure at a later age (Richardson *et al.*, 1998; Taylor *et al.*, 1998; Mikkola *et al.*, 2005).

Follow-up during the first 2 years of life showed the presence of neurodevelopmental disabilities such as cerebral palsy and mental retardation in 10 to 20 per cent of cases. Long-term follow-up to school age revealed an even higher frequency of developmental impairments.

These include motor performance problems, visual and auditory impairments, problems in cognitive and behavioural development, and school failure.

In several reports on the follow-up of VLBW infants, the need for special education increased from 19 per cent at age 9 to 28 per cent at age 14 years (de Kleine *et al.*, 2003). These findings make follow-up mandatory for timely identification of children with atypical development, with special regard to the cognitive aspects.

Cognitive development is usually conceptualized as the way by which the child gains access to the highest forms of mental reasoning. Thus cognitive development is identified with the concept of intelligence – that is, a function that can be assessed using standardized measures starting from 6 or 7 years of age. However, if we look at 'cognition' as a complex process that allows one to solve environmental questions, we can study cognitive development from the first months of life by assessing the strategies used for adaptive purposes. In this perspective, the assessment of early social communication skills is a useful tool, both for analysing affective development and for evaluating the development of the mentation and symbolic processes.

The development of the capacity to share or coordinate attention with a social partner is a major milestone of infancy (Bruner & Sherwood, 1983; Bakeman & Adamson, 1984; Tomasello, 1995; Mundy & Gomes, 1998). This broad capacity is often referred to as 'joint attention' skill development (Carpenter *et al.*, 1998). The study of joint attention skills is commonly associated with theory on social cognition or language acquisition and it has provided important new perspectives on the nature of atypical as well as typical early development (Baldwin, 1995; Ulvund & Smith, 1996; Carpenter *et al.*, 1998; Corkum & Moore, 1998; Morales *et al.*, 1998; Sigman & Ruskin, 1999; Mundy & Sigman, 2006). It is less well recognized, though, that research on joint attention skills may also contribute to a better understanding of the integration of social-emotional and cognitive processes in infancy, especially as these affect risk or vulnerability to psychopathology (Mundy & Willoughby, 1998).

This chapter describes a study aimed at assessing the predictability of joint attention behaviours in a sample of VLBW infants initially assessed at age 18 months and reassessed at age 5 years.

Methods

Two groups of children participated in the study. The target group consisted of VLBW infants recruited from various neonatal intensive care units in the Campania region. The inclusion criteria included:

- no history of seizure conditions or congenital and/or chromosomal abnormalities;
- absence of major neurological sequelae such as cerebral palsy;
- developmental quotient (DQ) > 80, taken from a standardized measure at age 18 months.

Using these inclusion criteria, the study subjects comprised 18 VLBW infants who supplied complete data relevant to this study at age 18 months and 5 years. A control group included 18 typically developing children drawn from a sample of 69 infants and families enrolled in a 9 to 36 month longitudinal study of social development (Militerni *et al.*, 2007). These children were matched pairwise with the VLBW subjects on the basis of chronological age (CA), DQ, and sex.

Measures

The following measures were administered:

Language

The MacArthur Communicative Development Inventory (CDI) (Caselli & Casadio, 1995) parent report measure was completed at 18 months. The raw totals of words produced and words comprehended were used in the analysis as measures of language expression and comprehension.

Developmental assessment

The Griffiths Mental Development Scales (Griffiths, 1996) were completed at 18 months.

Intelligence quotient

The Wechsler Preschool and Primary Scale of Intelligence (WIPPSI) (Wechsler, 1973) was completed at age 5 years. Full scale IQ (FIQ), verbal IQ (VIQ) and performance IQ (PIQ) standard scores were used as measures of cognitive outcome in the analysis.

Early social and communication behaviours

We used the Early Social Communication Scales (ESCS) (Mundy *et al.*, 2003). The ESCS is a 20 minute videotaped structured assessment designed to measure the development of a variety of non-verbal communication skills in the 6- to 30-month period. An experimenter and an infant, with the latter sitting in the caregiver's lap or independently in a child chair, were seated facing each other across a small table. A set of toys was visible to the child but out of reach, on the experimenter's side of the table. Posters were placed on the walls, 90 degrees to the child's left and right and 180 degrees behind the child. A video camera was positioned approximately 10 feet behind the experimenter. The camera was oriented to capture a three-quarter face image of the child with a profile view of the experimenter, as well as the position of the toys and posters. The experimenter presented the child with a sequence of activated wind-up toys (three trials), hand-operated mechanical toys (three trials), opportunities to play a tickle, turn-taking game (two trials), opportunities to play an object turn-taking game, such as catch with a ball (two trials), opportunities to take turns wearing a hat, comb, and glasses (three trials), and an opportunity to look at pictures in a book with the tester (one trial). The tester also presented the child with requests to give toys to the tester. Finally, the tester presented the child with two sets of three trials in which the tester attracted the child's attention, and then turned to visually fixate a wall poster, while pointing at the poster and saying the child's name three times with increasing emphasis. Trials to the left, right, and behind the child were conducted in each set.

Observations of the tester-child interaction in the ESCS yielded frequency of behaviour scores in three categories involving social attention coordination: Initiating Joint Attention (IJA); Responding to Joint Attention (RJA); and Initiating Behaviour Requesting/Regulation (IBR).

IJA scores refer to the frequency with which the child uses (a) eye contact, (b) alternating gaze, (c) pointing, and (d) showing, to share the experience of an active mechanical toy with the tester (IJA-Tot). We recorded the percentage of children who were able to use high-level communicative behaviours – that is, pointing and showing (IJA-Hi).

RJA refers to the percentage of trials on which a child correctly turns his/her gaze in the direction of the tester's gaze and pointing gesture.

IBR scores refer to the frequency with which the child uses eye contact, reaching, giving, and pointing to elicit aid in obtaining objects or reactivating objects (IBR-Tot). Also, we considered the percentage of children who were able to use high-level communicative behaviours – that is, pointing and giving (IBR-Hi).

Findings

Scores on the domain considered at the two time points are shown in Table 1 and data on the correlations among the different variables are presented in Table 2.

Table 1. DQ, Language, ESCS, and IQ scores at each assessment in the sample and control group

	VLBW	Normal	p Value
At age 18 months			
DQ	95 (9.4)	98 (9.7)	NS
MCDI	23.2 (30.9)	34.8 (29.6)	NS
ESCS IJA-T	17.3 (7.8)	21.5 (9.7)	NS
ESCS IJA-Hi	1.6 (1.8)	3.4 (3.3)	<0.05
ESCS RJA (%)	63.7 (19.3)	79.1 (20.2)	<0.05
ESCS IBR-T	27.9 (8.2)	29.8 (10.5)	NS
ESCS IBR-Hi	10.3 (2.5)	12.4 (3.3)	<0.05
At age 5 years			
FIQ	94 (14)	98 (12)	NS
VIQ	96 (18)	102 (15)	NS
PIQ	89 (19)	95 (16)	<0.05

Values are mean (SD).
DQ, developmental quotient; ESCS, Early Social Communication Scales; FIQ, full scale intelligence quotient; MCDI, Minnesota Child Development Inventory; PIQ, performance intelligence quotient; VIQ, verbal intelligence quotient.

Table 2. Within and across domain associations between 18 months measures and outcome at 5 years

	FIQ	VIQ	PIQ
DQ	0.43*	0.42*	0.41*
MCDI	0.18	0.19	0.18
ESCS IJA-Tot	0.47**	0.48**	0.46**
ESCS IJA-Hi	0.76**	0.77**	0.73**
ESCS RJA	0.49**	0.47**	0.49**
ESCS IBR-Tot	0.11	0.11	0.10
ESCS IBR-Hi	0.41*	0.42*	0.41*

* $p<0.05$; ** $p<0.01$.
DQ, developmental quotient; ESCS, Early Social Communication Scales; FIQ, full scale intelligence quotient; IBR, initiating behaviour requesting/regulation; IBR-Hi, IBR score for children using high-level communicative behaviours; IBR-Tot, IBR score for whole group; IJA, initiating joint attention; IJA-Hi, IJA score for children using high-level communicative behaviours; IJA-Tot, IJA score for whole group; MCDI, Minnesota Child Development Inventory; PIQ, performance intelligence quotient; VIQ, verbal intelligence quotient.

With these inclusion criteria, there were no differences in the mean DQ scores at 18 months of age between the sample group (95, SD 9.4) and the control group (98, SD 9.7). The language measures taken from the Minnesota Child Development Inventory (MCDI) showed that infants in the sample group had fewer words at 18 months (n=23.2, SD 30.9) than the infants in the control group (n=34.8, SD 29.6); however, the differences were not statistically significant. The mean IJA-Tot and IBR-Tot scores were similar in the sample and the control group. In contrast, IJA-Hi, IBR-Hi, and RJA scores in the sample group were higher than in the control group (1.6 vs. 3.4; 10.3 vs. 12.4; and 63.7 vs. 79.1, respectively). Data on the assessment at age 5 years showed that mean FIQ and VIQ did not differ between the groups. In contrast, the mean PIQ scores were significantly different between the sample group (89, SD 19) and the control group (95, SD 16).

To examine the predictability of the measures taken at age 18 months on the outcome at age 5 years, the correlations between the data at 18 months and 5 years were considered. All the measures related to joint attention – such as IJA-Tot, IJA-Hi, RJA, and IBR-Hi at age 18 months – were significantly correlated with the measures of the IQ at age 5 years. However, the MCDI scores were not significantly correlated with the measures of cognitive ability taken at age 5 years.

Comment

In this study we assessed the predictability of measures taken at age 18 months on the cognitive outcome as measured by the WIPPSI at age 5 years.

In contrast to the lack of predictability of the standard measures, such as MCDI, the measure of rate of joint attention behaviours, as measured by ESCS, predicted outcome in several domains of cognitive development. This is consistent with previous longitudinal studies where the developmental continuity between infant joint attention and later social and cognitive abilities is reasonably well supported (Mundy & Sigman, 2006; Vaughan et al., 2007).

One issue is what the predictive variable is an index of. The Social Cognitive Model (Tomasello, 1995) suggests that the joint attention reflects specific components of cognition – in particular, the development of infants' early understanding that others have intentions (that is, social cognition). The logic here is that if infants use gestures and eye contact to communicate intentionally with others, then they must have some awareness not only of the social signal value of their behaviours but also that others have powers of perception and intention that may be affected by the infant's behaviour. Thus, theory has come to suggest that early prelinguistic communication skills – especially joint attention development – reflect the emergence of social cognition, or the infants' understanding that others have intentions (Leslie & Happé, 1989; Baron-Cohen, 1995; Tomasello, 1995).

In turn, this epistemological component of joint attention provides a unique part of the cognitive foundation for advances in infants' referential communication and subsequent language development (Bruner, 1985; Bretherton, 1991; Tomasello, 1995; Brooks & Meltzoff, 2005; Tomasello et al., 2005). In language learning, for example, much of the early lexical acquisition takes place in unstructured or incidental social learning situations where parents provide learning opportunities by referring to a new object or event, but infants need to discriminate among a number of potential referents in the environment to focus on the correct object/event in order to acquire the appropriate new word-object/event association. The correct discrimination among potential referents allows infants to avoid possible referential mapping errors (Baldwin, 1995) and maximizes the opportunity to learn (Tomasello, 1995).

In this regard, Mundy & Sigman (2006) suggested that joint attention development should be thought of in terms of two phases: a 'learning to' phase and a 'learning from' phase. In the first year of development, several basic processes contribute to the capacity of infants to engage in IJA and RJA behaviours. Theoretically, the basic processes that support this 'learning to' phase of joint attention development include, but are not limited to, operant learning (Corkum & Moore, 1998), intrinsic biological motivation processes (Trevarthen & Aitken, 2001), and imitation (Lau et al., 2004; Meltzoff & Moore, 1997). With practice, the numerous processes involved in coordinating social attention become integrated and routinized, enabling infants gradually to move from the 'learning to' phase to the 'learning from' phase of joint attention development. Thus in the 'learning from' phase more resources become available to engage in integrative cognitive activities in the context of joint attention interactions with others – that is, the more frequently infants engage in episodes of joint attention with others, the more opportunities they have to expand their understanding of similarities and differences in the responses of self and other to external objects and events. From this perspective, joint attention may reasonably viewed as a special form of intent social engagement that contributes to self-constructivistic aspects of cognitive development (Piaget, 1966).

References

Bakeman, R. & Adamson, L. (1984): Coordinating attention to people and objects in mother-infant and peer-infant interaction. *Child Dev.* **55**, 1278–1289.

Baldwin, D.A. (1995): Understanding the link between joint attention and language. In: *Joint attention: its origins and role in development*, eds. C. Moore & P. Dunham, pp. 131–158. Hillsdale, NJ: Lawrence Erlbaum.

Baron-Cohen, S. (1995): *The mindblindness*. Cambridge, MA: MIT Press.

Bretherton, I. (1991): Intentional communication and the development of an understanding of mind. In: *Children's theories of mind: mental states and social understanding*, eds. D. Frye & C. Moore, pp. 49–75. Hillsdale, NJ: Lawrence Erlbaum.

Brooks, R. & Meltzoff, A. (2005): The development of gaze following and its relations to language. *Dev. Sci.* **8**, 535–543.

Bruner, J. (1985): *Child's talk: learning to use language*. New York: Norton.

Bruner, J. & Sherwood, V. (1983): Thought, language and interaction in infancy. In: *Frontiers in infant psychiatry*, eds. J. Call, E., Galenson & R. Tyson, pp. 38–55. New York: Basic Books.

Carpenter, M., Nagell, K. & Tomasello, M. (1998): Social cognition, joint attention, and communicative competence from 9 to 15 months of age. *Monographs of the Society for Research in Child Development*, vol. 63 (4, Serial No. 255).

Caselli M.C. & Casadio, P. (1995): *Il primo vocabolario del bambino. Guida all'uso del questionario MacArthur per la valuatazione della comunicazione e del linguaggio nei primi anni di vita*. Milan: Franco Angeli.

Corkum, V. & Moore, C. (1998): Origins of joint visual attention in infants. *Dev. Psychol.* **34**, 28–38.

de Kleine, M.J.K., den Ouden, A.L., Kollée, L.A.A., Nijhuis- van der Sanden, M.W.G., Sondaar, M., van Kessel-Feddema, B.J.M., Knuijt, S., van Baar, A.L., Ilsen, A., Breur-Pieterse, R., Briët, J.M., Brand, R. & Verloove-Vanhorick, S.P. (2003): Development and evaluation of a follow up assessment of preterm infants at 5 years of age. *Arch. Dis. Child.* **88**, 870–875.

Griffiths, R. (1996): *The Griffiths mental developmental scales*. Firenze: Organizzazioni Speciali (Italian translation).

Lau, H., Rogers, R., Haggard, P. & Passingham, R.E. (2004): Attention to intention. *Science* **303**, 1208–1209.

Leslie, A. & Happé, F. (1989): Autism and ostensive communication: the relavance of metarepresentation. *Dev. Psychopathol.* **1**, 205–212.

Meltzoff, A. & Moore, M. (1997): Explaining facial imitation: a theoretical model. *Early Dev. Parenting* **6**, 179–192.

Mikkola, K., Ritari, N., Tommiska, V., Salokorpi, T., Lehtonen, L., Tammela, O., Pääkkönen, L., Olsen, P., Korkman, M. & Fellman, V., for the Finnish ELBW Cohort Study Group (2005): Neurodevelopmental outcome at 5 years of age of a national cohort of extremely low birth weight infants who were born in 1996–1997. *Pediatrics* **116**, 1391–1400.

Militerni, R., Adinolfi, B., Esposito, M., Frolli, A., Militerni, G. & Sergi, L. (2007): Early predictors of social and adaptive outcomes in children with autistic disorder. Thirteenth International Congress of the European Society for Child and Adolescent Psychiatry (ESCAP), Florence, August 25-29.

Morales, M., Mundy, P. & Rojas, J. (1998): Following the direction of gaze and language development in 6-month-olds. *Infant Behav. Dev.* **21,** 373–377.

Mundy, P. & Gomes, A. (1998): Individual differences in joint attention skill development in the second year. *Infant Behav. Dev.* **21,** 469–482.

Mundy, P., & Sigman, M. (2006): Joint attention, social competence, and developmental psychopathology. In: *Developmental psychopathology, Vol. 1: Theory and methods*, eds. D. Cicchetti & D. Cohen, 2nd edition, pp. 293–332. Hoboken, NJ: John Wiley.

Mundy, P. & Willoughby, J. (1998): Nonverbal communication, affect, and social emotional development. In: *Transitions in prelinguistic communication: preintentional to intentional and presymbolic to symbolic*, eds. A. Wether by, S. Warren & J. Reichle, pp. 111–134. Baltimore: Brookes Publishing Co.

Mundy, P., Delgado, C., Block, J., Venezia, M., Hogan, A. & Seibert, J. (2003): A manual for the abridged early social communication scales (ESCS). Available through the University of Miami Psychology Department, Coral Gables, FL. Retrieved August 1, 1999, from http://www.psy.miami.edu/faculty/pmundy/main.phtml.

Piaget, J. (1966). *La rappresentazione del mondo nel fanciullo*. Torino: Boringhieri (Italian translation).

Richardson D.K., Gray J.E. & Gortmaker S.L. (1998): Declining severity adjusted mortality: evidence of improving neonatal intensive care. *Pediatrics* **102,** 893–899.

Sigman, M. & Ruskin, E. (1999): Continuity and change in the social competence of children with autism, Down syndrome, and developmental delays. *Monographs of the Society for Research in Child Development*, vol. 64 (1, Serial No. 256).

Taylor H.G., Klein N., Schatschneider C. & Hack M. (1998): Predictors of early school age outcomes in very low birth weight children. *J. Dev. Behav. Pediatr.* **19,** 235–243.

Tomasello, M. (1995): Joint attention as social cognition. In: *Joint attention: its origins and role in development*, eds. C. Moore & P. Dunham, pp. 103–130. Hillsdale, NJ: Lawrence Erlbaum.

Tomasello, M., Carpenter, M., Call, J., Behne, T. & Moll, H. (2005): Understanding sharing individual differences and joint attention intentions: the origins of cultural cognition. *Brain Behav. Sci.* **28,** 675–690.

Trevarthen, C. & Aitken, K. (2001): Infant intersubjectivity: research, theory and clinical applications. *J. Child Psychol. Psychiatry* **42,** 3–48.

Ulvund, S. & Smith, L. (1996): The predictive validity of nonverbal communicative skills in infants with perinatal hazards. *Infant Behav. Dev.* **19,** 441–449.

Vaughan, A., Mundy, P., Acra, F., Block, J., Delgado, C., Parlade, M., Meyer, J.A., Neal, A.R. & Pomares, Y.B. (2007): Infant joint attention, temperament, and social competence in preschool children. *Child Dev.* **78,** 53–69.

Wechsler, D. (1973): *Wechsler preschool and primary scale of intelligence (WIPPSI)*. Florence: Organizzazioni Speciali (Italian translation).

Chapter 19

The Neuronal Group Selection Theory: a framework to understand typical and atypical motor development

Mijna Hadders-Algra

Department of Neurology – Developmental Neurology, University Medical Centre Groningen, University of Groningen, Hanzeplein 1, 9713 GZ Groningen, The Netherlands
m.hadders-algra@med.umcg.nl

Summary

During the past decade, knowledge about brain development has increased substantially. Concurrently, insight into the epigenetic cascades governing motor development – that is, the complex interactions between genetically based and environmentally driven processes – has deepened. In particular the ideas contained in the Neuronal Group Selection Theory (NGST) have proven helpful in gaining an understanding of the mechanisms directing developmental motor disorders, such as cerebral palsy and developmental coordination disorder.

According to the NGST, normal motor development is characterized by two phases of variability. The variation is not random, but determined by criteria set by genetic information. Development starts with the phase of primary variability, during which variation in motor behaviour is not geared to external conditions. Next, the phase of secondary variability takes over, during which motor performance can be adapted to specific situations – that is, when the child learns to select the best motor solution for each situation on the basis of afferent information resulting from self-produced motor behaviour.

According to the NGST, children with developmental motor problems caused by a prenatally or perinatally acquired brain lesion suffer from stereotyped motor behaviour produced by a limited repertoire of (sub)cortical neuronal networks. In addition, children with an early lesion of the brain have problems with the selection of the most appropriately adapted strategy from the repertoire. The deficient capacity to select has a dual origin: it is related to deficits in the processing of sensory information and to the fact that the best solution may not be available because of repertoire reduction.

Introduction

During the last century, knowledge about mechanisms governing the functions of the central nervous system increased rapidly. This expansion in knowledge was brought about by the development of sophisticated genetic, physiological, neurochemical, and imaging techniques. In the field of motor control the augmented understanding of neurophysiology resulted in a gradual shift from the concept that motor behaviour is largely controlled by reflex mechanisms (Sherrington, 1906; Magnus & De Kleijn, 1912) towards the notion that motility is the net result of the activity of complex spinal or brain stem systems, which are subtly modulated by segmental afferent information and ingeniously controlled by supraspinal networks (Grillner et al., 1995; 2005). Essential elements in the reflex-based concepts of motor control are, first, that sensory input is essential for the generation of motor output, and second, that specific forms of input – acting through specific neural pathways ('reflex chains') – result in particular types of motor behaviour. Nowadays, it is realized that a fundamental feature of neural tissue is its ability to generate spontaneous, patterned activity (Droge et al., 1986; O'Donovan, 1999). In other words, motor behaviour may emerge in the absence of a sensory stimulus. In addition, it is currently recognized that motor behaviour is the net product of continuous interaction of multiple networks in which various neural pathways may mediate a motor action.

A good example of how motor control is organized is the control of rhythmic movements like locomotion, respiration, sucking, and mastication. The control of these movements is based on so-called central pattern generators (CPGs). CPGs are neural networks, usually located in the spinal cord or brain stem, which are able to coordinate the activity of many muscles autonomously – that is, without segmental sensory or supraspinal information. Of course, in typical conditions the CPG network does not work autonomously but is affected by segmental afferent signals and by information from cortical-subcortical circuitries. Activity in the latter is organized in large-scale networks in which cortical areas are functionally connected through direct recursive interaction or through intermediary cortical or subcortical (striatal, cerebellar) structures (Bressler, 1995; Hikosaka et al., 2002; Molinari et al., 2002). The cortical-subcortical networks expanded substantially during phylogeny and determine to a large extent human motor ontogeny.

Concurrently with the changes in insight into the neural mechanisms involved in motor control, knowledge about motor development has increased, if at a considerably slower pace. This has led to changes in the theoretical frameworks of the processes involved in the development of motor control. Initially, motor development was regarded as an innate, maturational process, but gradually it became clear that motor development is also affected considerably by experience. The Neuronal Group Selection Theory (NGST) is a recently developed theory allowing equally prominent roles for genetic endowment, epigenetic cascades, and experience, and thus might offer an excellent framework for the understanding of motor development (Edelman, 1989; 1993).

Neuronal group selection theory (NGST)

NGST and typical motor development

According to the NGST, motor development is characterized by two phases of variability: primary and secondary (Hadders-Algra, 2000a). The borders of variation are determined by genetic information, genetic instructions being the major driving forces behind the functional topography of the human brain (Krubitzer & Kaas, 2005). During the phase of primary variability, motor behaviour is characterized by abundant variation. Movement variation emerges early during fetal life, at 9 to 10 weeks' postmenstrual age. At that age, general movements – the most frequently used movement pattern in fetal and neonatal life – start to show variation and complexity (Lüchinger et al., 2008). The emergence of movement variation coincides with the emergence of synaptic activity in the cortical subplate (Molliver et al., 1973). The subplate, which is the earliest maturing cortical structure, is a transient structure lying between the intermediate zone – that is, the periventricular white matter – and the developing cortical plate (Kostovic & Rakic, 1990; Kostovic & Judas, 2006). The finding of the coincidence of the emergence of synaptic activity in the subplate and the emergence of movement variation inspired the hypothesis that variation of general movements is induced by the subplate. This means that movements of all parts of the body are brought about by the CPG networks in the spinal cord and brain stem, and that movement variation is the result of modulation of the CPG networks by activity of the cortical subplate (Hadders-Algra, 2007). Thus it seems that movement variation is brought about by exploratory activity of supraspinal networks, in which the subplate plays a crucial role during early phases of development. The networks explore all motor possibilities. The exploration generates a wealth of self-produced afferent information, which in turn is used for further shaping of the nervous system. Initially, however, the afferent information is not used for adaptation of motor behaviour to environmental constraints. In other words, the phase of primary variability is characterized by variable but non-adaptive motor behaviour (Hadders-Algra, 2000a).

At a certain point in time, the nervous system starts to use the afferent information produced by behaviour and experience for selection of the motor behaviour which fits the situation best: the phase of secondary or adaptive variability starts. The selection process is based on active trial-and-error experiences. Indeed, evidence is accumulating that self-produced sensorimotor experience plays a pivotal role in motor development (Bertenthal *et al.*, 1994; Higgins *et al.*, 1996).

The transition from primary to secondary variability occurs at function-specific ages. For instance, in the development of sucking behaviour the phase of secondary variability starts before full term, and in the development of foot placing during walking it starts between 12 and 18 months (Hadders-Algra, 2000a). Around the age of 18 months all basic motor functions have reached the first stages of secondary variability. Owing to the ingenious interaction between self-produced motor activities with trial-and-error learning and the long-lasting developmental processes in the brain – such as dendritic refinement, myelination, and extensive synapse rearrangement (De Graaf-Peters & Hadders-Algra, 2006) – it takes until the age of 18 to 20 years before the secondary neural repertoire has obtained its mature adult configuration. In the adult situation, human beings are equipped with a variable movement repertoire providing an efficient motor solution for each specific situation.

Motor development after a prenatal or perinatal lesion of the brain

A prenatal or perinatal lesion of the brain may be followed by atypical motor development, which can result in cerebral palsy or developmental coordination disorder. Note, however, that in general developmental coordination disorder cannot be attributed to a lesion of the brain (Hadders-Algra, 2002).

In terms of NGST, an early lesion of the brain has two major consequences (Hadders-Algra, 2000b). First, the repertoire of motor strategies is reduced. This results in less variable and more stereotyped motor behaviour. This is, for instance, very well reflected in the general movements of infants with a lesion of the brain (Prechtl *et al.*, 1997; Hadders-Algra, 2004). Recently it was shown that the presence of definitely abnormal general movements at 2 to 4 months of corrected age – that is, the presence of general movements which are virtually devoid of movement variation – is related in particular to lesions of the periventricular white matter (the area through which the motor efferents of the subplate run) (Hadders-Algra, 2007).

Children with an early lesion of the brain also have problems with the selection of the most appropriately adapted strategy from the repertoire. The deficient capacity for selection has a dual origin: it is related to deficits in the processing of sensory information, and it is related to the fact that the best solution may not be available owing to repertoire reduction.

The practical consequences of these problems are twofold. First, the limited motor repertoire may result in the absence of a specific motor strategy, which would be available as the best solution in a specific situation for a typically developing child. As a consequence of the absence of the 'best' solution, the child with an early lesion of the brain may have to choose a motor solution which differs from that of the typically developing child. Thus the different motor behaviour of a child with cerebral palsy should not always be regarded as deviant – that is, something which deserves to be 'treated away' – as it may be the child's best and most adaptive solution for the situation (Latash & Anson, 1996). Second, owing to the deficits in the processing of sensory information, which hamper the process of selection of the best strategy, children with an early lesion of the brain need a 10- or a 100-fold more active motor experience than typically developing children (Valvano & Newell, 1998). As children with brain dysfunction need more practice than their non-affected peers, it is important to reinforce the child's motivation by creating an ecological, playful setting with positive feedback.

Conclusions

According to the NGST, variation is the keyword of typical motor development. The variation is not random, but is determined by criteria set by genetic information. The variation has two forms: primary variability not geared to external conditions and secondary variability, in which motor performance can be adapted to specific situations.

Children with prenatally or perinatally acquired lesions of the brain, such as those with cerebral palsy and some children with developmental coordination disorder, suffer from stereotyped motor behaviour produced by a limited repertoire of the (sub)cortical neuronal networks. In addition, children with an early lesion of the brain have problems with the selection of the most appropriately adapted strategy out of the repertoire.

The above-mentioned principles of typical and atypical motor development might be helpful in diagnostics and intervention in children with developmental motor problems. Evaluation of the size of the child's motor repertoire – for instance, in young infants by means of the assessment of the quality of general movements (Hadders-Algra, 2004) and in older infants using the recently developed Infant Motor Profile (IMP, Heineman *et al.*, 2008) – may provide insight into the child's abilities and inabilities. Evaluation of children's ability to select the best motor strategy from their repertoire – a technique also applied in the IMP – may provide an indication of the amount of practice needed before a certain task is mastered. For intervention, the principles of the NGST suggest that the different motor behaviour of a child with a prenatal or perinatally acquired lesion of the brain should not immediately be regarded as deviant – that is, something which deserves to be 'treated away' – as it may be the child's best and most adaptive solution for the situation. In addition, NGST indicates that children with an early lesion of the brain need much more active motor experience than typically developing children. This stresses the need for practice in a motivating situation.

References

Bertenthal, B.I., Campos, J.J. & Kermoian, R. (1994): An epigenetic perspective on the development of self-produced locomotion and its consequences. *Curr. Dir. Psychol. Sci.* **3**, 141–145.

Bressler, S.L. (1995): Large scale cortical networks and cognition. *Brain Res. Rev.* **20**, 288–304.

De Graaf-Peters, V.B. & Hadders-Algra, M. (2006): Ontogeny of the human central nervous system: what is happening when? *Early Hum. Dev.* **82**, 257–266.

Droge, M.H., Gross, G.W., Hightower, M.H. & Czisny, L.E. (1986): Multielectrode analysis of coordinated, multisite, rhythmic bursting in cultured CNS monolayer networks. *J. Neurosci.* **6**, 1583–1592.

Edelman, G.M. (1989): *Neural Darwinism. The theory of neuronal group selection.* Oxford: Oxford University Press.

Edelman, G.M. (1993): Neural Darwinism: selection and reentrant signalling in higher brain function. *Neuron* **10**, 115–125.

Grillner, S., Deliagina, T.G., Ekeberg, O., El Manira, A., Hill, R.H., Lansner, A., Orlovsky, G.N. & Wallen, P. (1995): Neural networks that co-ordinate locomotion and body orientation in lamprey. *Trends Neurosci.* **18**, 270–279.

Grillner, S., Hellgren, J., Ménard, A., Saitoh, K. & Wikström, M.A. (2005): Mechanisms for selection of basic motor programs – roles for the striatum and pallidum. *Trends Neurosci.* **28**, 364–370.

Hadders-Algra, M. (2000a): The Neuronal Group Selection Theory: an attractive framework to explain variation in normal motor development. *Dev. Med. Child Neurol.* **42**, 566–572.

Hadders-Algra, M. (2000b): The Neuronal Group Selection Theory: promising principles for understanding and treating developmental motor disorders. *Dev. Med. Child Neurol.* **42**, 707–715.

Hadders-Algra, M. (2002): Two distinct forms of minor neurological dysfunction: perspectives emerging from a review of data of the Groningen Perinatal Project. *Dev. Med. Child Neurol.* **44**, 561–571.

Hadders-Algra, M. (2004): General movements: a window for early identification of children at high risk of developmental disorders. *J. Pediatr.* **145**, S12–S18.

Hadders-Algra, M. (2007): Putative neural substrate of normal and abnormal general movements. *Neurosci. Biobehav. Rev.* **31**, 1181–1190.

Heineman, K.R., Bos, A.F. & Hadders-Algra, M. (2008): The Infant Motor Profile: a standardized and qualitative method to assess motor behaviour in infancy. *Dev. Med. Child Neurol.* **50**, 275–282.

Higgins, C.I., Campos, J.J. & Kermoian, R. (1996): Effect of self-produced locomotion on infant postural compensation to optic flow. *Dev. Psychol.* **32**, 836–841.

Hikosaka, O., Makamura, K., Sakai, K. & Nakahara, H. (2002): Central mechanisms of motor skill learning. *Curr. Opin. Neurobiol.* **12**, 217–222.

Kostovic, I. & Rakic, P. (1990): Developmental history of the transient subplate zone in the visual and somatosensory cortex of the macaque monkey and human brain. *J. Comp. Neurol.* **297**, 441–470.

Kostovic, I. & Judas, M. (2006): Prolonged coexistence of transient and permanent circuitry elements in the developing cerebral cortex of fetuses and preterm infants. *Dev. Med. Child Neurol.* **48**, 388–393.

Krubitzer, L. & Kaas, J. (2005): The evolution of the neocortex in mammals: how is phenotypic diversity generated? *Curr. Opin. Neurobiol.* **15**, 444–453.

Latash, M.L. & Anson, J.G. (1996): What are 'normal movements' in atypical populations? *Behav. Brain Sci.* **19**, 55–68.

Lüchinger, A.B., Hadders-Algra, M., Van Kan, C.M. & De Vries, J.I.P. (2008): Fetal onset of general movements. *Pediatr. Res.* **63**, 191–195.

Magnus, R. & De Kleijn, A. (1912): Die abhängigkeit des Tonus der Extremitätenmuskeln von der Kopfstellung. *Pflüger's Arch.* **145**, 455–548.

Molinari, M., Filippini, V. & Leggio, M.G. (2002): Neuronal plasticity of the interrelated cerebellar and cortical networks. *Neuroscience* **111**, 863–870.

Molliver, M.E., Kostovic, I. & Van der Loos, H. (1973): Development of synapses in cerebral cortex of the human foetus. *Brain Res.* **50**, 403–407.

O'Donovan, M.J. (1999): The origin of spontaneous activity in developing networks of the vertebrate nervous system. *Curr. Opin. Neurobiol.* **9**, 94–104.

Prechtl, H.F.R., Einspieler, C., Cioni, G., Bos, A.F., Ferrari, F. & Sontheimer, D. (1997): An early marker of developing neurological handicap after perinatal brain lesions. *Lancet* **339**, 1361–1363.

Sherrington, C.S. (1906): The physiological position and dominance of the brain. In: *The integrative action of the nervous system,* ed. C.S. Sherrington, pp. 308–353. London: Constable.

Valvano, J. & Newell, K.M. (1998): Practice of a precision isometric grip-force task by children with spastic cerebral palsy. *Dev. Med. Child Neurol.* **40**, 464–473.

Chapter 20

Brain plasticity in newborn infants with brain lesions: the role of brain MRI

Eugenio Mercuri * °, Daniela Ricci * ° and Frances Cowan °

* Division of Child Neurology, Catholic University, Largo Gemelli, 00168 Rome, Italy;
° Departments of Paediatrics and Imaging Sciences, Imperial College Hammersmith Hospital, London, UK
mercuri@rm.unicatt.it

Summary

The concept of neonatal brain plasticity is relatively new for clinicians. We review our experience on how the use of an integrated clinical and magnetic resonance imaging (MRI) approach in infants with neonatal brain lesions can detect evidence of brain plasticity by identifying early prognostic signs of outcome and other markers that may enhance or reduce plasticity. In our experience even relatively large lesions have a greater chance of being associated with a relatively good outcome if they occur around term age and when there is no or little concomitant involvement of subcortical structures. Other variables such as the presence of early epilepsy or male sex appear to reduce the chances of brain plasticity.

Introduction

Brain plasticity refers to the brain's ability to adapt and change over time and in response to insults or environmental challenges. Several studies have described different possible mechanisms of brain plasticity in animal models, reporting how the brain can reorganize patterns of connectivity to recover from or compensate for injury incurred during development (Perretto *et al.*, 1999; Kitagawa *et al.*, 2001) by, for example, increasing neurogenesis and synaptogenesis or reorganizing existing circuitry (Alvarez-Buylla *et al.*, 2000; Hitoshi *et al.*, 2002; Rossini & Dal Forno, 2004).

The concept of neonatal brain plasticity is, however, relatively new for clinicians. Following the introduction of the routine use of cranial ultrasound, and more recently of brain magnetic resonance imaging (MRI), in newborns at risk of neurological abnormalities – such as term infants with neonatal encephalopathy or those born prematurely – there has been a sharp increase in the identification of neonatal brain lesions in the past 25 years. Clinical follow-up of these infants has revealed that not all neonates with lesions have an abnormal outcome and that neurological sequelae, when present, may seem disproportionate to the size and extent of the lesion, and are usually less severe than anticipated.

Neonates with relatively large focal lesions affecting language, motor, or visual areas may not show the functional impairment expected from experience in adults with similar lesions or from outcomes observed in experimental animal models (Staudt et al., 2002; Johansson, 2004; Fair et al., 2006; Jacobs et al., 2007; Kaas et al., 2007).

Brain plasticity is often proposed as an explanation for the usually better than expected outcome found in many neonates with brain injury of perinatal timing, with the implication that the neonatal brain is able to move functions to unaffected areas or to maintain connections that would usually be lost in the course of normal maturation and development (Lomber & Payne, 2001; Eyre, 2003; Yoshimura et al., 2003; Hensch, 2005; Seghier et al., 2006; Poo & Isaacson, 2007). Although it seems plausible that plasticity and reorganization of synaptic connections may occur in newborns, at a time when these are still being refined and modelled, the mechanisms underlying the processes of recovery from injury, the possible regeneration of nerve cells, and reconstruction and maintenance of circuitries are still unclear.

In the past few years the advent of newer MRI and electrophysiological techniques and more detailed clinical follow-up have significantly improved our knowledge of the correlations between lesions and functional impairment and of how to detect signs of possible reorganization of the neonatal brain following antenatal or perinatal lesions (Rutherford et al., 1997; Rutten et al., 2002; Krägeloh-Mann, 2004; Rutherford et al., 2005; Kostovic & Judas, 2006). In this chapter we will review our experience on how the use of an integrated clinical and MRI approach can help to detect evidence of brain plasticity by identifying early prognostic signs of outcome or other markers that may enhance or reduce plasticity in the neonatal brain.

Site and extent of the lesion on neonatal MRI as predictors of outcome

The study of focal, especially unilateral, lesions provides an excellent paradigm for studying the correlation between structure and function. In term-born infants the commonest focal unilateral brain lesions are strokes or ischaemic infarction caused by embolic or thrombotic events in an arterial distribution; the next commonest types of lesions are focal parenchymal haemorrhages.

While in the past neonatal strokes or other focal lesions were mainly diagnosed retrospectively in children who presented with hemiplegia or epilepsy, it is now well accepted that these lesions often occur in infants with normal Apgar scores and normal neurological examination at birth, who have convulsions within 2 to 3 days after birth. Follow-up of cohorts of infants with such neonatal diagnoses have shown that, although these lesions usually affect the motor areas, the incidence of contralateral hemiplegia is as low as 30 per cent (Mercuri et al., 2004a). At variance with what is reported in adults, the presence of hemiplegia is not therefore always related to the extent of the cortical involvement, and we have been able to show that the only children who develop hemiplegia are those who have concomitant involvement of the cerebral cortex, internal capsule, and basal ganglia (Mercuri et al., 1999). These findings, originally observed in a cohort of 24 infants followed for up to 2 years, have recently been updated and confirmed in a much larger cohort (previously unpublished data in Table 1) at 2 years and at school age (Mercuri et al., 2004a).

These findings are at variance with animal models of stroke and with studies in adults with similar lesions who have a much higher incidence of hemiplegia. In our cohort the abnormal outcome was not always related to the extent of cortical involvement, but the concomitant involvement of subcortical structures including the internal capsule appears to reduce the possibility that other areas of the brain may take over the function of the damaged area (Fig. 1).

Chapter 20 Brain plasticity in newborn infants with brain lesions: the role of brain MRI

Table 1. Comparison between MRI findings and motor outcome in infants with neonatal stroke (n = 47)

	n	Asymmetry	Hemiplegia
Hemispheric tissue only	19	–	–
Hemisphere and basal ganglia	5	–	–
Hemisphere and internal capsule	4	–	–
Basal ganglia and internal capsule	4	–	–
Hemisphere, basal ganglia, and internal capsule	2	2	13

MRI, magnetic resonance imaging.

Similar findings can also be observed in newborns with more diffuse lesions, such as those suffering from neonatal encephalopathy with low Apgar scores. In a cohort of 68 patients followed longitudinally from birth until school age (Barnett et al., 2002), we found that the severity of the motor outcome was not always related to the extent of cortical and white matter damage but rather to the severity of the concomitant involvement of the basal ganglia and thalami. More specifically, patients with diffuse bilateral white matter/cortical changes but with spared central grey matter had less severe motor sequelae than those with concomitant involvement of the basal ganglia, who often had mental retardation and severe dystonic cerebral palsy, and usually never achieved the ability to sit unsupported.

This holds true also for other aspects of development such as visual and perceptual abilities. Bilateral diffuse lesions involving both primary visual cortices and the optic radiations were not always associated with abnormal visual function if the lesions were localized in the hemispheric cortex and white matter and did not involve the basal ganglia and thalami (BGT). In contrast infants with concomitant involvement of cortex and BGT always had severe abnormalities of visual function (Mercuri et al., 1997) which persisted at school age (Mercuri et al., 2004b).

One of the possible hypotheses advocated to explain these findings is that the BGT, with their rich network of connections to different cortical areas and other subcortical structures, may represent a crucial centre that allows exchange of information from the affected cortex to other areas that may take over the function of the damaged area. An interruption of this network would therefore strongly reduce the chances of brain plasticity.

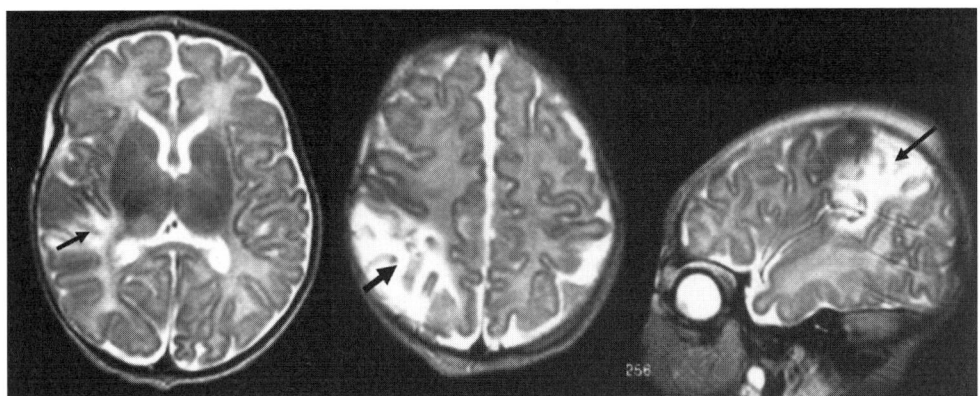

Fig. 1. Neonatal brain MRI showing left posterior branch MCA infarction with normal basal ganglia and PLIC. The child developed no hemiplegia.

Timing of the lesion: neonatal *vs.* acquired lesions

The findings reported so far are related mainly to infants with focal or diffuse neonatal lesions caused by perinatal insults, as demonstrated by early and serial brain MRI. The concomitant involvement of subcortical structures appears to be relevant in this cohort but does not always explain the variability in outcome in patients with similar lesions, so other variables should be taken into account.

Comparing the neonatal stroke data with other published data in older children or adult patients with similar lesions that were, however, acquired after the neonatal period, it is obvious that the incidence of hemiplegia in acquired strokes is much higher than in neonatal strokes, and that the timing of the insult appears to play a significant role in determining the outcome. We recently compared our neonatal MRI data with those collected in older children with acquired strokes, mainly caused by lesions in the middle cerebral artery territory (Boardman *et al.*, 2005). Hemiparesis was more common after childhood onset stroke (56 per cent) than in those with neonatal onset (24 per cent), with lesions matched for site and extent. In children with neonatal onset, concomitant involvement of basal ganglia, cerebral cortex and internal capsule predicts the development of hemiparesis, while no child with only one or two of these structures involved developed hemiparesis (Table 2). In contrast, in childhood onset this adverse outcome was seen also among patients with only one- or two-site involvement.

Table 2. Comparison of outcome in neonatal and childhood stroke

	Neonatal	Childhood
Infarct site(s)	Number with hemiparesis / total number with lesion distribution	Number with hemiparesis / total number with lesion distribution
BG & CC & PLIC	7/8	9/11
BG & CC	0/2	5/6
BG only	0/3	4/13
PLIC & CC	0/3	0/0
CC only	0/12	1/2
BG & PLIC	0/0	5/11
Total	7/28	24/43

BG, basal ganglia; CC, cerebral cortex; PLIC, posterior limbs of the internal capsule.

Timing of the lesion: perinatal *vs.* antenatal

The advent of new MRI techniques, such as diffusion weighted imaging (DWI), has helped us to a better understanding of the timing and the evolution of neonatal lesions, and has enabled us to investigate the association between the timing of the lesion and the outcome in infants who have lesions on the neonatal scans but in whom the insults may have also occurred prenatally. In our own cohort of infants with neonatal stroke the great majority of lesions had occurred perinatally, showing a typical MRI pattern that can be detected using early and serial conventional MRI and DWI. Early brain changes may be difficult to visualize on early scans done soon after the onset of seizures but are best visualized on DWI, which highlights the infarcted areas. The abnormalities on DWI become less obvious by the end of the first week, by which time the abnormalities are more obvious on the conventional T1- and T2-weighted imaging.

In infants with evidence of perinatal lesions, signs of Wallerian degeneration are generally not obvious on the early scans, and are usually more obvious on the follow-up scans done after at least 6 weeks. DWI can better identify early signs of Wallerian degeneration (de Vries et al., 2005).

In our cohort only a few children had infarcts occurring before term age with clear signs of Wallerian degeneration on the early scans and they all had a different evolution of clinical signs and a more severe outcome compared to those with perinatal lesions. While the term infants with perinatal lesions who developed hemiplegia showed minimal signs of asymmetry of tone and movements in the first months, and signs of increased flexor tone in the arms were only obvious after 6 months, in the two children with antenatal lesions flexion of the arm was already present before 3 months after term age. One of the two also developed West syndrome which is not frequent in infants with focal neonatal stroke. Antenatal lesions were therefore not only associated with a more severe outcome but the abnormal clinical signs occurred earlier than generally observed in infants with similar lesions occurring in the perinatal period.

Preterm infants

The previous findings suggest that lesions occurring antenatally or in preterm infants before term age have a greater chance of being associated with an abnormal outcome than when the same lesions occur perinatally in term infants. In preterm infants, however, the pattern of lesions is often different from those described in full term infants with neonatal encephalopathy.

Most of the studies correlating imaging and outcome in preterm infants are based mainly on cranial ultrasound findings but a few recent studies have reported the value of brain MRI.

There are fewer systematic studies establishing plasticity in preterm infants. Cystic periventricular leucomalacia (PVL), which has recently become much less frequent, is generally associated with cerebral palsy, the severity of which increases according to the extent and the site of the lesion. Almost all infants with grade III PVL develop cerebral palsy and only a small percentage achieve independent walking. Most of the infants with grade II PVL also develop cerebral palsy but it is less severe and they often achieved independent walking (Ricci et al., 2006a). In addition, some of these infants can have a normal outcome. Grade II PVL is often unilateral while grade III always shows bilateral cysts, frequently located in the parieto-occipital periventricular white matter (Pierrat et al., 2001). It is noteworthy that even when the posterior limb of the internal capsule is not involved, motor outcome is usually poor, suggesting less plasticity in preterm infants than in term infants with similar bilateral white matter injury.

Several studies in infants with PVL have shown a significant correlation between the impairment of optic radiations and abnormal visual function: the severity of visual impairment appeared to be correlated with the severity of the involvement of optic radiations (Cioni et al., 1997; Lanzi et al., 1998; Fazzi et al., 2004) but we have recently reported that, as observed in full term infants with neonatal encephalopathy, the concomitant involvement of the thalami was always associated with the most severe visual abnormalities (Ricci et al., 2006b).

Other variables

Combined clinical and imaging studies have also suggested that, although the extent and the timing of the lesion may allow one to identify early markers of plasticity, other clinical variables should be considered. The role of early epilepsy as an additional risk factor for abnormal neurodevelopmental outcome has been reported for both preterm and full term infants. In full term infants with encephalopathy, the presence of epilepsy in the first two years was always associated with abnormal outcome, irrespective of the extent of the lesion (Mercuri et al., 1998). There are similar findings in full term and preterm infants with antenatal post-haemorrhagic ventricular dilatation (Ricci et al., 2007).

Conclusions

Brain MRI appears to provide important prognostic information and can often identify markers of plasticity of the brain. In our experience even relatively large lesions have a greater chance of being associated with a relatively good outcome when occurring around term age and when there is no or little concomitant involvement of subcortical structures. Other variables such as the presence of early epilepsy or male sex appear to reduce the chances of brain plasticity. Structural brain MRI is therefore a valuable tool in identifying early indicators of possible plasticity but has a limited value in identifying the mechanisms underlying it. Newer techniques such as functional MRI (fMRI), tractography, and magnetoencephalography (MEG) may allow a better understanding of how these children cope with their lesions. Such studies are important both for recognizing the difficulties these children have and for designing time-appropriate interventions and coping strategies.

References

Alvarez-Buylla, A., Herrera, D.G. & Wichterle, H. (2000): The subventricular zone: source of neuronal precursors for brain repair. *Prog. Brain Res.* **127**, 1–11.

Barnett, A., Mercuri, E., Rutherford, M., Haataja, L., Frisone, M.F., Henderson, S., Cowan, F. & Dubowitz, L. (2002): Neurological and perceptual-motor outcome at 5–6 years of age in children with neonatal encephalopathy: relationship with neonatal brain MRI. *Neuropediatrics* **33**, 242–248.

Boardman, J.P., Ganesan, V., Rutherford, M.A., Saunders, D.E., Mercuri, E. & Cowan, F. (2005): Magnetic resonance image correlates of hemiparesis after neonatal and childhood middle cerebral artery stroke. *Pediatrics* **115**, 321–326.

Cioni, G., Fazzi, B., Coluccini, M., Bartalena, L., Boldrini, A. & van Hof-van Duin, J. (1997): Cerebral visual impairment in preterm infants with periventricular leucomalacia. *Pediatr. Neurol.* **17**, 331–338.

de Vries, L.S., Van der Grond, J., Van Haastert, I.C. & Groenendaal, F. (2005): Prediction of outcome in new-born infants with arterial ischaemic stroke using diffusion-weighted magnetic resonance imaging. *Neuropediatrics* **36**, 12–20.

Eyre, J.A. (2003): Development and plasticity of the corticospinal system in man. *Neural Plast.* **10**, 93–106.

Fair, D.A., Brown, T.T., Petersen, S.E. & Schlaggar, B.L. (2006): fMRI reveals novel functional neuroanatomy in a child with perinatal stroke. *Neurology* **67**, 2246–2249.

Fazzi, E., Bova, S.M., Uggetti, C., Signorini, S.G., Bianchi, P.E., Maraucci, I., Zoppello, M. & Lanzi, G. (2004): Visual-perceptual impairment in children with periventricular leucomalacia. *Brain Dev.* **26**, 506–512.

Hensch, T.K. (2005): Critical period plasticity in local cortical circuits. *Nat. Rev. Neurosci.* **6**, 877–888.

Hitoshi, S., Tropepe, V., Ekker, M. & van der Koov, D. (2002): Neural stem cell lineages are regionally specified, but not committed, within distinct compartments of the developing brain. *Development* **129**, 233–244.

Jacobs, R., Harvey, A.S. & Anderson, V. (2007): Executive function following focal frontal lobe lesions: impact of timing of lesion on outcome. *Cortex* **43**, 792–805.

Johansson, B.B. (2004): Brain plasticity in health and disease. *Keio J. Med.* **53**, 231–246.

Kaas, J.H., Qi, H.X., Burish, M.J., Gharbawie, O.A., Onifer, S.M. & Massey, J.M. (2007): Cortical and subcortical plasticity in the brains of humans, primates, and rats after damage to sensory afferents in the dorsal columns of the spinal cord. *Exp. Neurol.* **6** [Epub ahead of print].

Kitagawa, K., Matsumotor, M. & Hori, M. (2001): Protective and regenerative response endogenously induced in the ischemic brain. *Can. J. Physiol. Pharmacol.* **79**, 262–265.

Kostovic, I. & Judas, M. (2006): Prolonged coexistence of transient and permanent circuitry elements in the developing cerebral cortex of fetuses and preterm infants. *Dev. Med. Child. Neurol.* **48,** 388–393.

Krägeloh-Mann, I. (2004): Imaging of early brain injury and cortical plasticity. *Exp. Neurol.* **190,** S84–S90.

Lanzi, G., Fazzi, E., Uggetti, C., Cavallini, A., Danova, S., Egitto, M.G., Ginevra, O.F., Salati, R. & Bianchi, P.E. (1998): Cerebral visual impairment in periventricular leucomalacia. *Neuropediatrics* **29,** 145–150.

Lomber, S.G. & Payne, B.R. (2001): Perinatal-lesion-induced reorganization of cerebral functions revealed using reversible cooling deactivation and attentional tasks. *Cereb. Cortex* **11,** 194–209.

Mercuri, E., Atkinson, J., Braddick, O., Anker, S., Cowan, F., Rutherford, M., Pennock, J. & Dubowitz, L. (1997): Visual function in full-term infants with hypoxic-ischaemic encephalopathy. *Neuropediatrics* **28,** 155–161.

Mercuri, E., Braddick, O., Atkinson, J., Cowan, F., Anker, S., Andrew, R., Wattam-Bell, J., Rutherford, M., Counsell, S. & Dubowitz, L. (1998): Orientation-reversal and phase-reversal visual evoked potentials in full-term infants with brain lesions: a longitudinal study. *Neuropediatrics* **29,** 169–174.

Mercuri, E., Rutherford, M., Cowan, F., Pennock, J., Counsell, S., Papadimitriou, M., Azzopardi, D., Bydder, G. & Dubowitz, L. (1999): Early prognostic indicators of outcome in infants with neonatal cerebral infarction: a clinical, electroencephalogram, and magnetic resonance imaging study. *Pediatrics* **103,** 39–46.

Mercuri, E., Barnett, A., Rutherford, M., Guzzetta, A., Haataja, L., Cioni, G., Cowan, F. & Dubowitz, L. (2004a): Neonatal cerebral infarction and neuromotor outcome at school age. *Pediatrics* **113,** 95–100.

Mercuri, E., Anker, S., Guzzetta, A., Barnett, A.L., Haataja, L., Rutherford, M., Cowan, F., Dubowitz, L., Braddick, O. & Atkinson, J. (2004b): Visual function at school age in children with neonatal encephalopathy and low Apgar scores. *Arch. Dis. Child. Fetal Neonat. Ed.* **89,** F258–F262.

Peretto, P., Merighi, A., Fasolo, A. & Bonfanti, L. (1999): The subependymal layer in rodents: a site of structural plasticity and cell migration in the adult mammalian brain. *Brain Res. Bull.* **49,** 221–243.

Pierrat, V., Duquennoy, C., van Haastert, I.C., Ernst, M., Guilley, N. & de Vries, L.S. (2001): Ultrasound diagnosis and neurodevelopmental outcome of localised and extensive cystic periventricular leucomalacia. *Arch. Dis. Child. Fetal Neonat. Ed.* **84,** F151–F156.

Poo, C. & Isaacson, J.S. (2007): An early critical period for long-term plasticity and structural modification of sensory synapses in olfactory cortex. *J. Neurosci.* **27,** 7553–7558.

Ricci, D., Cowan, F., Pane, M., Gallini, F., Haataja, L., Luciano, R., Cesarini, L., Leone, D., Donvito, V., Baranello, G., Rutherford, M., Romagnoli, C., Dubowitz, L. & Mercuri, E. (2006a): Neurological examination at 6 to 9 months in infants with cystic periventricular leucomalacia. *Neuropediatrics* **37,** 247–252.

Ricci, D., Anker, S., Cowan, F., Pane, M., Gallini, F., Luciano, R., Donvito, V., Baranello, G., Cesarini, L., Bianco, F., Rutherford, M., Romagnoli, C., Atkinson, J., Braddick, O., Guzzetta, F. & Mercuri, E. (2006b): Thalamic atrophy in infants with PVL and cerebral visual impairment. *Early Hum. Dev.* **82,** 591–595.

Ricci, D., Luciano, R., Baranello, G., Veredice, C., Cesarini, L., Bianco, F., Pane, M., Gallini, F., Vasco, G., Savarese, I., Zuppa, A.A., Masini, L., Di Rocco, C., Romagnoli, C., Guzzetta, F. & Mercuri, E. (2007): Visual development in infants with prenatal post-haemorrhagic ventricular dilatation. *Arch. Dis. Child. Fetal Neonat. Ed.* **92,** F255–F258.

Rossini, P.M. & Dal Forno, G. (2004): Integrated technology for evaluation of brain function and neural plasticity. *Phys. Med. Rehabil. Clin. North Am.* **15,** 263–306.

Rutherford, M.A., Pennock, J.M., Cowan, F.M., Dubowitz, L.M., Hajnal, J.V. & Bydder, G.M. (1997): Does the brain regenerate after perinatal infarction? *Eur. J. Paediatr. Neurol.* **1,** 13–17.

Rutherford, M.A., Ward, P. & Malamatentiou, C. (2005): Advanced MR techniques in the term-born neonate with perinatal brain injury. *Semin. Fetal Neonat. Med.* **10,** 445–460.

Rutten, G.J., Ramsey, N.F., van Rijen, P.C., Franssen, H. & van Veelen, C.W. (2002): Interhemispheric reorganization of motor hand function to the primary motor cortex predicted with functional magnetic resonance imaging and transcranial magnetic stimulation. *J. Child Neurol.* **17,** 292–297.

Seghier, M.L., Lazeyras, F. & Huppi, P.S. (2006): Functional MRI of the newborn. *Semin. Fetal Neonat. Med.* **11,** 479–488.

Staudt, M., Lidzba, K., Grodd, W., Wildgruber, D., Erb, M. & Krageloh-Mann, I. (2002): Right-hemispheric organization of language following early left-sided brain lesions: functional MRI topography. *Neuroimage* **16,** 954–967.

Yoshimura, Y., Ohmura, T. & Komatsu, Y. (2003): Two forms of synaptic plasticity with distinct dependence on age, experience, and NMDA receptor subtype in rat visual cortex. *J. Neurosci.* **23,** 6557–6566.

Chapter 21

Perinatal brain damage: from pathogenesis to neuroprotection

Géraldine Favrais * ° ^, Luigi Titomanlio * ° ¶, Vincent Degos * ° ^
and Pierre Gressens * ° ^ ¶

Inserm U676, Paris, France;
° *Université Paris 7, Faculté de Médecine Denis-Diderot, IFR02 and IFR25, Paris;*
^ *PremUp, Paris, France;*
¶ *AP-HP, Hôpital Robert Debré, Service de Neurologie Pédiatrique, 48 Blvd Sérurier, 75019 Paris, France*
pierre.gressens@inserm.fr

Summary

Human preterm infants are at risk of developing cerebral palsy and cognitive or behavioural impairments. The most recognized underlying brain lesion in preterm infants is periventricular white matter damage, which can be focal, multifocal, or diffuse. Periventricular leucomalacia is the best described type of periventricular white matter damage. Clinical, epidemiological, and experimental studies have demonstrated the multifactorial origin of these types of white matter damage in preterm infants, generating more than one potential target for neuroprotection. These studies have permitted some key factors to be unravelled, such as inflammation and excess production of cytokines, oxidative stress, hypoxic-ischaemic insults, excess release of glutamate, and the excitotoxic cascade. Animal models have also shown that pre-oligodendrocytes, macrophage-microglia, and sub-plate neurons are key cells in the pathophysiology of periventricular white matter damage. One key safety issue for potential neuroprotective strategies in premature infants is the demonstration of the lack of interference with normal brain development. Several neuroprotective approaches are currently tested in animal models of white matter damage, including drugs targeting glutamate receptors, drugs targeting inflammation, cytokines or macrophage activation, anti-oxidant molecules, and strategies such as growth factors and cell replacement aiming at improving post-lesional plasticity and tissue repair. Finally, some clinical trials using magnesium sulphate in preterm infants have been completed or are in progress, raising the hope that effective treatments will eventually be available to protect the newborn brain.

Introduction

The frequency of motor or cognitive handicaps linked to perinatal brain injury increased during the 1990s but currently seems to be remaining stable (Vincer *et al.*, 2006; Robertson *et al.*, 2007; Wilson-Costello *et al.*, 2007). These data can be explained by progress in the field of neonatal intensive care, leading to an increase in survival of very preterm neonates to nearly 70 per cent, but without significant improvement in their neurological outcome. Ten per cent of preterm neonates of birth weight less than 1,500 g later develop cerebral palsy, and about 50 per cent develop cognitive and behavioural deficits (Wilson-Costello *et al.*, 2005).

Periventricular white matter is preferentially affected in preterm infants, while cortico-subcortical lesions are observed after perinatal hypoxic-ischaemic insults in term babies. The incidence of hypoxic-ischaemic encephalopathy has remained essentially unchanged (Himmelmann *et al.*, 2005). Epidemiological and experimental studies highlight potential therapeutic targets, but there is a lack of pharmaceutical company investment in this domain because of lack of knowledge about the long-term effects of drugs, ethical dilemmas, and the cost and safety of clinical trials. Thus the prevention and treatment of these neurodevelopmental impairments remain a major challenge.

Pathogenesis of perinatal brain damage

Owing to epidemiologic and experimental studies, neonatal brain susceptibility to perinatal insults is well known. Periventricular white matter damage (PWMD) affects preterm neonates born between 23 and 32 weeks of gestation and follows successive pathological events from the prenatal to the postnatal period (Fig. 1). In parallel, brain lesions proceeding from acute hypoxia-ischaemia in term neonates involve an apoptotic/necrotic process, leading to early or delayed neuronal cell death in the grey matter, mainly at thalamic level (Perlman, 2007).

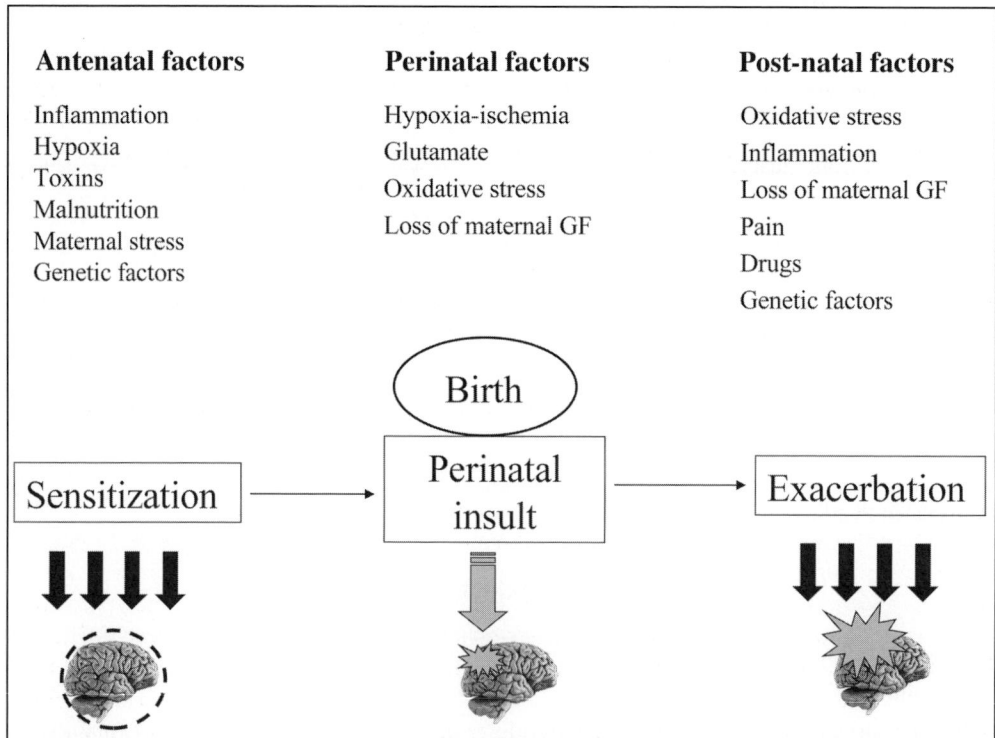

Fig. 1. Risk factors leading to the development of periventricular white matter damage. This schematic representation illustrates the multiple-hit hypothesis including pre-, peri-, and postnatal factors. GF, growth factor.

Pathophysiology of PWMD

PWMD comprises two histopathological forms, 'focal' and 'diffuse'. The focal form appears as necrotic cysts within the white matter. This subtype is now less often seen, because of improvements in neonatal care, and will not be considered in this review. The diffuse form is linked to premyelinating oligodendrocyte vulnerability and leads to a global myelination delay and deep grey matter damage (Volpe, 2001).

Premyelinating oligodendrocytes are the main component of white matter between 23 and 32 weeks' post-conceptional age. Findings from animal models show a maturation-dependent vulnerability of oligodendrocyte lineage to the detriment of premyelinating oligodendrocytes, acting through several cytotoxic pathways. Premyelinating oligodendrocytes are vulnerable to excitotoxic stress because of the presence on their surface of the glutamatergic receptors α-3-amino-hydroxy-5-methyl-4-isoxazole propionic acid (AMPA)-kainate (Follett *et al.*, 2000) and N-methyl-D-aspartate (NMDA) (Salter & Fern, 2005; Micu *et al.*, 2006). In parallel, at this developmental stage, premyelinating oligodendrocytes are the victims of oxidative stress because of a transient deficiency of the superoxide dismutase antioxidant enzymes, causing a lack of cellular defence against free-radical attacks (Kinney, 2006; Back *et al.*, 2007).

Moreover, a strong correlation between the increase in brain pro-inflammatory cytokines and PWMD development has been proven (Yoon *et al.*, 1997). *In vitro*, tumour necrosis factor α (TNFα) has a cytotoxic effect on oligodendrocytes (Feldhaus *et al.*, 2004), and interleukin 1β (IL-1β) disrupts physiological proliferative and maturational processes of the oligodendroglial lineage (Vela *et al.*, 2002). These pro-inflammatory cytokines are produced mainly by activated microglia, which is also involved in free radical synthesis (Pearson *et al.*, 1999). Microglia/macrophages can be activated by different stimuli including hypoxic-ischaemic insult, excitotoxic insult through transient NMDA receptor expression, and systemic infections through, for example, the toll-like receptor 4 (TLR) for *E. Coli* lipopolysaccharide (Olson & Miller, 2004).

In addition, a selective cell death of subplate neurons has been observed in experimental PWMD models, without any clear pathophysiological explanation at present. These subplate neurons play an important role in axonal guidance and cortical organization (McQuillen & Ferriero, 2004; Robinson *et al.*, 2006).

Up to a few years ago, PWMD was thought to result only from a hypoxic-ischaemic mechanism, caused by a decrease in cerebral blood flow and poor development of the vasculature (Volpe, 2001). However, it is now conceded that in animal models several risk factors are implicated and are frequently associated with PWMD pathogenesis. These comprise prenatal risk factors, such as inflammation/cytokine release and maternal stress; perinatal factors, such as hypoxic-ischaemic stimuli; and postnatal factors, such as growth factor deprivation, inflammation/cytokine release, drug side effects, and pain. Each can represent a potential neuroprotective target. Furthermore, a combination of noxious factors in experimental models has resulted in the emergence of a multiple-hit hypothesis, which consists of a sensitization state created by a mild first event, leading to an increased susceptibility to a second injury (Fig. 1). For example, in a mouse model of excitotoxic periventricular leucomalacia, exposure to pro-inflammatory cytokines (such as IL-1β, TNFα, or IL-6) did not produce detectable clastic brain lesions, while a similar cytokine pretreatment followed by a mild excitotoxic insult induced severe PWMD (Dommergues *et al.*, 2000).

Pathophysiology of hypoxic-ischaemic brain injury

In the pathophysiology of hypoxic-ischaemic brain injury, two successive haemodynamic phases have been described. The initial ischaemic phase is characterized by a fall in cerebral blood flow and partial pressure of oxygen, inducing a dramatic cerebral energy failure associated with early neuronal cell death. The second phase is initiated during reperfusion, which brings blood-derived inflammatory cells and inflammatory mediators to the site of brain damage. This latter phase is accompanied by a delayed energy failure (6 to 48 hours after the injury) which leads to delayed apoptotic neuronal cell death.

Mitochondrial dysfunction is the key regulator of the apoptotic event through the release of proapoptotic proteins (such as caspase-2, caspase-9, and apoptosis-inducible factor (AIF)). This mitochondrial failure is linked to certain events. First, an accumulation of calcium is observed in the cytosol. This has three causes – an extracellular influx induced by NMDA receptor overstimulation; release of intracellular calcium from mitochondria; and perturbation of calcium efflux. In parallel, oxygen free radicals are produced, causing cell membrane fragmentation (Perlman, 2007). Second, cytokines and microglial activation play a key role in brain damage and are induced within 1 to 4 hours after hypoxia-ischaemia (Hagberg et al., 1996). The precise mechanisms whereby these inflammatory mediators participate in brain damage remain to be determined. From a clinical viewpoint, an increase in IL-1β in the cerebrospinal fluid seems to be correlated with a poor neurological outcome (Aly et al., 2006).

Remote from the acute phase of brain damage, mechanisms of brain repair and plasticity take place, though their precise contribution to long term neuronal function remains to be established. Trophic factors such as brain-derived neurotrophic factor (BDNF) have been identified as potential mediators of post-lesional plasticity. Surprisingly, activated microglia and blood-derived macrophages seem to play a beneficial role at this delayed stage of post-lesional plasticity (Ueno et al., 2006). Part of the positive effects of microglial activation could be linked to BDNF production (Hohlfeld et al., 2000) (Fig. 2).

Potential targets for neuroprotection

Current understanding of the pathophysiology of perinatal brain injury has allowed the identification of potential targets for neuroprotection, including excitotoxicity, oxidative stress, inflammation, apoptosis, and plasticity/repair processes. Accordingly, experimental and clinical trials have been undertaken to test several drugs or new therapeutic and preventive strategies.

Antenatal neuroprotection

All clinical studies show that administration of betamethasone to the mother before preterm delivery causes a decrease in PWMD incidence (Baud et al., 1999; Canterino et al., 2001; Lee et al., 2006) whereas dexamethasone, whether in prenatal multiple courses or in postnatal therapy, leads to neurological impairment (Spinillo et al., 2004). Based on animal models, several hypotheses have been proposed to explain the effects of glucocorticoids on the developing brain but are beyond the scope of the present review (Matthews, 2001; Baud & Sola, 2007).

Magnesium sulphate ($MgSO_4^+$) interacts with NMDA receptors (Hoffman et al., 1994) and has anti-inflammatory (Shogi et al., 2003) and anti-oxidative properties (Fig. 2). In acute brain injury, there is a decrease in magnesium sulphate concentration in the CSF, and magnesium sulphate supplementation has neuroprotective effects in murine models (Heath & Vink, 1997;

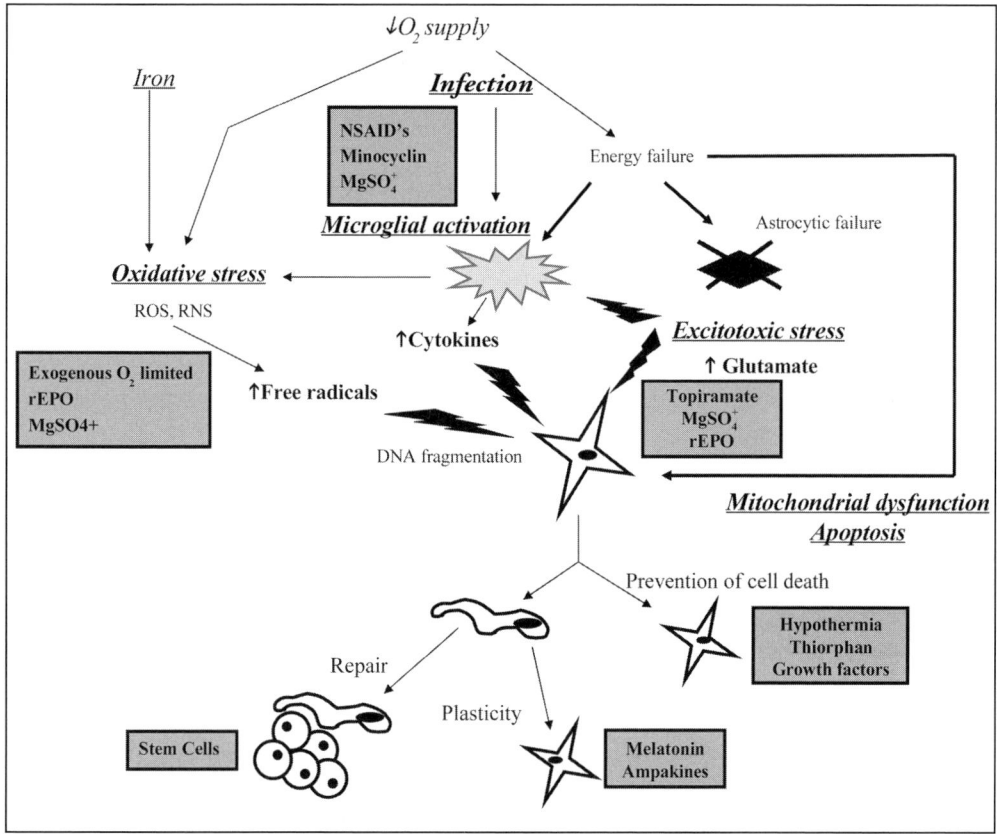

Fig. 2. Schematic representation of the major pathophysiological pathways leading to perinatal brain damage and of some potential neuroprotective strategies.

Vink et al., 2003). Thus current adult traumatic brain injury management includes $MgSO_4^+$ supplementation. It was hoped that $MgSO_4^+$, which has been used for decades as a tocolytic agent, would have a neuroprotective effect in preterm neonates (Nelson & Grether, 1995; Schendel et al., 1996). The first multicentre controlled clinical trial where mothers at risk of preterm birth before 30 weeks' gestation were given magnesium has been completed (Crowther et al., 2003). The results showed a lack of significant perinatal side effects and some benefit for the neurodevelopment of survivors examined at the age of 2 years. A more recent trial showed similar trends (Marret et al., 2007a; Marret et al., 2007b).

Excitotoxic processes

The NMDA receptor plays a major role in neuronal migration, proliferation, survival, and differentiation during brain development (Lujan et al., 2005). Dizocilpine (MK-801), a specific antagonist of the NMDA receptor, has two opposite effects according to the context (physiological or post-injury). Thus in an excitotoxic mouse model, MK-801 has a neuroprotective effect after an intracranial injection of ibotenate, an NMDA and metabotropic receptor agonist (Husson et al., 2004). In contrast, in the absence of brain damage, MK-801 along with some anaesthetic drugs such as ketamine and other NMDA receptor antagonists triggers apoptotic neurodegeneration (Ikonomidou, 1999; Scallet *et al.*, 2004; Wang *et al.*, 2005). In conclusion, a brief and partial blockade of the NMDA receptor during the course of excitotoxicity seems to be neuroprotective without adverse neurodevelopmental effects.

In parallel, such duality is not so clear for the AMPA-kainate glutamatergic receptor. Blockade of this receptor by topiramate, an anti-epileptic drug, has a neuroprotective effect after excitotoxic stress (Sfaello *et al.*, 2005) or in association with hypothermia after hypoxic-ischaemic injury (Liu *et al.*, 2004) (Fig. 2). While topiramate has a beneficial action at therapeutic dosage, apoptotic neuronal cell death is observed at high doses in neonatal rats (Glier *et al.*, 2004). Currently, the safety of topiramate for neonates has not been established and administration of this drug is authorized in France only for children over 2 years of age. In the same way, anandamide – which belongs to the endocannabinoid family – reduces the size of brain lesions caused by an AMPA-kainate receptor agonist. However, the cannabinoid system has been implicated in brain development and in psychiatric disorders such as schizophrenia (Shouman *et al.*, 2006) and this could limit its clinical use in preterm infants.

Inflammatory processes

Microglial or astrocytic production of pro-inflammatory cytokines during the acute phase of brain damage has deleterious effects acting through the autocrine/paracrine loop and a direct cytotoxic effect. Furthermore, systemic infectious/inflammatory processes leading to a more strongly activated microglia have been shown to be very damaging for preterm white matter.

Chloroquine, an antimalarial drug, in association with colchicine targets specifically the phagocytic function of macrophages. In an excitotoxic murine model, these drugs significantly reduce microglial activation and the size of brain lesions induced by a glutamate agonist (Dommergues *et al.*, 2003). By the same mechanism, minocycline – which belongs to the tetracycline family – inhibits microglial activation (Dommergues *et al.*, 2003), subsequently decreasing brain IL-1β synthesis and oxidative stress after acute brain damage (Fig. 2). Apoptotic neuronal cell death is thereby reduced. Furthermore, myelination and the mature oligodendrocyte population are restored (Cai *et al.*, 2006). The same protector effects are observed after systemic neonatal infection induced by intraperitoneal lipopolysaccharide injections (Fan *et al.*, 2005). However, the toxicity of these drugs seems to compromise their use in neonates.

Tianeptine (Stablon®) is a well tolerated antidepressive drug. Chronic high levels of brain IL-1β lead to clinical depressive symptoms. In a murine PWMD model, tianeptine shows neuroprotective properties only if inflammation caused by systemic IL-1β administration is present (Plaisant *et al.*, 2003a). The way in which this agent reduces the risk of neurodevelopmental damage is not yet known, but it does not seem to involve glutamate receptors directly. Currently, no neonatal trials are ongoing.

IL-10, a Th2 anti-inflammatory cytokine, shows marked suppressive effects on the production of pro-inflammatory cytokines by activated microglia-macrophages. Clinical trials based on IL-10 administration to adult patients suffering from autoimmune diseases such as psoriasis are currently in progress. Such studies may provide some preliminary information on the safety profile of IL-10 in humans. Similarly, a soluble TNFα receptor (Etanercept®) is currently being used in humans with Crohn's disease or other inflammatory diseases. IL-10 and Etanercept® have been shown to block the deleterious effects of inflammatory cytokines on murine neonatal excitotoxic brain damage models.

Non-steroidal anti-inflammatory drugs (NSAIDs) could have beneficial effects on perinatal brain damage, as has been demonstrated in adult hypoxia-ischaemia and neurodegenerative diseases (Candelario-Jalil et al., 2005). They are already widely used at low dosage in human preterm babies for closure of patent ductus arteriosus, and they seem to cause a reduction in cerebral intraventricular haemorrhage (Ment et al., 2004). Recently, it has been shown that cyclo-oxygenase-2 (COX-2) blockade by indomethacin (a COX-1 and COX-2 inhibitor) and nimesulide (a specific COX-2 inhibitor) abolishes the sensitizing effect of IL-1β on excitotoxic brain lesions in newborn mice (Favrais et al., 2007) (Fig. 2). This effect is dose-dependent.

Oxidative processes

Neonates, and especially preterm infants, are highly vulnerable to oxidative or nitrosative stress, as they are relatively deficient in the cellular machinery required to detoxicate reactive oxygen and nitrogen species. Thus the classic means of reducing oxidative and nitrosative stresses may be considered as potential therapeutic strategies. Allopurinol, a free radical inhibitor targeting xanthine production, reduces blood free radical concentration and protects the immature rat brain from hypoxic-ischaemic damage (Vanucci & Perlman, 1997). It has also been tested in clinical trials (Van Bel et al., 1998). Deferoxamine, an iron chelating agent, prevents the formation of hydroxyl radical from free iron during reperfusion and limits brain damage in an animal model (Peeters-Scholte et al., 2003). Neither of these antioxidants had a beneficial effect on neuronal cells in vitro (Peeters et al., 2003), and allopurinol has been used in human neonates with asphyxia without resulting in clinical improvement (Benders et al., 2006). Another free radical scavenger, N-acetylcysteine, can reduce oxidative stress and inflammation and shows neuroprotective properties in an inflammatory sensitization model, particularly if it is employed before hypoxic-ischaemic stress (Wang et al., 2007). It is well tolerated by pregnant women and could be a good candidate for neuroprotection in preterm births evolving in an infectious context. Many other compounds interfering with the oxidative stress cascade have been tested successfully in animal models (Marret et al., 1999; Largeron et al., 2001; Plaisant et al., 2003b; Vamecq et al., 2003).

Another way to minimize oxidative stress is to limit the amount of pro-oxidative molecules given in the neonatal period, particularly oxygen and iron. Oxygen can be a major source of oxidative stress, especially during the reperfusion phase, and several studies have clearly identified the risk of an excess of inhaled oxygen for the preterm brain (Saugstad et al., 2005). Similarly, free iron induces the formation of reactive oxygen species and exogenous iron has been shown to significantly exacerbate excitotoxic PWMD in newborn mice (Dommergues et al., 1998). However, this toxic effect might be compensated in the clinical settings by the co-administration of erythropoietin which has trophic properties (Siren et al., 2001). Further experimental and clinical studies are necessary to clarify this issue.

Prevention of delayed neuronal cell death

Hypothermia has been shown to be highly neuroprotective during the second energy failure pathway which follows hypoxia-ischaemia in several experimental settings (Adachi et al., 2001; Tomimatsu et al., 2003) by preventing apoptotic neuronal cell death (Ohmura et al., 2005). Multicentre controlled clinical trials have been completed, showing a significant reduction in neurological handicap at 18 months of age in infants with a moderate neonatal insult, without any significant clinical side effects during the neonatal procedure (Gunn et al., 1998; Battin et al., 2001; Shankaran et al., 2005).

Growth factors such as insulin-like growth factor 1 (IGF-1), nerve growth factor (NGF), and brain derived neurotrophic factor (BDNF) have anti-apoptotic and trophic properties. They prevent hypoxic neuronal death (Johnston *et al.*, 1996; Cheng *et al.*, 1997; Sizonenko *et al.*, 2003) and IGF-1 prevents oligodendrocytic death (Lin *et al.*, 2005) in animal models of perinatal damage. Interestingly, neuroprotective effects of BDNF in the neonatal murine neocortex are highly stage-dependent (Husson *et al.*, 2005): at postnatal day 5 (P5), BDNF was neuroprotective through TrkB receptors and the MAPK pathway, reducing apoptosis, thus mimicking protective effects observed in the P7 rat model; in contrast, BDNF exacerbated ibotenate-induced neuronal apoptotic death at P0 through the $p75^{NTR}$ pathway, and had no detectable effect on lesions at P10. Some neuroprotective agents induce these anti-apotopic factors. For example, a high dose of recombinant erythropoietin (r-EPO), which interferes with oxidative pathways, counteracts neuronal cell death by partially restoring the expression of neurotrophic factors such as BDNF and glial cell line-derived neurotrophic factor (GDNF) (Dzietko *et al.*, 2004) (Fig. 2).

In humans, and in several animal models, mutations in mitochondrial genes are known to be involved in neurological disorders, and mitochondria are clearly involved in many apoptotic processes. No treatments are focused on these targets. Recent studies suggest that some trophic factors might target mitochondrial function through an unknown mechanism. Indeed, BDNF, but not NGF, increases rat and mouse brain mitochondrial respiratory coupling at complex I *in vitro* (Markham *et al.*, 2004). Further studies will be necessary to confirm this effect *in vivo* and to determine its relevance in BDNF-mediated neuroprotection.

Neuropeptides are modulators of neuronal activity and could therefore modulate glutamate-induced neuronal cell death. They undergo enzymatic proteolysis which leads to their inactivation. Inhibition of this degradation is a potential alternative therapeutic approach. Among the various peptidases identified, neutral endopeptidase (NEP or neprilysin) is the prototypical member of the M13 family of metalloproteases and is widely distributed in various tissues. NEP is involved in the regulation and metabolism of a variety of biologically active peptides including tachykinins/neurokinins (Roques *et al.*, 1993). Interestingly, racecadotril (Tiorfan®), an NEP inhibitor, is used in clinical practice for diarrhoea, with a remarkable safety profile (Schwartz, 2000). Racecadotril is quickly and entirely metabolized to its active metabolite thiorphan. A recent study showed that systemic administration of thiorphan was neuroprotective against excitotoxic neuronal cell death in newborn mice (Medja *et al.*, 2006) (Fig. 2). This neuroprotective effect was long lasting and was still observed when thiorphan was administered 12 hours after the insult, showing a good window for therapeutic intervention.

Caspases are effectors of apoptotic cell death. Caspase inhibitors may be an attractive approach to preserving neuronal function by extending the therapeutic window and providing long-term neuroprotection. Currently, several inhibitors are in preclinical drug development (Legos *et al.*, 2001).

Plasticity and repair processes

Neuroprotective strategies can certainly stop lesions from getting worse, but agents which have neurotrophic properties can also affect repair in a developing brain. Although prevention and treatment of brain lesions at an early stage are desirable, post-lesion plasticity is the only available target in many cases, because of the lack of early detectors of perinatal brain lesions.

This property has been highlighted for melatonin in excitotoxic models of neonatal PWMD (Husson *et al.*, 2002). Although melatonin did not prevent the initial appearance of PWMD, it promoted repair of secondary lesions with axonal regrowth or sprouting. Behavioural studies support the hypothesis that melatonin-induced white matter repair is accompanied by improved learning capabilities. Melatonin is a safe compound (Penev & Zee, 1997), in neonates as well as in adults (Gitto et al., 2001) (Fig. 2). Thus melatonin derivatives (Valdoxan®, Roserem®) should be evaluated in controlled trials in the future.

In a similar excitotoxic model of neonatal PWMD, post-lesion plasticity was also induced by BDNF (Husson et al., 2005). However, its clinical use is limited by its low capacity to cross the blood-brain barrier and by its central role in multiple steps of brain development, raising legitimate concerns about its use in neonates. Potential substitute agents could be ampakines (positive allosteric modulators of AMPA receptors) (Lauterborn et al., 2000) or vasoactive intestinal peptide (VIP) (Moody et al., 2003), which lead to an increase in brain BDNF production and may be given systemically. In the same way, BDNF expression induced by viral vectors could follow a single intracerebral injection over a protracted period of time. These agents were shown experimentally to mimic the neuroprotective properties of BDNF (Gressens et al., 1998; Dicou et al., 2003). Although promising, these data require confirmation in other preclinical models.

In the past decade, many reports demonstrated successful *in vitro* culture of neural stem cells and their subsequent differentiation into specific cell populations (McKay, 2004). Recent studies showed potential for cellular therapy in degenerative brain pathologies (Lindvall et al., 2004), raising the hope of being able to graft these cells into a damaged brain. Two major stem cell sources have proved suitable for generating neuronal and glial cell subpopulations: multipotent embryonic stem (ES) cells (cells derived from the inner mass of early stage embryos) and neural stem cells (derived from early embryonic neural tissues). *In vitro*, ES cells can spontaneously differentiate into various cell lineages. Addition of specific soluble factors in the culture medium results in enrichment of specific cellular populations, including neural lineage. For instance, addition of VIP in the culture medium of murine ES cells enhanced the neuronal differentiation of these ES cells (Cazillis et al., 2004). Similarly, neural stem cells can differentiate *in vitro* into various neuronal and glial lineages, according to culture conditions.

To our knowledge, there are no reports addressing experimentally the feasibility and the potential benefits of grafting stem cells following perinatal brain damage.

A potential alternative to grafting exogenous stem cells is to stimulate the endogenous production of neural progenitors from resident stem cells. It was recently shown that an enhanced proliferation of neural stem/progenitor cells occurs in response to neonatal hypoxia-ischaemia in newborn rats (Felling et al., 2006). Although very promising, this approach requires, first, the demonstration that these newly formed neural cells survive and integrate into the existing neuronal network and improve brain function, and second, the ability to stimulate the proliferation and survival of newly produced neural cells pharmacologically.

Conclusions

The pathophysiology of perinatal brain damage is now better understood, allowing the identification of targets for neuroprotection. Based on this knowledge, several compounds have been shown to be neuroprotective in relevant animal models of perinatal brain damage. However, safety is a major issue before treating human neonates, and this slows down pharmaceutical investment in this area. Recent improvements in neurological outcome of neonates have largely been due to changes in neonatal care, including more adequate use of drugs in the perinatal period. For example, Wilson-Costello et al. (2007) linked the decrease in neurological impairment in preterm neonates to the generalized use of prenatal betamethasone, the withdrawal of postnatal dexamethasone, and the prevention of sepsis during neonatal intensive care.

Some recent studies have focused on the cerebral effects of caffeine, erythropoietin, ibuprofen, $MgSO_4^+$, and inhaled nitric oxide (NO) – agents currently used in neonatology units. In addition, hypothermia seems to be the most promising advance in neuroprotective care for term infants suffering from hypoxic-ischaemic injury. A further step would be to explore the potential benefits of combining multiple neuroprotective agents. However, such combinations could increase the risk of potential toxic effects.

Acknowledgments: Supported by Inserm, Université Paris Diderot, PremUp, Société Française de Pédiatrie, Fondation Motrice, and Fondation Grace de Monaco.

References

Adachi, M., Sohma, O., Tsuneishi, S., Takada, S. & Nakamura, H. (2001): Combination effect of systemic hypothermia and caspase inhibitor administration against hypoxic-ischemic brain damage in neonatal rats. *Pediatr. Res.* **50**, 590–595.

Aly, H., Khashaba, M.T., El-Ayouty, M., El-Sayed, O. & Hasanein, B.M. (2006): IL-1beta, IL-6 and TNF-alpha and outcomes of neonatal hypoxic ischemic encephalopathy. *Brain Dev.* **28**, 178–182.

Back, S.A., Riddle, A. & McClure, M.M. (2007): Maturation-dependent vulnerability of perinatal white matter in premature birth. *Stroke* **38**, 724–730.

Battin, M.R., Dezoete, J.A., Gunn, T.R., Gluckman, P.D. & Gunn, A.J. (2001): Neurodevelopmental outcome of infants treated with head cooling and mild hypothermia after perinatal asphyxia. *Pediatrics* **107**, 480–484.

Baud, O., Foix-L'Helias, L., Kaminski, M., Audibert, F., Jarreau, P., Papiernik, E., Huon, C., Lepercq, J., Dehan, M. & Lacaze-Masmonteil, T. (1999): Antenatal glucocorticoid treatment and cystic periventricular leucomalacia in very premature infants. *N. Engl. J. Med.* **341**, 1190–1196.

Baud, O. & Sola, A. (2007): Corticosteroids in perinatal medicine: how to improve outcomes without affecting the developing brain? *Semin. Fetal Neonat. Med.* **12**, 273–279.

Benders, M.J., Bos, A.F., Rademaker, C.M., Rijken, M., Torrance, H.L., Groenendaal, F. & Van Bel, F. (2006): Early postnatal allopurinol does not improve short term outcome after severe birth asphyxia. *Arch. Dis. Child. Fetal Neonat. Ed.* **91**, 163–165.

Candelario-Jalil, E., Mhadu, N.H., Gonzalez-Falcon, A., Garcia-Cabrera, M., Munoz, E., Leon, O.S. & Fiebich, B.L. (2005): Effects of cyclooxygase-2 inhibitor nimesulide on cerebral infarction and neurological deficits induced by permanent middle cerebral artery occlusion in the rat. *J. Neuroinflammation* **2**, 3.

Cai, Z., Lin, S., Fan, L.W., Pang, Y. & Rhodes, P.G. (2006): Minocycline alleviates hypoxic-ischemic injury to developing oligodendrocytes in the neonatal rat brain. *Neuroscience* **137**, 425–435.

Canterino, J.C., Verma, U., Visintainer, P.F., Elimian, A., Klein, S.A. & Tejani, N. (2001): Antenatal steroids and neonatal periventricular leucomalacia. *Obstet. Gynecol.* **97**, 135–139.

Cazillis, M., Gonzalez, B.J., Billardon, C., Lombet, A., Fraichard, A., Samarut, J., Gressens, P., Vaudry, H. & Rostene, W. (2004): VIP and PACAP induce selective neuronal differentiation of mouse embryonic stem cells. *Eur. J. Neurosci.* **19**, 798–808.

Cheng, Y., Gidday, J.M., Yan, Q., Shah, A.R. & Holtzman, D.M. (1997): Marked age-dependent neuroprotection by brain-derived neurotrophic factor against neonatal hypoxic-ischemic brain injury. *Ann. Neurol.* **41**, 521–529.

Crowther, C.A., Hiller, J.E., Doyle, L.W., Haslam, R.R. for Australasian Collaborative Trial of Magnesium Sulphate (ACTOMg SO4) Collaborative Group (2003): Effect of magnesium sulfate given for neuroprotection before preterm birth: a randomized controlled trial. *JAMA* **290**, 2669–2676.

Dicou, E., Rangon, C.M., Guimiot, F., Spedding, M. & Gressens, P. (2003): Positive allosteric modulators of AMPA receptors are neuroprotective against lesions induced by an NMDA agonist in neonatal mouse brain. *Brain Res.* **970**, 221–225.

Dommergues, M.A., Gallego, J., Evrard, P. & Gressens, P. (1998): Iron supplementation aggravates periventricular cystic white matter lesions in newborn mice. *Eur. J. Paediatr. Neurol.* **2**, 313–318.

Dommergues, M.A., Patkai, J., Renauld, J.C., Evrard, P. & Gressens, P. (2000): Proinflammatory cytokines and interleukin-9 exacerbate excitotoxic lesions of the newborn murine neopallium. *Ann. Neurol.* **47**, 54–63.

Dommergues, M.A., Plaisant, F., Verney, C. & Gressens, P. (2003): Early microglial activation following neonatal excitotoxic brain damage in mice: a potential target for neuroprotection. *Neuroscience* **121**, 619–628.

Dzietko, M., Felderhoff-Mueser, U., Sifringer, M., Krutz, B., Bittigau, P., Thor, F., Heumann, R., Buhrer, C., Ikonomidou, C. & Hansen, H.H. (2004): Erythropoietin protects the developing brain against N-methyl-D-aspartate receptor antagonist neurotoxicity. *Neurobiol. Dis.* **15**, 177–187.

Fan, L.W., Pang, Y., Lin, S., Tien, L.T., Ma, T., Rhodes, P.G. & Cai, Z. (2005): Minocycline reduces lipopolysaccharide-induced neurological dysfunction and brain injury in the neonatal rat. *J. Neurosci. Res.* **82**, 71–82.

Favrais, G., Schwendimann, L., Gressens, P. & Lelievre, V. (2007): Cyclooxygenase-2 mediates the sensitizing effects of systemic IL-1-beta on excitotoxic brain lesions in newborn mice. *Neurobiol. Dis.* **25**, 496–505.

Feldhaus, B., Dietzel, I.D., Heumann, R. & Berger, R. (2004): Effects of interferon-gamma and tumor necrosis factor-alpha on survival and differentiation of oligodendrocyte progenitors. *J. Soc. Gynecol. Invest.* **11**, 89–96.

Felling, R.J., Snyder, M.J., Romanko, M.J., Rothstein, R.P., Ziegler, A.N., Yang, Z., Givogri, M.I., Bongarzone, E.R. & Levison, S.W. (2006): Neural stem/progenitor cells participate in the regenerative response to perinatal hypoxia/ischemia. *J. Neurosci.* **26**, 4359–4369.

Follett, P.L., Rosenberg, P.A., Volpe, J.J. & Jensen, F.E. (2000): NBQX attenuates excitotoxic injury in developing white matter. *J. Neurosci.* **20**, 9235–9241.

Gitto, E., Karbownik, M., Reiter, R.J., Tan, D.X., Cuzzocrea, S., Chiurazzi, P., Cordaro, S., Corona, G., Trimarchi, G. & Barberi, I. (2001): Effects of melatonin treatment in septic newborns. *Pediatr. Res.* **50**, 756–760.

Glier, C., Dzietko, M., Bittigau, P., Jarosz, B., Korobowicz, E. & Ikonomidou, C. (2004): Therapeutic doses of topiramate are not toxic to the developing rat brain. *Exp. Neurol.* **187**, 403–409.

Gressens, P., Marret, S., Martin, J.L., Laquerriere, A., Lombet, A. & Evrard, P. (1998): Regulation of neuroprotective action of vasoactive intestinal peptide in the murine developing brain by protein kinase C and mitogen-activated protein kinase cascades: in vivo and in vitro studies. *J. Neurochem.* **70**, 2574–2584.

Gunn, A.J., Gluckman, P.D. & Gunn, T.R. (1998): Selective head cooling in newborn infants after perinatal asphyxia: a safety study. *Pediatrics* **102**, 885–892.

Hagberg, H., Gilland, E., Bona, E., Hanson, L.A., Hahin-Zoric, M., Blennow, M., Holst, M., McRae, A. & Soder, O. (1996): Enhanced expression of interleukin (IL)-1 and IL-6 messenger RNA and bioactive protein after hypoxia-ischemia in neonatal rats. *Pediatr. Res.* **40**, 603–609.

Heath, D.L. & Vink, R. (1997): Magnesium sulphate improves neurologic outcome following severe closed head injury in rats. *Neurosci. Lett.* **228**, 175–178.

Himmelmann, K., Hagberg, G., Beckung, E., Hagberg, B. & Uvebrant, P. (2005): The changing panorama of cerebral palsy in Sweden. IX. Prevalence and origin in the birth-year period 1995-1998. *Acta Paediatr.* **94**, 287–294.

Hoffman, D.J., Marro, P.J., McGowan, J.E., Mishra, O.P. & Delivoria-Papadopoulos, M. (1994): Protective effect of MgSO4 infusion on NMDA receptor binding characteristics during cerebral cortical hypoxia in the newborn piglet. *Brain Res.* **644**, 144–149.

Hohlfeld, R., Kerschensteiner, M., Stadelmann, C., Lassmann, H. & Wekerle, H. (2000): The neuroprotective effect of inflammation: implications for the therapy of multiple sclerosis. *J. Neuroimmunol.* **107**, 161–166.

Husson, I., Mesples, B., Bac, P., Vamecq, J., Evrard, P. & Gressens, P. (2002): Melatoninergic neuroprotection of the murine periventricular white matter against neonatal excitotoxic challenge. *Ann. Neurol.* **51**, 82–92.

Husson, I., Mesples, B., Medja, F., Leroux, P., Kosofsky, B. & Gressens, P. (2004): Methylphenidate and MK-801, an N-methyl-d-aspartate receptor antagonist: shared biological properties. *Neuroscience* 125, 163–170.

Husson, I., Rangon, C.M., Lelievre, V., Bemelmans, A.P., Sachs, P., Mallet, J., Kosofsky, B.E. & Gressens, P. (2005): BDNF-induced white matter neuroprotection and stage-dependent neuronal survival following a neonatal excitotoxic challenge. *Cereb. Cortex* **15**, 250–261.

Ikonomidou, C., Bosch, F., Miksa, M., Bittigau, P., Vockler, J., Dikranian, K., Tenkova, T.I., Stefovska, V., Turski, L & Olney, J.W. (1999): Blockade of NMDA receptors and apoptotic neurodegeneration in the developing brain. *Science* **283**, 70–74.

Johnston, B.M., Mallard, E.C., Williams, C.E. & Gluckman, P.D. (1996): Insulin-like growth factor-1 is a potent neuronal rescue agent after hypoxic-ischemic injury in fetal lambs. *J. Clin. Invest.* **97**, 300–308.

Kinney, H.C. (2006): The near-term (late preterm) human brain and risk for periventricular leucomalacia: a review. *Semin. Perinatol.* **30**, 81–88.

Largeron, M., Mesples, B., Gressens, P., Cecchelli, R., Spedding, M., Le Ridant, A. & Fleury, M. (2001): The neuroprotective activity of 8-alkylamino-1,4-benzoxazine antioxidants. *Eur. J. Pharmacol.* **424**, 189–194.

Lauterborn, J.C., Lynch, G., Vanderklish, P., Arai, A. & Gall, C.M. (2000): Positive modulation of AMPA receptors increases neurotrophin expression by hippocampal and cortical neurons. *J. Neurosci.* **20**, 8–21.

Lee, B.H., Stoll, B.J., McDonald, S.A., Higgins, R.D., for the National Institute of Child Health and Human Development Neonatal Research Network (2006): Adverse neonatal outcomes associated with antenatal dexamethasone versus antenatal betamethasone. *Pediatrics* **117**, 1503–1510.

Legos, J.J., Lee, D. & Erhardt, J.A. (2001): Caspase inhibitors as neuroprotective agents. *Expert Opin. Emerg. Drugs* **6**, 81–94.

Lin, S., Fan, L.W., Pang, Y., Rhodes, P.G., Mitchell, H.J. & Cai, Z. (2005): IGF-1 protects oligodendrocyte progenitor cells and improves neurological functions following cerebral hypoxia-ischemia in the neonatal rat. *Brain Res.* **1063**, 15–26.

Lindvall, O., Kokaia, Z. & Martinez-Serrano, A. (2004): Stem cell therapy for human neurodegenerative disorders – how to make it work. *Nat. Med.* **10**, S42–S50.

Liu, Y., Barks, J.D., Xu, G. & Silverstein, F.S. (2004): Topiramate extends the therapeutic window for hypothermia-mediated neuroprotection after stroke in neonatal rats. *Stroke* **35**, 1460–1465.

Lujan, R., Shigemoto, R. & Lopez-Bendito, G. (2005): Glutamate and GABA receptor signalling in the developing brain. *Neuroscience* **130**, 567–580.

McQuillen, P.S. & Ferriero, D.M. (2004): Selective vulnerability in the developing central nervous system. *Pediatr. Neurol.* **30**, 227–235.

Markham, A., Cameron, I., Franklin, P. & Spedding, M. (2004): BDNF increases rat brain mitochondrial respiratory coupling at complex I, but not complex II. *Eur. J. Neurosci.* **20**, 1189–1196.

Marret, S., Bonnier, C., Raymackers, J.M., Delpech, A., Evrard, P. & Gressens, P. (1999): Glycine antagonist and NO synthase inhibitor protect the developing mouse brain against neonatal excitotoxic lesions. *Pediatr. Res.* **45**, 337–342.

Marret, S., Doyle, L.W., Crowther, C.A. & Middleton, P. (2007a): Antenatal magnesium sulphate neuroprotection in the preterm infant. *Semin. Fetal Neonat. Med.* **12**, 311–317.

Marret, S., Marpeau, L., Zupan-Simunek, V., Eurin, D., Leveque, C., Hellot, M.F., Benichou, J. for PREMAG trial group (2007b): Magnesium sulphate given before very-preterm birth to protect infant brain: the randomised controlled PREMAG trial*. *Br. J. Obstet. Gynaecol.* **114**, 310–318.

Matthews, S.G. (2001): Antenatal glucocorticoids and the developing brain: mechanisms of action. *Semin. Neonatol.* **6**, 309–317.

McKay, R.D. (2004): Stem cell biology and neurodegenerative disease. *Phil. Trans. R. Soc. Lond. B Biol. Sci.* **359**, 851–856.

Medja, F., Lelievre, V., Fontaine, R.H., Lebas, F., Leroux, P., Ouimet, T., Saria, A., Rougeot, C., Dournaud, P. & Gressens, P. (2006): Thiorphan, a neutral endopeptidase inhibitor used for diarrhoea, is neuroprotective in newborn mice. *Brain* **129**, 3209–3223.

Ment, L.R., Vohr, R., Makuch, R.W., Westerveld, M., Katz, K.H., Scheinder, K.C., Duncan, C., Ehrenkranz, R.D., Oh, W., Philip, A.G.S., Scott, D.T. & Allan, A.C. (2004): Prevention of intraventricular hemorrhage by indomethacin in male preterm infants. *J. Pediatr.* **145**, 832–834.

Micu, I., Jiang, Q., Coderre, E., Ridsdale, A., Zhang, L., Woulfe, J., Yin, X., Trapp, B.D., McRory, J.E., Rehak, R., Zamponi, G.W., Wang, W. & Stys, P.K. (2006): NMDA receptors mediate calcium accumulation in myelin during chemical ischaemia. *Nature* **439**, 988–992.

Moody, T.W., Hill, J.M. & Jensen, R.T. (2003): VIP as a trophic factor in the CNS and cancer cells. *Peptides* **24**, 163–177.

Nelson, K.B. & Grether, J.K. (1995): Can magnesium sulfate reduce the risk of cerebral palsy in very low birthweight infants? *Pediatrics* **95**, 263–269.

Ohmura, A., Nakajima, W., Ishida, A., Yasuoka, N., Kawamura, M., Miura, S. & Takada, G. (2005): Prolonged hypothermia protects neonatal rat brain against hypoxic-ischemia by reducing both apoptosis and necrosis. *Brain Dev.* **27**, 517–526.

Olson, J.K. & Miller, S.D. (2004): Microglia initiate central nervous system innate and adaptive immune responses through multiple TLRs. *J. Immunol.* **173**, 3916–3924.

Pearson, V.L., Rothwell, N.J. & Toulmond, S. (1999): Excitotoxic brain damage in the rat induces interleukin-1 beta protein in microglia and astrocytes: correlation with the progression of cell death. *Glia* **25**, 311–323.

Peeters, C., Hoelen, D., Groenendaal, F., van Bel, F. & Bar, D. (2003): Deferoxamine, allopurinol and oxypurinol are not neuroprotective after oxygen/glucose deprivation in an organotypic hippocampal model, lacking functional endothelial cells. *Brain Res.* **963**, 72–80.

Peeters-Scholte, C., Braun, K., Koster, J., Kops, N., Blomgren, K., Buonocore, G., van Buul-Offers, S., Hagberg, H., Nicolay, K., van Bel, F. & Groenendaal, F. (2003): Effects of allopurinol and deferoxamine on reperfusion injury of the brain in newborn piglets after neonatal hypoxia-ischemia. *Pediatr. Res.* **54**, 516–522.

Penev, P.D. & Zee, P.C. (1997): Melatonin: a clinical perspective. *Ann. Neurol.* **42**, 545–553.

Perlman, J.M. (2007): Pathogenesis of hypoxic-ischemic brain injury. *J. Perinatol.* **27,** S39–S46.

Plaisant, F., Dommergues, M.A., Spedding, M., Cecchelli, R., Brillault, J., Kato, G., Muñoz, C. & Gressens, P. (2003a): Neuroprotective properties of tianeptine: interactions with cytokines. *Neuropharmacology* **44,** 801–809.

Plaisant, F., Clippe, A., Vander Stricht, D., Knoops, B. & Gressens, P. (2003b): Recombinant peroxiredoxin 5 protects against excitotoxic brain lesions in newborn mice. *Free Radic. Biol. Med.* **34,** 862–872.

Robertson, C.M., Watt, M.J. & Yasui, Y. (2007): Changes in the prevalence of cerebral palsy for children born very prematurely within a population-based program over 30 years. *JAMA* **297,** 2733–2740.

Robinson, S., Li, Q., Dechant, A. & Cohen, M.L. (2006): Neonatal loss of gamma-aminobutyric acid pathway expression after human perinatal brain injury. *J. Neurosurg.* **104,** 396–408.

Roques, B.P., Noble, F., Dauge, V., Fournie-Zaluski, M.C. & Beaumont, A. (1993): Neutral endopeptidase 24.11: structure, inhibition, and experimental and clinical pharmacology. *Pharmacol. Rev.* **45,** 87–146.

Salter, M.G. & Fern, R. (2005): NMDA receptors are expressed in developing oligodendrocyte processes and mediate injury. *Nature* **438,** 1167–1171.

Saugstad, O.D., Ramji, S. & Vento, M. (2005): Resuscitation of depressed newborn infants with ambient air or pure oxygen: a meta-analysis. *Biol. Neonate* **87,** 27–34.

Scallet, A.C., Schmued, L.C., Slikker, W., Grunberg, N., Faustino, P.J., Davis, H., Lester, D., Pine, P.S., Sistare, F. & Hanig, J.P. (2004): Developmental neurotoxicity of ketamine: morphometric confirmation, exposure parameters, and multiple fluorescent labeling of apoptotic neurons. *Toxicol. Sci.* **81,** 364–370.

Schendel, D.E., Berg, C.J., Yeargin-Allsopp, M., Boyle, C.A. & Decoufle, P. (1996): Prenatal magnesium sulfate exposure and the risk for cerebral palsy or mental retardation among very low-birth-weight children aged 3 to 5 years. *JAMA* **276,** 1805–1810.

Schwartz, J.C. (2000): Racecadotril: a new approach to the treatment of diarrhoea. *Int. J. Antimicrob. Agents* **14,** 75–79.

Sfaello, I., Baud, O., Arzimanoglou, A. & Gressens, P. (2005): Topiramate prevents excitotoxic damage in the newborn rodent brain. *Neurobiol. Dis.* **20,** 837–848.

Shankaran, S., Laptook, A.R., Ehrenkranz, R.A., Tyson, J.E., McDonald, S.A., Donovan, E.F., Fanaroff, A.A., Poole, W.K., Wright, L.L., Higgins, R.D., Finer, N.N., Carlo, W.A., Duara, S., Oh, W., Cotton, C.M., Stevenson, D.K., Stoll, B.J., Lemons, J.A., Guillet, R., Jobe, A.H. & National Institute of Child Health and Human Development Neonatal Research Network (2005): Whole-body hypothermia for neonates with hypoxic-ischemic encephalopathy. *N. Engl. J. Med.* **353,** 1574–1584.

Shogi, T., Miyamoto, A., Ishiguro, S. & Nishio, A. (2003): Enhanced release of IL-1beta and TNF-alpha following endotoxin challenge from rat alveolar macrophages cultured in low-mg(2+) medium. *Magnes. Res.* **16,** 111–119.

Shouman, B., Fontaine, R.H., Baud, O., Schwendimann, L., Keller, M., Spedding, M., Lelievre, V. & Gressens, P. (2006): Endocannabinoids potently protect the newborn brain against AMPA-kainate receptor-mediated excitotoxic damage. *Br. J. Pharmacol.* **148,** 442–451.

Siren, A.L., Fratelli, M., Brines, M., Goemans, C., Casagrande, S., Lewczuk, P., Keenan, S., Gleiter, C., Pasquali, C., Capobianco, A., Mennini, T., Heumann, R., Cerami, A., Ehrenreich, H. & Ghezzi, P. (2001): Erythropoietin prevents neuronal apoptosis after cerebral ischemia and metabolic stress. *Proc. Natl. Acad. Sci. USA* **98,** 4044–4049.

Sizonenko, S.V., Sirimanne, E., Mayall, Y., Gluckman, P.D., Inder, T. & Williams, C. (2003): Selective cortical alteration after hypoxic-ischemic injury in the very immature rat brain. *Pediatr. Res.* **54,** 263–269.

Spinillo, A., Viazzo, F., Colleoni, R., Chiara, A., Maria Cerbo, R. & Fazzi, E. (2004): Two-year infant neurodevelopmental outcome after single or multiple antenatal courses of corticosteroids to prevent complications of prematurity. *Am. J. Obstet. Gynecol.* **191,** 217–224.

Tomimatsu, T., Fukuda, H., Endoh, M., Mu, J., Kanagawa, T., Hosono, T., Kanzaki, T., Doi, K., Kubo, T. & Murata, Y. (2003): Long-term neuroprotective effects of hypothermia on neonatal hypoxic-ischemic brain injury in rats, assessed by auditory brainstem response. *Pediatr. Res.* **53,** 57–61.

Ueno, M., Katayama, K., Yamauchi, H., Yasoshima, A., Nakayama, H. & Doi, K. (2006): Repair process of fetal brain after 5-azacytidine-induced damage. *Eur. J. Neurosci.* **24,** 2758–2768.

Vamecq, J., Maurois, P., Bac, P., Bailly, F., Bernier, J.L., Stables, J.P., Husson, I. & Gressens, P. (2003): Potent mammalian cerebroprotection and neuronal cell death inhibition are afforded by a synthetic antioxidant analogue of marine invertebrate cell protectant ovothiols. *Eur. J. Neurosci.* **18,** 1110–1120.

Van Bel, F., Shadid, M., Moison, R.M., Dorrepaal, C.A., Fontijn, J., Monteiro, L., Van De Bor, M. & Berger, H.M. (1998): Effect of allopurinol on postasphyxial free radical formation, cerebral hemodynamics, and electrical brain activity. *Pediatrics* **101,** 185–193.

Vanucci, R.C. & Perlman, J.M. (1997): Interventions for perinatal hypoxic-ischemic encephalopathy. *Pediatrics* **100,** 1004–1014.

Vincer, M.J., Allen, A.C., Joseph, K.S., Stinson, D.A., Scott, H. & Wood, E. (2006): Increasing prevalence of cerebral palsy among very preterm infants: a population-based study. *Pediatrics* **118**, 1621–1626.

Vela, J.M., Molina-Holgado, E., Arévalo-Martín, A., Almazán, G. & Guaza, C. (2002): Interleukin-1 regulates proliferation and differentiation of oligodendrocytes progenitor cells. *Mol. Cell. Neurosci.* **20**, 489–502.

Volpe, J.J. (2001): Neurobiology of periventricular leucomalacia in the premature infant. *Pediatr. Res.* **50**, 553–562.

Vink, R., O'Connor, C.A., Nimmo, A.J. & Heath, D.L. (2003): Magnesium attenuates persistent functional deficits following diffuse traumatic brain injury in rats. *Neurosci. Lett.* **336**, 41–44.

Wang, C., Sadovova, N., Fu, X., Schmued, L., Scallet, A., Hanig, J. & Slikker, W. (2005): The role of the N-methyl-D-aspartate receptor in ketamine-induced apoptosis in rat forebrain culture. *Neuroscience* **132**, 967–977.

Wang, X., Svedin, P., Nie, C., Lapatto, R., Zhu, C., Gustavsson, M., Sandberg, M., Karlsson, J.O., Romero, R., Hagberg, H. & Mallard, C. (2007): N-acetylcysteine reduces lipopolysaccharide-sensitized hypoxic-ischemic brain injury. *Ann. Neurol.* **61**, 263–271.

Wilson-Costello, D., Friedman, H., Minich, N., Fanaroff, A.A. & Hack, M. (2005): Improved survival rates with increased neurodevelopmental disability for extremely low birth weight infants in the 1990s. *Pediatrics* **115**, 997–1003.

Wilson-Costello, D., Friedman, H., Minich, N., Siner, B., Taylor, G., Schluchter, M. & Hack, M. (2007): Improved neurodevelopmental outcomes for extremely low birth weight infants in 2000-2002. *Pediatrics* **119**, 37–45.

Yoon, B.H., Romero, R., Kim, C.J., Koo, J.N., Choe, G., Syn, H.C. & Chi, J.G. (1997): High expression of tumor necrosis factor-alpha and interleukin-6 in periventricular leucomalacia. *Am. J. Obstet. Gynecol.* **177**, 406–411.

Chapter 22

Caring for the preterm infant: earliest brain development and experience

Heidelise Als

Harvard Medical School and Children's Hospital, 320 Longwood Avenue, Boston, MA 02115, USA
heidelise.als@childrens.harvard.edu

Summary

The prematurely born infant exchanges the womb for the newborn intensive care unit (NICU) at a time of rapid brain development. Avoidance of overstimulation and stress, and support for self-regulation, enhances preterm neurodevelopment. The presence of reliable caregivers in support of parents as the infant's nurturers is critical. Four historical and six randomized controlled trials report the effectiveness of the Newborn Individualized Developmental Care and Assessment Program (NIDCAP) model. Consistent findings are: improved lung function, feeding behaviour, and growth; reduced length of hospital admission; and improved neurodevelopmental function. Enhanced parent competence and lower stress have also been reported. Magnetic resonance imaging studies show enhanced fibre tract development in the frontal lobe and internal capsule. Better Bayley mental and psychomotor performance at 3, 5, and 9 months corrected age (CA), as well as improved regulation attention, play, planning, affect, and communication, and at 3 years CA better auditory processing and speech, have been documented. At age 6 years, functioning free of developmental disability, mental retardation, or attention deficits is more frequent. Thus NIDCAP improves early brain development, functional competence, and quality of life for preterm infants and their families. It is cost-effective for health care and education systems. Introduction of NIDCAP requires commitment and resources at the organizational level. Sixteen NIDCAP training centres in several countries, certified by the NIDCAP Federation International (NFI), are available to other nurseries for education and consultation in implementing NIDCAP care. NIDCAP rapidly is becoming the standard for all newborn intensive care.

Introduction

Need for developmental NICU care

The prematurely born infant provides an opportunity to improve our understanding of early experience and brain development. In the last decade, prematurity rates have been on the rise worldwide. In the USA, they are currently at 12 per cent, and for African Americans, 18 per cent. Prematurely born children require early intervention and a disproportionate provision of community preschool services (Blair *et al.*, 1995; Hack *et al.*, 2005; Behrman, 2007). When reaching school age, preterm children contribute overwhelmingly to the learning disabled and poorly achieving student population (McCormick *et al.*, 1992;

McCormick et al., 1993). Up to 52 per cent have school problems and emotional disabilities because of central processing deficits which hamper integrative problem solving, planning, and prioritizing abilities, affecting many areas. The gap between expected and actual achievement widens as the children become older and the demands for complex processing and performance increase (Hack et al., 2002). Compensatory educational efforts, begun after hospital discharge, have been disappointing. This is especially true for the infants born before 32 weeks' gestation (Ramey et al., 1992; Brooks-Gunn et al., 1994; McCormick et al., 1998). Increasing evidence points to the mismatch of the preterm brain's expectation for continued intrauterine experience and the contrasting experience of the newborn intensive care unit (NICU) (Als & Brazelton, 1981; Als, 1982). The dual stress experience of isolation from the mother and simultaneous repeated experience of pain leads to cascading neurotoxic sequelae and altered brain outcomes (Anand & Scalzo, 2000).

The goal of individualized developmental NICU care for the preterm infant is to improve brain development and developmental outcome by preventing unexpected sensory overload for the immature, rapidly developing nervous system. The individualized approach is geared to support professional caregivers and parents in understanding the immature infant from a brain developmental perspective, as expressed in the infant's continuously observable behaviour. The approach aims to modify NICU care in accordance with each infant's neurobehavioural thresholds from modulation to disorganization and stress, as inferred from the infant's behaviour. The goal is to provide security, protection, and nurture for the infant as a unique person (Als, 1977; Als, 1986; Als 1988; Als, 1989; Als, 1992).

Behavioural infant individuality

The infant's behaviour is understood as the child's means of communication (Als, 1977). The behavioural repertoire is conceptualized in a model of three continuously interactive subsystems of functioning, which in turn continuously interact with the infant's environment (Als, 1982). As infants experience the world directly through their senses, without the cognitive buffering that older children and adults employ, their behaviour provides a continuous, accurate reflection of the appropriateness of current sensory experience. If an experience is appropriate for the infant in terms of complexity or intensity, the infant will attempt to approach and move towards the experience, which will become developmentally supportive. If an experience is currently inappropriate in timing, complexity, or intensity for the infant's thresholds of functioning, the infant will actively attempt to defend against and move away from such an experience, which in turn is stressful and costly. The infant's behaviour thus indicates the current appropriateness or inappropriateness of an experience. Should the infant be unsuccessful in self-regulation or should the stimulus continue to remain inappropriate, the cost will steadily increase, reflected in the infant's deteriorating behaviour. The infant's behaviour in terms of autonomic function (respiration, colour, and visceral function), motor function (tone, movement, and posture), and state organization (range, robustness, and transition modulation of states) constitutes their communication with their caregivers about their experience of the environment and care that are currently provided. Infant behaviours which reflect stress, defence, and avoidance indicate inappropriate experiences. The respective situations require modification of environment and care. Infant behaviours which reflect approach, interest, wellbeing, and integration indicate appropriate and supportive environments and care. The respective situations should be maintained and enhanced (Als, 1999). The caregiver's goal and responsibility is the continuous adaptation and adjustment of environment and care for each infant, in order to reduce and eliminate stressful experiences and promote experiences and circumstances that increase the infant's capacity for self-regulation and the development of strengths. The implementation of such an individualized approach to care requires staff training and leadership support (Als & Gilkerson, 1995; Als, 2004; Als & Butler, 2005). A formal training programme (www.NIDCAP.org) is well established. Its focus is the education and formal training of multidisciplinary developmental specialist teams in NICUs. These teams in turn support and educate the bedside professionals, including neonatologists, nurses, therapists, and consultants, about the importance of individualizing care, and the teams help the caregivers recognize the central role that parents play in their NICU infants' lives, wellbeing, and development.

Short- and long-term outcome of NIDCAP care

There are currently four historical (Als et al., 1986; Parker et al., 1992; Becker et al., 1993; Petryshen et al., 1997) and six randomized controlled trials (Als et al., 1994; Buehler et al., 1995; Fleisher et al., 1995; Westrup et al., 2000; Als et al., 2003; Als et al., 2004) that have reported on the effectiveness of individualized developmental care in the Newborn Individualized Developmental Care and Assessment Program (NIDCAP) model. A recent ambivalent interpretation aside (Jacobs et al., 2002), the results of the studies provide consistent evidence of beneficial effects in terms of improved lung function, feeding behaviour, growth, and reduced length of hospital stay. They also show improved neurodevelopmental outcome. This includes improved neurobehaviour as well as improved neurophysiology. Most recently (Als et al., 2004), diffusion tensor imaging (MR-DTI) has shown regionally enhanced fibre tract development in the frontal lobe and internal capsule in infants receiving NIDCAP care. These brain structural findings may at least partly account for the demonstrated behavioural enhancement in complex attention and cognitive processing, as well as improved motor system competency. A three-centre trial (Als et al., 2003), which involved two transport and one inborn NICU, showed medical outcome and growth results consistent with those of the earlier studies quoted above for infants who were born at and before 29 weeks' gestational age – namely improved lung function, feeding behaviour, growth, and reduced length of hospital stay. Evaluation of family functioning measured in the three-centre trial identified significantly lower parental stress for the experimental group families, with an enhanced sense of parental competence and higher infant individualization scores. Outcome studies into the first year showed significantly better Bayley mental developmental (MDI) (Bayley, 1969; Bayley, 1993) and psychomotor developmental (PDI) scores at 3 and 5 months (Parker et al., 1992) and at 9 months corrected age (Als et al., 1986; Als et al., 1994; Als et al., 2004), as well as significantly improved behavioural regulation – including attention, social and object interaction, cognitive planning, affect regulation, fine and gross motor modulation, and vocal communication, as measured in a complex unstructured videotaped play paradigm (Kangaroo-Box paradigm) (Als et al., 1986; Als et al., 1994). Outcome at 3 years corrected age in a Swedish study (Kleberg et al., 2000) documented significantly better performance in auditory processing and speech (Griffiths Developmental Scales (Griffiths, 1970)). Furthermore, the children in the experimental group had significantly fewer behaviourally worrisome symptoms (Höök-Cedarblad Child Behaviour Interview) (Kleberg et al., 2000) and better communication skills in mother-child interaction (Parent-Child Early Relational Assessment Scale, ERA) (Clark et al., 1993). Outcome at age 6 years (Westrup et al., 2004) showed continued advantage in terms of survival without developmental disability, specifically without mental retardation and attention deficits. Improvement in general cognition approached statistical significance.

The importance of NIDCAP and the challenges of system-wide implementation

Based on this growing body of research evidence, one may conclude with confidence that individualized developmentally supportive care in the NICU, as delivered in the NIDCAP model, is scientifically sound. NIDCAP has also been shown to save costs in the NICU system (Als *et al.*, 1994; Fleisher *et al.*, 1995; Stevens *et al.*, 1996; Petryshen *et al.*, 1997). It is likely to be similarly cost-effective for other agencies such as the early intervention system, as well as for educational and special rehabilitative service systems.

None of the studies so far has calculated the cost of the implementation of the NIDCAP model *per se*. A developmental team consisting of two NIDCAP trained and certified developmental specialists typically implemented the intervention as tested in the various NIDCAP studies. A team usually consisted of a medical professional, such as a nurse or a neonatologist, and a developmental professional, such as a psychologist, an early childhood educator, or a physical/ occupational therapist. These specially trained and well prepared developmental specialists, as they are termed in the NIDCAP education model, conducted detailed weekly bedside observations of the experimental group infants. They followed the observations with written documentation in the form of a detailed written report formulated in collaboration with the infant's care team, including the parents. This report contained a detailed description of the infant's current strengths and thresholds to stress and vulnerability; the infant's apparent current goals and next steps; and suggestions and recommendations for strengthening the infant's competencies and reducing further the stressful events. The reports served as the basis for discussion and support for the family and the infant's caregivers on how best to support the infant's current strengths and reduce stress and sensory overstimulation. Daily check-in and problem solving with the parents and the care teams was part of the intervention. Environmental modifications typically included reduction in lighting and the creation of quiet surroundings for much of the 24-hour day; support for the parents for prolonged periods of skin-to-skin holding and nurturing, as well as support for successful breast pumping and breast feeding. Comfortable recliner bedchairs, attractive bedside screens, comfortable and soft infant clothing and bedding, specially designed buntings, sheepskins, incubator covers, canopies for infants in open cribs, and various other facilitative items were created and made available to the parents and the care team as indicated. The main ingredient of the intervention success was the consistency and continuity of support to the care teams and the families provided by the developmental specialists. Consistency in individualizing support and care assures steadiness of small, incremental steps of progress for the infant. It provides the opportunity to build continuously on the infant's newly emerging strengths, and to prevent even minor setbacks, which so often occur because of lack of continuity and up-to-date information concerning the infant's strengths and thresholds of current sensitivity and reactivity.

Given the encouraging results in terms of medical and neurodevelopmental advantages, preventive neuroanatomical remodelling, and enhanced parental confidence, it behoves those responsible for the quality of NICU care to be knowledgeable about the NIDCAP model. Introduction of NIDCAP into a system is not a trivial process and involves a considerable investment of funds, time, and energy at all levels of the organization. In some situations, NIDCAP may require physical changes and adaptations in the NICU. However, these are never barriers for the changes in care implementation carried out by the caregivers, as NIDCAP first and foremost requires a significant shift in mind, attitude, and role definition for those in the system. Such a shift and paradigm change in turn requires substantial educational efforts and the creation and support of a climate and culture of reflection. Only in such a reflection- and relationship-based system will there occur significant changes in the practice of care. Once the culture has embraced such change, the likelihood of fallback and slippage to the former task orientation or action-oriented model of care diminishes markedly. An NICU will grow in the NIDCAP model of care implementation and transaction when two well trained developmentalists are on the staff and salaried by the NICU system, with the charge of guiding and nurturing, coaching, and supporting the daily hands-on staff, and the emotional interactive attitudinal stance of the NICU. Then infants and families truly will have the chance to thrive, and the staff will show a healthy and competent self-image and great professional satisfaction. NIDCAP is highly compelling from an ethical human perspective and is in direct keeping with the best principles of family-centred care. It holds high promise as best practice and standard of NICU care for all nurseries (Als & Gilkerson, 1995).

A well established training programme focuses on the education and formal training and certification of a multidisciplinary developmental specialist team. The NIDCAP Federation International (NFI), a non-profit professional membership organization, is the certifying organ for all NIDCAP professionals and NIDCAP trainers. There are currently 16 NIDCAP training centres worldwide; of these 10 are in the USA, five in Europe (in Sweden, France, the Netherlands, the United Kingdom, and Belgium), and one in South America (Argentina). Several further centres are in development in various countries, including Norway, Italy, Portugal, Spain, and Ireland, as well as Canada and Israel. The NFI website (www.nidcap.org) provides further information. There are more than 1000 NIDCAP certified professionals in various NICUs around the world, who provide the support for institutional change, as well as the required continuous leadership and organizational support. The support necessary includes regularly provided opportunities for continuing education and development for professional as well as personal and emotional growth, enhancement of self-awareness, and the capacity to be present in the moment, to connect, and to 'hold' the complex relationships and interactions involved in all NICU work. The self-definition of the developmentally skilled NICU professional in a NIDCAP nursery includes the highest technical skill embedded in the highest relational skill. All NICU work involves human interaction and relationships at many levels. NICU work occurs in the most complex interface of physical and emotional vulnerability and development. At its core is a tiny, immature, fully dependent, yet rapidly developing human being with a highly sensitive nervous system. This small human being, as well as his or her parents and family, trust and count on the caregivers' full attention, affective attunement, and unwavering faith and investment. Therein lies the challenge and the opportunity of all developmental NICU care.

Acknowledgments: Supported by Grant Sponsor: NIH/ NICHD; grant number: R01 HD047730 and R01 HD046855 (H.A.). Grant Sponsor: US Department of Education/OSEP; grant number: H324CO40045 (H.A.). Grant sponsor: I. Harris Foundation (H.A.). Grant Sponsor: NIH/MRDDRC; grant number: P01HD18655 (M. Greenberg).

References

Als, H. (1977): The newborn communicates. *J. Commun.* **27,** 66–73.

Als, H. (1982): Toward a synactive theory of development: promise for the assessment of infant individuality. *Infant Mental Health J.* **3,** 229–243.

Als, H. (1986): A synactive model of neonatal behavioral organization: framework for the assessment and support of the neurobehavioral development of the premature infant and his parents in the environment of the neonatal intensive care unit. *Phys. Occup. Ther. Pediatr.* **6,** 3–53.

Als, H. (1988): Neurobehavioral development of the premature infant and the environment of the neonatal intensive care unit. In: *Pediatric Medicine*, eds. M.E. Avery & L.R. First, pp. 125–130. Baltimore: Williams and Wilkins.

Als, H. (1989): Caring for the preterm infant. In: *Neurological lesions in infancy: early diagnosis and intervention*, eds. M. Bottos, T.B. Brazelton, A. Ferrari & F. Zacchello, pp. 201–216. Padova: Liviana Editrice.

Als, H. (1992): Individualized, family-focused developmental care for the very low birthweight preterm infant in the NICU. In: *Advances in applied developmental psychology*, vol. 6, eds. S.L. Friedman & M.D. Sigman, pp. 341–388. Norwood, NJ: Ablex Publishing Company.

Als, H. (1999): Reading the premature infant. In: *Developmental interventions in the neonatal intensive care nursery*, ed. E. Goldson, pp. 18–85. New York: Oxford University Press.

Als. H. (2004): Individualized developmental care for preterm infants. In: *Encyclopedia on early childhood development* (pp. http://www.excellence-earlychildhood.ca/liste_theme.asp): Centre of Excellence for Early Childhood Development Website.

Als, H. & Brazelton, T.B. (1981): A new model of assessing the behavioral organization in preterm and fullterm infants: two case studies. *J. Am. Acad. Child Psychiatry* **20**, 239–263.

Als, H. & Gilkerson, L. (1995): Developmentally supportive care in the neonatal intensive care unit. *Zero to Three* **15**, 1–10.

Als, H. & Butler, S. (2005): Neurobehavioral development of the preterm infant. In: *Fanaroff and Martin's Neonatal-Perinatal Medicine: diseases of the fetus and infant*, 8th edition, eds. R. Martin, A. Fanaroff & M. Walsh, vol 2, pp. 1051–1068. St. Louis: C.V. Mosby.

Als, H., Lawhon, G., Brown, E., Gibes, R., Duffy, F.H., McAnulty, G.B. & Blickman, J.G. (1986): Individualized behavioral and environmental care for the very low birth weight preterm infant at high risk for bronchopulmonary dysplasia: neonatal intensive care unit and developmental outcome. *Pediatrics* **78**, 1123–1132.

Als, H., Lawhon, G., Duffy, F.H., McAnulty, G.B., Gibes-Grossman, R. & Blickman, J.G. (1994): Individualized developmental care for the very low birthweight preterm infant: medical and neurofunctional effects. *JAMA* **272**, 853–858.

Als, H., Gilkerson, L., Duffy, F.H., McAnulty, G.B., Buehler, D.M., VandenBerg, K.A., Sweet, N., Sell, E., Parad, R.B., Ringer, S.A., Butler, S., Blickman, J.G. & Jones, K.J. (2003): A three-center randomized controlled trial of individualized developmental care for very low birth weight preterm infants: medical, neurodevelopmental, parenting and caregiving effects. *J. Dev. Behav. Pediatr.* **24**, 399–408.

Als, H., Duffy, F.H., McAnulty, G.B., Rivkin, M.J., Vajapeyam, S., Mulkern, R.V., Warfield, S., Hüppi, P.S., Butler, S., Conneman, N., Fischer, C. & Eichenwald, E. (2004): Early experience alters brain function and structure. *Pediatrics* **113**, 846–857.

Anand, K.J.S. & Scalzo, F.M. (2000): Can adverse neonatal experiences alter brain development and subsequent behavior? *Biol. Neonat.* **77**, 69–82.

Bayley, N. (1969): *Bayley scales of infant development*. New York: The Psychological Corporation.

Bayley, N. (1993): *Bayley scales of infant development, 2nd ed*. San Antonio, Texas: The Psychological Corporation.

Becker, P.T., Grunwald, P.C., Moorman, J. & Stuhr, S. (1993): Effects of developmental care on behavioral organization in very-low-birth-weight infants. *Nurs. Res.* **42**, 214–220.

Behrman, R. (2007): *Preterm birth: causes, consequences, and prevention*. Washington, DC: The National Academies Press.

Blair, C., Ramey, C.T. & Hardin, J.M. (1995): Early intervention for low birthweight, premature infants: participation and intellectual development. *Am. J. Ment. Retard.* **99**, 542–554.

Brooks-Gunn, J., McCarton, C.M., Casey, P.H., McCormick, M.C., Bauer, C.R., Bernbaum, J.C., Tyson, J., Swanson, M., Bennett, F.C., Scott, D.T., et al. (1994): Early intervention in low birth weight premature infants: results through age 5 years from the Infant Health and Development Program. *JAMA* **272**, 1257–1262.

Buehler, D.M., Als, H., Duffy, F.H., McAnulty, G.B. & Liederman, J. (1995): Effectiveness of individualized developmental care for low-risk preterm infants: behavioral and electrophysiological evidence. *Pediatrics* **96**, 923–932.

Clark, R., Paulson, A. & Colin, S. (1993): Assessment of developmental status and parent-infant relationship: the therapeutic process of evaluation. In: *Handbook of infant mental health*, ed. C. Zeanah. New York: Guilford Press.

Fleisher, B.F., VandenBerg, K.A., Constantinou, J., Heller, C., Benitz, W.E., Johnson, A., Rosenthal, A. & Stevenson, D.K. (1995): Individualized developmental care for very-low-birth-weight premature infants. *Clin. Pediatr.* **34**, 523–529.

Griffiths, R. (1970): *The abilities of young children*. London: Child Development Research Centre.

Hack, M., Flanner, D.J., Schluchter, M., Cartar, L., Borawski, E. & Klein, N. (2002): Outcomes in young adulthood for very-low-birth-weight infants. *N. Engl. J. Med.* **346**, 149–157.

Hack, M., Taylor, H.G., Drotar, D., Schluchter, M., Cartar, L., Andreias, L., Wilson-Costello, D. & Klein, N. (2005): Chronic conditions, functional limitations, and special health care needs of school-aged children born with extremely low-birth-weight in the 1990s. *JAMA* **294**, 318–325.

Jacobs, S., Sokol, J. & Ohlsson, A. (2002): The newborn individualized developmental care and assessment program is not supported by meta-analyses of the data. *J. Pediatr.* **140**, 699–706.

Kleberg, A., Westrup, B. & Stjernqvist, K. (2000): Developmental outcome, child behavior and mother-child interaction at 3 years of age following Newborn Individualized Developmental Care and Intervention Program (NIDCAP) intervention. *Early Hum. Dev.* **60**, 123–135.

McCormick, M.C., Brooks-Gunn, J., Workman-Daniels, K., Turner, J. & Peckman, G.J. (1992): The health and developmental status of very low-birthweight children at school age. *JAMA* **267**, 2204–2208.

McCormick, M.C., Workman-Daniels, K., Brooks-Gunn, J. & Peckham, G.J. (1993): Hospitalization of very low birthweigth children at school age. *J. Pediatr.* **122**, 360–365.

McCormick, M.C., McCarton, C., Brooks-Gunn, J., Belt, P. & Gross, R.T. (1998): The infant health and development program: interim summary. *J. Dev. Behav. Pediatr.* **19**, 359–370.

Parker, S.J., Zahr, L.K., Cole, J.G. & Brecht, M. (1992): Outcome after developmental intervention in the neonatal intensive care unit for mothers of preterm infants with low socioeconomic status. *J. Pediatr.* **120**, 780–785.

Petryshen, P., Stevens, B., Hawkins, J. & Stewart, M. (1997): Comparing nursing costs for preterm infants receiving conventional vs. developmental care. *Nurs. Econ.* **15**, 138–150.

Ramey, C.T., Bryant, D.M., Wasik, B.H., Sparling, J.J., Fendt, K.H. & LaVange, L.M. (1992): Infant Health and Development Program for Low Birthweight, Premature Infants: program elements, family participation, and child intelligence. *Pediatrics* **89**, 454–465.

Stevens, B., Petryshen, P., Hawkins, J., Smith, B. & Taylor, P. (1996): Developmental versus conventional care: a comparison of clinical outcomes for very low birth weight infants. *Can. J. Nurs. Res.* **28**, 97–113.

Westrup, B., Kleberg, A., von Eichwald, K., Stjernqvist, K. & Lagercrantz, H. (2000): A randomized controlled trial to evaluate the effects of the Newborn Individualized Developmental Care and Assessment Program in a Swedish setting. *Pediatrics* **105**, 66–72.

Westrup, B., Bohm, B., Lagercrantz, H. & Stjernqvist, K. (2004): Preschool outcome in children born very prematurely and cared for according to the Newborn Individualized Developmental Care and Assessment Program (NIDCAP). *Acta Paediatr.* **93**, 498–507.

Chapter 23

Neonatal seizures: monitoring and treatment

Licia Lugli, Maria Pina Guerra, Maria Federica Roversi and Fabrizio Ferrari

Neonatology Unit, University of Modena and Reggio Emilia, via del Pozzo 71, 41100 Modena, Italy
ferrarif@unimore.it

Summary

Neonatal seizures are a common neurological emergency and still represent a diagnostic and therapeutic challenge to clinicians. They are an expression of neural compromise, with many different aetiologies. The main causes are perinatal hypoxia-ischaemia, intracranial haemorrhage or infarction, meningitis, congenital abnormalities of the brain, and inborn or acquired metabolic disorders. Estimates of the incidence of clinical neonatal seizures range from 0.7 to 3 per 1,000 live term births, though the incidence of clinically silent seizures is unknown. Neonatal seizures are usually 'subtle' and clinical diagnosis may be unreliable; thus EEG recordings are imperative when seizures are suspected. Prolonged or continuous EEG or video-EEG monitoring provides an excellent opportunity to study neonatal seizures, and modern digital equipment makes such monitoring feasible in the neonatal intensive care unit. As seizures can be dangerous for the developing brain, there is general consensus that they should be treated, particularly if they are frequent or prolonged. Seizures on their own can cause neuronal injury, as they increase the metabolic demands of the central nervous system, cause release of excitatory neurotransmitters, and may lead to fluctuations in systemic blood pressure. There is no evidence that prophylactic antiepileptic treatment in neonates with perinatal asphyxia is beneficial. Treatment of neonatal seizures has changed little over the past 50 years and phenobarbital remains the first-line drug, with a loading dose up to 40 mg/kg, and is effective in about one-third of cases. Infants responding to phenobarbital have a smaller seizure burden, relatively normal background EEG, and a better prognosis than babies requiring second-line treatment. Neonates who fail to respond to phenobarbital are more likely to have hypoxic-ischaemic encephalopathy, an abnormal EEG background activity, and a worse prognosis. Most benzodiazepines have been tried in the newborn period, and midazolam – a new short-acting benzodiazepine effective in treating status epilepticus in older children – is often used as second-line treatment. Some clinicians consider that phenytoin, with a loading dose of 15–20 mg/kg, is more effective than benzodiazepines as a second-line drug, but hypotension and arrhythmias have been reported. There is little published experience with other antiepileptic drugs (valproic acid, vigabatrin, carbamazepine) in the newborn period. The treatment of neonatal seizures remains a challenge and the search for an effective antiepileptic regimen needs to continue.

Introduction

During the neonatal period seizures represent the main sign of neural compromise. The incidence of seizures in newborn infants is considerably higher than at any other time of life. Recent epidemiological studies report seizures in 0.7 to 3 per 1,000 term neonates, but this may be an underestimate as data are based on the clinical diagnosis, which can be unreliable in the neonate. In practice, electroclinical dissociation is often observed, as neonates may have abnormal electrographic activity not accompanied by any obvious clinical signs, particularly after antiepileptic drug treatment. Conversely, normal motor or autonomic behaviour in healthy babies may appear 'seizure-like' or resemble the paroxysmal movements of encephalopathic infants (Evans & Levene, 1998; Rennie & Boylan, 2007; Silverstein & Jensen, 2007).

The reason for the increased susceptibility of the immature brain to seizure activity is related to the development of neuroexcitatory and neuroinhibitory activity. In early life the γ-amino butyric (GABA) receptor system is functionally more active than the N-methyl-D-aspartate (NMDA) system and it provides an excitatory effect instead of the inhibition of neural activation that is typical of later life. In particular, GABA receptors have an activating function on neurons and facilitate cell depolarization. This situation changes with nervous system development and the sensitivity to seizures progressively diminishes in later life. The seizure susceptibility of newborn infants is also attributable to the phenomenon of 'kindling', which is more pronounced in the immature than in the mature brain; kindling refers to the effect of a brief but repetitive stimulation of a susceptible area of the brain, which may produce an accelerating and prolonged convulsive effect, with the possibility of generalized seizures. Repetition of seizure activity leads to an increase of duration and a decrease of latency between seizures, resulting in a reduction in the convulsion threshold and also making the brain more vulnerable to seizures in later life (Sanchez *et al.*, 2005; Dzhala *et al.*, 2006; Rennie & Boylan, 2007).

Aetiology

The aetiology of neonatal seizures is varied. Improvements in neuroimaging techniques have revealed previously unsuspected cerebral lesions, and the proportion of cases with an unknown underlying cause has diminished in recent years (Volpe, 1989; Tekgul *et al.*, 2006; Silverstein & Jensen, 2007).

The main cause of neonatal seizures remains perinatal hypoxic-ischaemic injury, and seizures represent a typical manifestation of neonatal encephalopathy (isolated seizures or repeated seizures comprising status epilepticus). Intracranial haemorrhage or infarction often causes seizures, as do cerebral malformations and venous sinus thrombosis (Ferriero, 2004). Seizures also often occur in cases of meningitis or meningoencephalitis. Inborn errors of metabolism or acquired metabolic abnormalities (hypocalcaemia, hypoglycaemia, hypomagnesaemia) are possible causes as well. Sometimes seizures have a genetic origin (mutations of the potassium channel genes KCNQ2 and KCNQ3), and rarely they are manifestations of the neonatal epileptic syndrome (neonatal epileptic encephalopathy or neonatal onset epilepsy).

Aetiology-specific treatment is critical as it may prevent further brain injury. This is particularly true for seizures associated with metabolic disorders such as hypoglycaemia, hypocalcaemia, or hypomagnesaemia, and in cases of central nervous system (CNS) or systemic infections. Neonatal seizures may not be effectively controlled by antiepileptic drugs unless their underlying cause is treated.

Metabolic disturbances which need to be corrected include the following:

- Hypoglycaemia: give 2 ml/kg of 10 per cent glucose in water intravenously (0.2 g/kg) as a bolus, followed by a continuous infusion at up to 8 mg/kg/min.

- Hypocalcaemia: give 2 ml/kg of 10 per cent calcium gluconate intravenously over 1 to 3 minutes, followed by maintenance of 6 ml/kg/24 h intravenously or orally.
- Hypomagnesaemia: give 0.8 ml/kg/dose of 10 per cent magnesium sulphate intravenously.
- Pyridoxine-dependent seizures are responsive to treatment with vitamin B-6 (pyridoxine), with a loading dose of 50 to 100 mg/kg intravenously, followed by a maintenance dose of 50 to 100 mg daily orally throughout life; high doses may be required during periods of intercurrent illness. Treatment should be started with EEG monitoring as the effect of pyridoxine becomes evident immediately, confirming the diagnosis. In rare cases seizures are not controlled by pyridoxine but are responsive to pyridoxal 5'-phosphate, the active form of pyridoxine (Evans & Levene, 1998; Ferrari et al., 2006; Hoffmann et al., 2007).

Adverse effects of seizures on the brain

Although the prognosis of neonates with seizures depends mainly on the underlying cause, there is increasing evidence that the seizure burden can affect the outcome (Tekgul et al., 2006). As the duration and frequency of seizures may have an additional adverse effect on outcome, there is general consensus that seizures must be treated and an aggressive therapeutic strategy is often used. There are increasing data indicating that seizures have an adverse effect on developmental outcome and predispose to cognitive, behavioural, or epileptic complications (McBride et al., 2000; Levene, 2002; Rennie & Boylan, 2007).

Animal studies have shown that seizures impair neurogenesis and alter neural structure, function, and connections. Seizures cause synaptic reorganization with aberrant growth or sprouting of cell axons, and lead to neuronal apoptosis and sclerosis in the hippocampal regions. Seizures can inhibit brain growth, modify neuronal circuits, and increase neural excitability. Recurrent convulsions during early development may lead to impairment of visual-spatial learning and memory and predispose to seizures in later life. They also cause an increase in cerebral blood flow velocity to meet the increased demands, but a mismatch between energy supply and demand can be generated and the pathologically exaggerated requirements may not be satisfied. Convulsive activity increases the metabolic rate and this is particularly dangerous for an already metabolically compromised brain and after a hypoxic-ischaemic injury (Mizrahi, 1999; McBride et al., 2000; Wirrel, 2005; Rennie & Boylan, 2007). Magnetic resonance spectroscopy studies have shown areas of metabolic dysfunction in babies with seizures (Miller et al., 2002). Indeed seizures add further insult after a hypoxic-ischaemic injury, and status epilepticus may be particularly harmful (Wirrel, 2005). Consequently, seizures in the context of asphyxia need to be treated, but this goal remains a challenge, as seizure control can be achieved in no more than 60 per cent of neonates with seizures caused by hypoxic-ischaemic injury (Hunt & Inder, 2005). Moreover, there is concern that undiagnosed and untreated subclinical seizures, which may be equally damaging to the brain – one study showed that the outcome was worse in newborns with subclinical untreated electrographic seizures (McBride et al., 2000).

Diagnosis and monitoring of seizures

Seizures are traditionally classified as clonic, tonic, myoclonic, and subtle, according to the Volpe classification (Figs. 1 and 2) (Volpe, 1989). In the neonate the most common seizures are subtle and include blinking, chewing, eye movements, motor automatisms, apnoea, and autonomic phenomena. Such manifestations are similar to physiological phenomena in healthy newborn infants and may be missed by clinical observations. Moreover, there is poor concordance between the clinical manifestations and the electrographic features of neonatal seizures, mostly after antiepileptic drug administration. Thus the clinical phenomena may resolve with treatment, but EEG discharges can continue without any appreciable clinical manifestations (Biagioni *et al.*, 1998; Scher *et al.*, 2003). It is not unusual to find neonates with clinically unsuspected epileptic activity during EEG monitoring (Clancy, 2006a). Thus in the neonatal period the clinical diagnosis of seizures is unreliable and EEG recording is mandatory in infants with suspected seizures or who are at risk of seizures (hypoxic-ischaemic injury, cerebral lesions, metabolic derangement). Continuous and prolonged EEG polygraphic monitoring or video-EEG monitoring affords the possibility of evaluating the seizure burden (the number and duration of seizures per hour), electro-clinical correlations, the effect of treatment, and any modification of seizure pattern after antiepileptic drug administration. Moreover, EEG background activity, a strong prognostic indicator, can be recorded and analysed (Ferrari *et al.*, 2001).

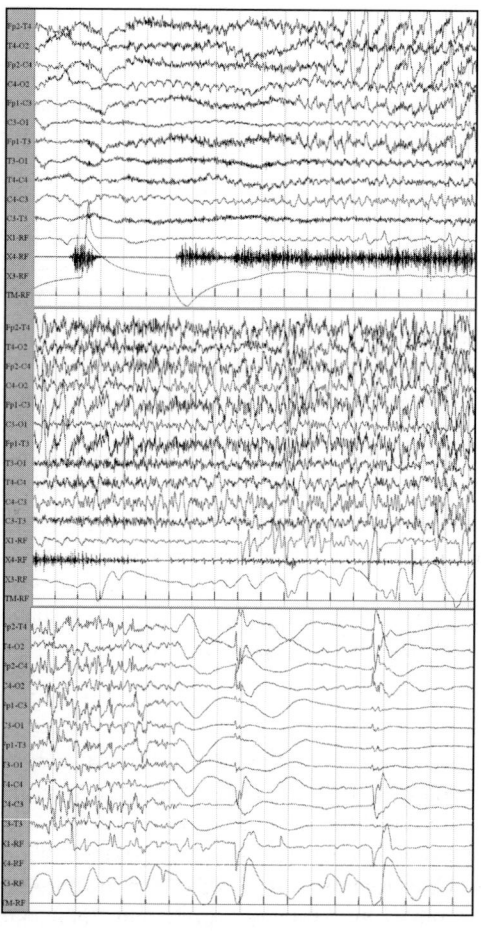

Fig. 1. Tonic seizure and apnoea followed by EEG background depression.

Chapter 23 Neonatal seizures: monitoring and treatment

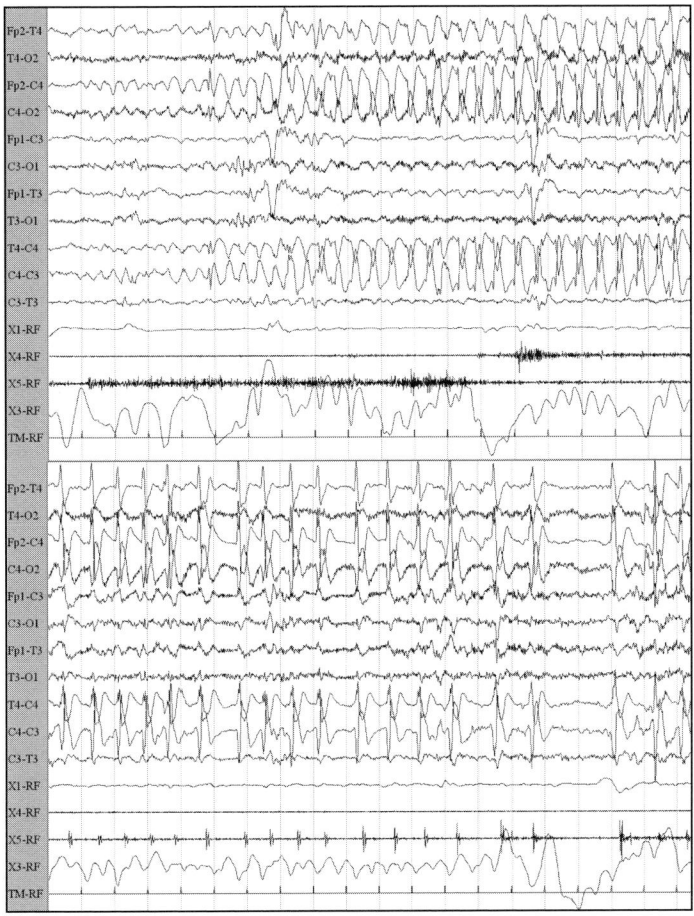

Fig. 2. Clonic seizure starting with a tonic phase.

Improvements in recording techniques and the development of digital instrumentation make EEG monitoring more feasible in the intensive unit care. Modern digital EEG and video-EEG equipment can record signals for long periods without the constant attention of a technician (Rennie & Boylan, 2003; Clancy, 2006a; Rennie & Boylan, 2007).

The cerebral function monitor (CFM) is a simplified EEG device, providing an amplitude-integrated EEG (aEEG). The use of CFM is widespread in neonatal intensive care units, as it is considered to be an easy-to-use monitoring system for neonates with seizures. This technology cannot replace the traditional EEG, as CFM misses localized seizures and those of short duration or low voltage. CFM should be considered as a readily available bedside monitoring instrument that can be applied and interpreted by non-neurologists with modest training (Rennie et al., 2004; De Vries & Hellstrom-Westas, 2005). The traditional EEG remains the gold standard for establishing the presence of seizures, quantifying them, and evaluating the efficacy of antiepileptic treatment (Rennie & Boylan, 2007).

Antiepileptic treatment in newborn infants with perinatal asphyxia

Seizures are common after perinatal asphyxia and they may exacerbate secondary neuronal injury by increasing cerebral metabolic demands, causing fluctuations in oxygenation and perfusion, and triggering the release of excitatory neurotransmitters. Anticonvulsant therapy has been used in infants with perinatal asphyxia in order to prevent seizures (Hall et al., 1998; Guillet & Kwon, 2007). However, long-term anticonvulsant therapy may lead to inhibition of brain development (Marsh et al., 2006). The use of anticonvulsant therapy to prevent seizures following perinatal asphyxia has been evaluated in a recent Cochrane review (Evans et al., 2007). Seven randomized or quasi-randomized controlled trials were considered. No studies were of sufficient methodological quality and size to demonstrate a valid, clinically significant change in the risk of mortality or severe neurodevelopmental disability. A meta-analysis combining five studies comparing barbiturates with conventional therapy following perinatal asphyxia showed no difference in risk of death, severe neurodevelopmental disability, or the combined outcome of death and severe neurodevelopmental disability. The authors concluded that, at the present time, anticonvulsant therapy for term infants in the immediate period following perinatal asphyxia cannot be recommended in routine clinical practice other than in the treatment of prolonged or frequent clinical seizures.

Treatment of neonatal seizures

There is increasing evidence that seizures are dangerous for the developing brain, and the prognosis is not solely dependent on the aetiology. Thus the treatment of seizures is recommended, with the goal of eliminating electro-clinical and electrographic seizures (Mizrahi, 1999). There is no evidence that prophylactic antiepileptic treatment in babies with perinatal asphyxia is of benefit, although one small randomized study reported a reduction in disability after early high dose of phenobarbital (Hall et al., 1998; Guillet & Kwon, 2007).

Neonatal seizures require urgent treatment to prevent brain injury. It must be emphasized that both the seizures and their subsequent treatment may be associated with changes in respiration, heart rate, and blood pressure. Thus the therapeutic strategy needs to ensure an adequate airway and access to the circulatory system early in the course of treatment. Anticonvulsant drugs should be given after adequate ventilation, perfusion, and a normal glucose concentration have been established. Metabolic disturbances should be corrected if present.

Antiepileptic therapy for neonatal seizures has changed little in the past 50 years and few clinical trials have been done on the management of the neonate with seizures (Levene, 2002; Hunt & Inder, 2005; Sankar & Painter, 2005). Phenobarbital (phenobarbitone) and phenytoin have been the mainstays of treatment, and benzodiazepines have been used more recently. Some clinicians have also used lidocaine (lignocaine) with encouraging results, while there is little published experience with any other antiepileptic drugs (valproic acid, vigabatrin, carbamazepine, and so on) (Rennie & Boylan, 2003; Booth & Evans, 2004; Rennie & Boylan, 2007).

Phenobarbital

Phenobarbital is a central nervous system depressant which is an effective anticonvulsant. It appears to increase the seizure threshold and to limit the spread of seizure activity. The mechanism of its pharmacological action is not fully known but it may involve an increase in inhibitory neurotransmission through enhancement of the GABAergic systems (Evans & Levene, 1998). It is widely distributed, with a higher distribution volume in neonates and infants than in adults. It has low binding to plasma proteins, is metabolized by the liver, and is excreted by the kidneys. The pharmacokinetics in the neonatal period are variable (the elimination half-life ranges from 40 to 200 hours). It is administered in a loading dose of 20 mg/kg by slow intravenous infusion over 30 minutes. Additional 5–10 mg/kg loading doses may be given if seizures are not controlled, the maximum loading dose being 40 mg/kg. Maintenance is 3 to 5 mg/kg daily intravenously or orally, with the first dose given no earlier than 12 hours after the loading dose (Painter et al., 1981). Phenobarbital is the traditional antiepileptic drug and is used worldwide to treat neonatal seizures, but its efficacy remains uncertain. Its widespread clinical use is not founded on a firm scientific basis: no formal, prospective, randomized, placebo-controlled trial has ever shown the efficacy of phenobarbital in treating neonatal seizures, and published reports fail to provide clear support for its use. However, it continues to be the first-line drug for treatment of neonatal seizures (Booth & Evans, 2004; Clancy, 2006b). Approximately one-third to one-half of babies with seizures respond to phenobarbital (Boylan et al., 2002). A recent study using EEG monitoring to diagnose seizures and to measure the response to therapy compared phenobarbital with phenytoin and showed that 43 per cent of subjects (13/30) responded to phenobarbital, while 45 per cent (13/29) responded to phenytoin. In another study, continuous seizures were controlled by phenobarbital in 50 per cent of subjects (11/22) (Boylan et al., 2004). Phenobarbital is likely to be effective in neonates with isolated seizures rather than with status epilepticus, and in cases with mild to moderate EEG background abnormalities. Phenobarbital causes electro-clinical dissociation, as babies are sedated by the drug and cease to make abnormal movements, though electrographic seizures may continue (Scher et al., 2003; Hahn & Riviello, 2004). There is concern about the safety of phenobarbital and other CNS-depressant drugs in newborn infants. Like other antiepileptic drugs, phenobarbital has several side-effects, such as sedation and respiratory and cardiac depression. Moreover, in immature animal models phenobarbital has a measurable adverse impact on brain growth and development (Rennie & Boylan, 2003; Marsh et al., 2006).

Phenytoin

Phenytoin is an anticonvulsant drug whose primary site of action is the motor cortex. It causes an efflux of sodium from neurons and therefore stabilizes the threshold against overactivity of neurons, particularly in the brain stem centres responsible for the tonic phase of seizures. The pharmacokinetics are dose-dependent over the therapeutic range and are poorly predictable in the neonate. It has high binding to plasma proteins and it is eliminated by the kidney (Painter et al., 1981).

Phenytoin is generally used as a second-line drug in newborn infants who fail to respond to phenobarbital. It is given in a loading dose of 15 to 20 mg/dl by slow intravenous infusion, followed by a maintenance dose of 2 to 4 mg/kg/dose twice a day by slow intravenous infusion or orally. The maintenance dose needs to be monitored and adjusted according to blood levels. In newborns phenytoin has not been reported to cause the skin rashes, coarse facial appearance, and gum hypertrophy that are reported in paediatric patients, but it can cause hypotension and arrhythmias, mostly when there is occult myocardial damage (Rennie & Boylan, 2003; Riviello, 2004; Sankar, 2004).

In a randomized trial, Painter and colleagues (Painter et al., 1999) evaluated phenytoin as an alternative to phenobarbital as a first line drug. Infants enrolled were at risk of seizures because of various historical factors, and an EEG was done on those infants considered to be eligible. Neonates with seizures were randomly assigned to receive intravenous phenobarbital or phenytoin; if the infant continued to have seizures the second drug was added. The primary end point of the study was complete control of seizure activity with one or both drugs, based on interpretation of the EEG recordings. Fifty-nine neonates were included. About 65 per cent had a gestational age of at least 37 weeks and most had seizures secondary to birth asphyxia, haemorrhage, or infarction. Twenty-nine were initially given phenytoin and 30 initially received phenobarbital. Of those receiving phenobarbital, 13 (43 per cent) had complete control of seizures. After adding phenytoin to those who failed single-drug treatment, four more children had control of seizures, for an overall seizure-free rate of 57 per cent. Among the group randomized to receive phenytoin first, 13 (45 per cent) had complete control of seizures. Following the addition of phenobarbital, five more infants were seizure-free, for an overall rate of 62 per cent. The severity of the seizures was inversely related to control by one or both drugs. No adverse events related to the drugs were reported. The investigators concluded that phenytoin and phenobarbital were equally but not completely effective in the treatment of neonatal seizures (Painter et al., 1999).

Benzodiazepines

Benzodiazepines have anxiolytic, sedative, muscle relaxant, and anticonvulsant actions. They provide their anticonvulsive effect by facilitating the action of GABA in the brain. Benzodiazepines cause sedation, respiratory depression, hypotonia, hypotension, hypersalivation, and increased bronchial secretions (Riviello, 2004).

Several different benzodiazepines have been employed in newborns. Diazepam can be used in single doses of 0.3 to 1 mg/kg, but is not suitable for continuous infusion. Lorazepam can be used intravenously in a dose of 0.05 to 0.15 mg/kg. Clonazepam can be given as an infusion, but a bolus dose of 0.1 mg/kg every 24 hours is more appropriate.

Midazolam is a newer benzodiazepine, a short-acting GABA antagonist with a good safety profile and is effective for treating status epilepticus in children. It is given in a loading dose of 50 to 150 µg/kg as a slow push, followed by a continuous infusion of 50 to 200 µg/kg/hour. It has been used as second-line treatment in neonates with seizures. Midazolam has been reported to cause seizures or seizure-like activity such as myoclonic jerks and dystonic posturing; moreover, there are concerns about its use in preterm babies as the outcome was better in babies sedated with morphine than when midazolam was used (Rennie & Boylan, 2003).

Benzodiazepine therapy in newborn infants with seizures has had variable results, probably because of differences in case selection, in the definition of seizures and seizure control, and in the type and dose of the drugs administered.

Boylan and colleagues (Boylan et al., 2004) conducted a randomized trial of second-line anticonvulsant treatment for neonates, assessing the response to treatment using continuous video-EEG monitoring. Of 22 neonates with EEG-confirmed seizures included in the study, 11 did not respond to phenobarbital and required a second line drug. Six neonates were treated with benzodiazepines (three with clonazepam and three with midazolam) as second-line treatment. None responded and their neurodevelopmental outcome was poor.

Sheth and colleagues (Sheth et al., 1996) evaluated six neonates with persisting seizures despite high-dose phenobarbital therapy, with or without the addition of phenytoin. Midazolam was then given by continuous intravenous infusion. Within one hour of initiation of midazolam, seizures were controlled in all six neonates, and electroencephalographic seizures were abolished in four of the six; however, two continued to have electrographic seizures without clinical manifestations for a further 12 hours.

Another recent study reported that midazolam controlled seizures in 100 per cent of treated cases (Castro Conde et al., 2005). The investigators analysed the outcome with respect to treatment in 45 neonates with EEG-confirmed seizures. Electroencephalographic seizures persisted in 17 of 32 neonates receiving phenobarbital/phenytoin, of whom 13 had a poor outcome and four died. In contrast, electroencephalographic seizures were controlled in all of 13 non-responders to phenobarbital/phenytoin who were treated with midazolam (four had a poor outcome and two died). The investigators concluded that midazolam was effective in controlling seizures in non-responders to phenobarbital/phenytoin, and that non-responders to phenobarbital/phenytoin had a significantly worse outcome than responders.

As more than one third of all neonatal seizures are refractory to high-dose phenobarbital and phenytoin, midazolam given by continuous intravenous infusion may be a valuable adjunct (Castro Conde et al., 2005).

Lidocaine

Lidocaine is a membrane-stabilizing agent with local anaesthetic and antiarrhythmic effects. It also alters depolarization in neurons by blocking the fast-voltage gated sodium (Na^+) channels in the cell membrane, and stabilizes the neuronal membrane, preventing the initiation and transmission of depolarization. Consequently it has an anticonvulsive action and it may be used to treat seizures. It can be administered as a loading dose followed by a continuous infusion. It has a narrow therapeutic range and it accumulates; consequently infusions should be limited in time. One of the most common side effects is cardiac arrhythmia, but it can also induce seizures. Lidocaine is an effective drug for the treatment of neonatal convulsions unresponsive to traditional anticonvulsant therapy, and it has often been used in Europe (Rennie & Boylan, 2003; Riviello, 2004).

Malingré and colleagues (Malingré et al., 2006) studied the treatment of neonatal seizures with lidocaine and tried to develop an optimal dosing strategy with minimal risk of cardiac arrhythmias. They studied 20 neonates during routine treatment of neonatal seizures with lidocaine. All were given a loading dose of 2 mg/kg in 10 minutes, followed by a continuous infusion of 6 mg/kg/hour for 12 hours, 4 mg/kg/hour for 12 hours, and finally 2 mg/kg/hour for 12 hours. No cardiac arrhythmias were observed, and lidocaine was effective in 76 per cent of the treatments. In most of the treatments, maximum plasma concentrations were > 9 mg/l and plasma levels of this order have been associated with cardiac toxicity when the agent is used as an anti-arrhythmic drug in adults. The investigators therefore developed an optimal dosing regimen, which was defined as an infusion regimen during which maximum plasma concentrations did not exceed 9 mg/l. This was achieved by reducing the infusion duration at the dose of 6 mg/kg/hour from 12 hours to 6 hours. This dosing regimen was effective in 78 per cent of cases. Preterm infants showed relatively high plasma lidocaine concentrations. This new lidocaine-dosing regimen should carry a lower risk of cardiac arrhythmias and appears to be as effective in term infants as regimens that led to higher plasma concentrations. For preterm infants the optimum regimen remains to be determined.

A recent study (Shany et al., 2007) compared the effectiveness of lidocaine and midazolam in the treatment of intractable seizures in newborn infants born at or after 36 weeks of gestation who suffered from hypoxic-ischaemic encephalopathy and who had monitoring of cerebral activity; 77 per cent had a good or a partial response to lidocaine and 50 per cent had a partial response to midazolam. These findings suggest that lidocaine may be more effective than midazolam in reducing or controlling refractory neonatal seizures. The lower response rate to midazolam was more evident in infants with severe hypoxic-ischaemic encephalopathy.

Other drugs

There is little published experience with other antiepileptic drugs in the newborn period. Valproic acid may sometimes be effective as it acts on GABA receptors, but it can cause liver damage. Moreover, it is toxic for the developing brain, as evidenced by the fetal-valproate syndrome. Vigabatrin and lamotrigin are not available in an intravenous form and they are not very useful in the emergency treatment of seizures. Some reports have suggested that they may be used as adjunctive therapy in babies with partial seizures or infantile spasms. Carbamazepine is rarely used in partial seizures. New agents such as topiramate and levetiracetam look promising in neonatal seizure therapy, and there is no experimental evidence for neurotoxicity at anticonvulsant concentrations. Topiramate has the advantage of extending the therapeutic window during which therapeutic post-ischaemic hypothermia is effective (Levene, 2002; Rennie & Boylan, 2003; Booth & Evans, 2004; Sankar & Painter, 2005).

There are some reports of the use of levetiracetam in neonates and older infants. This agent is a commonly prescribed oral anticonvulsant for use as adjunctive therapy for partial seizures in adults, with favourable tolerability, and it has recently been approved for children older than 4 years. There are no published studies on the safety and efficacy of this drug in the infant population. In a recent paper, Shoemaker & Rotenberg (2007) describe the use of levetiracetam in three infants, aged 2 days to 3 months, for refractory seizures or intolerance of other anticonvulsants. Each patient was seizure-free on levetiracetam monotherapy and there were no adverse effects.

Antiepileptic drugs and brain development

Seizures and antiepileptic drugs affect brain development and have long-term neurological consequences (Holmes & Ben-Ari, 2001; Holmes, 2004). The specific molecular and cellular changes, the precise timing of their influence during brain development, and the full extent of the long-term consequences of seizures and antiepileptic drug exposure have not been fully established. There is evidence from both clinical and animal studies that many of the antiepileptic drugs used to treat seizures in children may themselves interfere with normal brain development (Marsh et al., 2006). The effects of antiepileptic drug exposure *in utero* on the occurrence of malformations in the offspring have recently been reviewed (Holmes et al., 2001; Artama et al., 2005). Numerous studies of the older antiepileptic drugs (phenobarbital, carbamazepine, phenytoin, and valproic acid) suggest that exposure during pregnancy increases the risk of minor or major malformations two- to threefold (Holmes et al., 2001). Cognitive function in children exposed *in utero* to antiepileptic drugs has not been extensively studied (Meador & Zupanc, 2004), but there is some evidence that exposure to such drugs *in utero* increases the risk of cognitive dysfunction later in life. For ethical and practical reasons, most studies of antiepileptic drug effects on cognitive development have been carried out on children with epilepsy. An exception was a study of children with febrile seizures who were randomized to placebo or phenobarbital and underwent neuropsychological testing while undergoing treatment; the study found a decrease in the mean IQ of the phenobarbital-treated group (Farwell et al., 1990). These findings suggest that exposure to phenobarbital in early childhood may result in mild but lasting differences in some cognitive abilities. Valproate has been shown to have variable effects, with the most severe cognitive changes associated with polytherapy (Adab *et al.*, 2001). As with the link between seizures and development, animal studies can address the issue of the cognitive effects of antiepileptic drugs in a more controlled fashion. There are several potential mechanisms whereby such drugs may affect the developing brain, including chronic alterations in gene regulation and protein expression. During development, neurotransmitter receptor signalling plays a role in neuroblast migration, proliferation, and differentiation. Altered neuroblast migration during development may contribute to the cognitive changes that have been reported after *in utero* exposure to antiepileptic drugs such as GABAergic modulators. Normal programmed cell death apoptosis during development is essential for network formation in the brain and has been found to be influenced by several antiepileptic drugs. Moreover, antiepileptic drugs alter synaptic transmission and therefore could theoretically affect synapse formation and stability (Marsh *et al.*, 2006).

In summary, there is ample evidence that antiepileptic drug exposure during early life in rodents, especially with the older drugs such as phenobarbital, phenytoin, and valproic acid, alters neuronal development, including gene expression, neuronal migration, differentiation, and survival. What is lacking is a better understanding of the long-term cognitive and memory consequences of exposure to antiepileptic drugs during different developmental periods, especially those that correlate with term infants and young children. Therefore further studies are required (Marsh *et al.*, 2006).

The best anticonvulsion regimen

There is wide variation in clinical practice in both diagnosis and treatment of neonatal seizures, and this reflects the lack of clear evidence of the relative benefits and harm of the anticonvulsants used (Table 1).

Standardized approaches to the treatment of neonatal seizures remain undeveloped and a recent study highlighted a multicentre variability in current treatment practices. The type and number of anticonvulsants were assessed among five neonatal intensive care units in the USA between 2000 and 2003. Almost all of the 480 neonates (94 per cent) with seizures were treated, initially with phenobarbital (82 per cent), lorazepam (nine per cent), phenytoin (two per cent), other anticonvulsants (one per cent), or a combination of the first two drugs (six per cent). While the majority of neonates were treated with one drug (59 per cent), the number of anticonvulsants varied. The wide therapeutic variability reflects the lack of standardized diagnostic and treatment approaches, particularly for seizures refractory to initial phenobarbital therapy (Bartha *et al.*, 2007). There is also a variable approach to therapy between neonatologists and paediatric neurologists: neonatologists use phenobarbital, phenytoin, or a benzodiazepine for second and third episodes of seizures, while neurologists tend not to use benzodiazepines; neonatologists use larger total doses of phenobarbital than neurologists in pursuit of seizure control; neonatologists discontinue antiepileptic drugs earlier than neurologists (Carmo & Barr, 2005).

The routine use of anticonvulsants has been evaluated in a Cochrane review (Booth & Evans, 2004), with the aim of assessing and comparing different anticonvulsants administered to neonates to treat seizures. All randomized or quasi-randomized controlled clinical trials were considered in order to evaluate mortality, neurodevelopmental disability, the need for additional anticonvulsants, the need for maintenance anticonvulsants at discharge, and any adverse events in neonates treated for seizures with systemic anticonvulsants, compared with placebo, no drug, or alternative anticonvulsants. Only two randomized controlled trials published in full could be identified. Painter and colleagues (Painter *et al.*, 1999) showed that the two most commonly

Table 1. Therapeutic strategies

PAPER	First line AED	Second line AED	Third line AED
Sheth et al., 1996	Pb 20 mg/kg followed by 5 mg/kg (maximum 40 mg/kg total)	Phe 20 mg/kg	MDZ 100–400 µg/kg/h
Evans & Levene, 1998	Pb 20 mg/kg followed by 5 mg/kg (maximum 40 mg/kg total)	CNZ 100–200 µg/kg followed by 10–30 µg/kg/h	Phe 20 mg/kg
Kuban & Filiano, 1998	Pb 15–20 mg/kg followed by 10 mg/kg	Phe 15–25 mg/kg	DZP 100–300 µg/kg LZP 50 µg/kg MDZ 20–100 µg/kg followed by 60–400 µg/kg/h
Painter et al., 1999	Phe 15–20 mg/kg (rate < 1 mg/kg/min) followed by 2 mg/kg every 8 h Pb 20 mg/kg followed by 5 mg/kg	Pb 20 mg/kg followed by 5 mg/kg Phe 15–20 mg/kg (rate < 1 mg/kg/min) followed by 2 mg/kg every 8 h	–
Volpe, 2000	Pb 20 mg/kg followed by 5 mg/kg (maximum 40 mg/kg total)	Phe 20 mg/kg	LZP 50–100 µg/kg
Rennie & Boylan, 2003	Pb 40 mg/kg (if newborn artificially ventilated) Pb 20 mg/kg (if newborn breathing spontaneously) followed by 5–10 mg/kg	Phe 20 mg/kg	DZP 0.3–1.0 mg/kg LZP 50–150 µg/kg MDZ 150–200 µg/kg followed by 30–60 µg/kg/h CNZ 100–200 µg/kg followed by 4–10 µg/kg/h
Zupanc, 2004	Pb 20 mg/kg followed by 5–10 mg/kg (maximum 40 mg/kg total) Phe 20 mg/kg (if newborn has respiratory depressed/HIE) LZP 50–100 µg/kg (if NSE)	Phe 20 mg/kg Pb 20 mg/kg	–
Boylan et al., 2004	Pb up to 40 mg/kg followed by 5 mg/kg	Lid 2 mg/kg followed by 2 mg/kg/h (maximum 6 mg/kg/h) DZP 0.3–1.0 mg/kg LZP 50–150 µg/kg CNZ 100–200 µg/kg followed by 4–10 µg/kg/h	–
Castro Conde et al., 2005	Pb 20 mg/kg followed by 10 mg/kg (maximum 40 mg/kg total)	MDZ 150 µg/kg followed by 1 µg/kg/min increasing by 0.5–1 µg/kg/min every 2 min (maximum 18 µg/kg/min)	MDZ 100–150 µg/kg
Malingré et al., 2006	Pb 20 mg/kg followed by 5 mg/kg (maximum 40 mg/kg total)	MDZ 200 µg/kg followed by 30–60 µg/kg/h (full term) CNZ 100 µg/kg followed by 4 µg/kg/h (preterm)	Lid 2 mg/kg followed by 6 mg/kg/h during the first 12 h, 4 mg/kg/h during 12 h, and 2 mg/kg/h for the last 12 h

AED, antiepileptic drug; CNZ, clonazepam; DZP, diazepam; HIE, hypoxic-ischaemic encephalopathy; Lid, lidocaine; LZP, lorazepam; MDZ, midazolam; NSE, neonatal status epilepticus; Pb, phenobarbital; Phe, phenytoin.

used anticonvulsants (phenobarbital and phenytoin) had similar efficacy, but they controlled seizures in less than fifty per cent of the infants. The investigators did not report mortality or neurodevelopmental outcome. Boylan and colleagues (Boylan et al., 2004) randomized infants who failed to respond to phenobarbital to receive either lidocaine or midazolam as second-line agents. There was a trend for lidocaine to be more effective in reducing seizure burden but both groups had a similarly poor long-term outcome assessed at one year. The reviewers concluded that there is little evidence from randomized controlled trials to support the use of any of the anticonvulsants currently employed in the neonatal period (Booth & Evans, 2004). In the literature, there remains a body of opinion that seizures should be treated because of the concern that they may themselves be harmful, although this is supported only by relatively low-grade evidence. The development of safe and effective treatment strategies relies on future studies of high quality (randomized controlled trials with methodology that assures validity) and of sufficient size to have the power to detect clinically important reductions in mortality and severe neurodevelopmental disability (Levene, 2002; Clancy, 2006b).

Until common guidelines for the treatment of neonatal seizures are available, it is at least advisable that each neonatal unit develops a drug protocol based on its own experience and on analysis of previous cases (Levene, 2002). Our own therapeutic strategy is based on the administration of phenobarbital as the first-line drug, followed by a second-line drug (phenytoin or midazolam) in case of refractory seizures. In the management of seizures we consider EEG monitoring to be fundamental, both to confirm the diagnosis of seizures and to evaluate the effect of therapy on the EEG (seizure activity and EEG background). The aim of treatment should be complete seizure control, which means eliminating both electro-clinical and electrographic seizures. We believe that therapy should be driven by the EEG and adjusted in relation to the response of each individual patient, in order to obtain control of seizures as soon as possible with the minimum dosage of antiepileptic drugs (Ferrari et al., 2002).

Discontinuation of therapy

Taking into account the potential toxicity of anticonvulsant drugs, it seem good practice to stop medication as soon as possible. Our practice is to withdraw antiepileptic drugs before discharge in newborns with no further seizure activity, even in those with cerebral lesions or who are at risk of subsequent epilepsy. There is in fact no evidence that continuation of antiepileptic therapy prevents future epilepsy. This approach makes it mandatory to follow up those subjects with cerebral lesions or neurological abnormalities who are at risk of seizure recurrence and epilepsy, mostly in the first years of life. If babies are discharged home with anticonvulsants, withdrawal should be undertaken at the earliest opportunity if they are seizure-free, and a subsequent epilepsy follow-up is required.

Therapy should be continued in subjects with persistence of seizures after the neonatal period and with neonatal epileptic encephalopathy.

In a recent study the majority (75 per cent) of survivors received anticonvulsant treatment after discharge. These neonates were more likely to have had abnormal electroencephalography or brain imaging, or to have needed a second anticonvulsant, compared with neonates whose drug therapy was discontinued (Bartha et al., 2007). Another study investigated treatment patterns at discharge in infants with neonatal seizures and evaluated the impact of phenobarbital prophylaxis on the frequency of seizure recurrence and the long-term neurodevelopmental outcome. Phenobarbital prophylaxis did not improve neurological outcome, either with respect to seizure recurrence or with respect to neurological development (Guillet & Kwon, 2007).

New antiepileptic drugs: 'mechanism-based therapy'

Basic science has provided new insights into the mechanism of neuron activation and seizure generation; moreover, there is increasing interest of research on 'mechanism-based' therapeutic strategies (Dzhala et al., 2006).

The mechanisms of seizure generation, propagation, and termination are different early in development compared with more mature ages; these age-related mechanisms are relevant clinically, as the existing drugs used to treat neonatal seizures are not fully adequate (Ben-Ari, 2006; Dzhala et al., 2006; Shany et al., 2007). Understanding the developmental mechanisms of seizure generation may improve therapeutic strategies. The seizure susceptibility of the developing brain is attributable to the excitatory effect of GABA, the primary inhibitory neurotransmitter in the mature brain. This paradoxical action of GABA is due to age-related differences in chloride homeostasis. Early in development the $Na^+,K^+,2Cl^-$ co-transporter (NKCC1) imports Cl^- into the neuron; when the $GABA_A$ receptor is activated, Cl^- flows out of the neuron, thus depolarizing it. Over time, NKCC1 expression diminishes and another Cl^- transporter, KCC2, is expressed. KCC2 has an opposite effect: it extrudes Cl^- out of the neuron and $GABA_A$ receptor activation allows extracellular Cl^- to flow into the neuron, thus hyperpolarizing it, the net result being inhibitory action. This developmental 'switch' in Cl^- homeostasis might influence the seizure susceptibility of the neonatal brain, shifting the excitation/inhibition balance toward excessive excitation and thus toward seizure activity. Blocking NKCC1 function with a commonly used diuretic, bumetanide, prevents the accumulation of intracellular Cl^-, thereby averting the depolarizing action of $GABA_A$ receptor activation. In animal studies bumetanide reduces kainic-acid-induced seizures in neonatal rats and burst firing in hippocampal slices. Bumetanide is therefore a promising antiepileptic drug with a novel target, the immature chloride cotransporter NKCC1. Its long-term safety profile needs to be established more fully, but it offers an alternative to $GABA_A$ receptor agonists for the treatment of neonatal seizures (Sanchez et al., 2005; Dzhala et al., 2006).

Nevertheless, it is unclear why some GABAergic agents (for example, phenobarbital, benzodiazepines) do not routinely aggravate human neonatal seizures. While the efficacy of these agents is limited, they do stop seizures in a definite percentage of neonates. Interestingly, GABA signalling develops in a caudo-rostral direction; thus phenobarbital and benzodiazepines may increase GABA-mediated inhibition in the spinal cord and brain stem, but may be ineffective in more rostral structures (persistent GABA excitatory effect). Consequently, in some cases barbiturates and benzodiazepines inhibit motor manifestations of neonatal seizures but not cortical seizure activity (Dzhala et al., 2006).

Conclusions

The risk of seizures is greatest in the neonatal period. Currently used treatments have limited efficacy. Although the treatment of neonatal seizures has not changed significantly in the past several decades, there has been substantial progress in understanding developmental mechanisms that influence seizure generation and the responsiveness to anticonvulsants (Rennie & Boylan, 2007). Anticonvulsant therapy is used in the majority of neonates with seizures, mostly with phenobarbital; phenytoin may be an alternative drug, while benzodiazepines and lidocaine are generally used as second-line treatment. The observed wide therapeutic variability may reflect a lack of standardized diagnostic and treatment approaches, particularly for seizures refractory to initial phenobarbital therapy. Trials of anticonvulsants with long-term neurodevelopmental follow-up are needed to develop evidence-based treatment guidelines. Understanding the pathophysiology of neonatal seizures may provide the foundation for better treatment (Silverstein & Jensen, 2007).

References

Adab, N., Jacoby, A., Smith, D. & Chadwick, D. (2001): Additional educational needs in children born to mothers with epilepsy. *J. Neurol. Neurosurg. Psychiatry* **70**, 15–21.

Artama, M., Auvinen, A., Raudaskoski, T., Isojarvi, I. & Isojarvi, J. (2005): Antiepileptic drug use of women with epilepsy and congenital malformations in offspring. *Neurology* **64**, 1874–1878.

Bartha, A.I., Shen, J., Katz, K.H., Mischel, R.E., Yap, K.R., Ivacko, J.A., Andrews, E.M., Ferriero, D.M., Ment, L.R. & Silverstein, F.S. (2007): Neonatal seizures: multicenter variability in current treatment practices. *Pediatr. Neurol.* **37**, 85–90.

Ben-Ari, Y. (2006): Seizures beget seizures: the quest for GABA as a key player. *Crit. Rev. Neurobiol.* **18**, 135–144.

Biagioni, E., Ferrari, F., Boldrini, A., Roversi, M.F. & Cioni, G (1998): Electroclinical correlation in neonatal seizures. *Eur. J. Paediatr. Neurol.* **2**, 117–125.

Booth, D. & Evans, D.J. (2004): Anticonvulsant for neonates with seizures. *Cochrane Database of Systematic Reviews* **18**, CD004218.

Boylan, G.B., Rennie, J.M., Pressler, R.M., Wilson, G., Morton, M. & Binnie, C.D. (2002): Phenobarbitone, neonatal seizures, and video-EEG. *Arch. Dis. Child. Fetal Neonat. Ed.* **86**, F165–F170.

Boylan, G.B., Rennie, J.M., Chorley, G., Pressler, R.M., Fox, G.F., Farrer, K., Morton, M. & Binnie, C.D. (2004): Second-line anticonvulsant treatment of neonatal seizures: a video-EEG monitoring study. *Neurology* **62**, 486–488.

Carmo, K.B. & Barr, P. (2005): Drug treatment of neonatal seizures by neonatologists and paediatric neurologists. *J. Paediatr. Child Health* **41**, 311–312.

Castro Conde, J.R., Hernandez Borges, A.A., Martinez, E.D., Campo, C.G. & Soler, R.P. (2005): Midazolam in neonatal seizures with no response to phenobarbital. *Neurology* **64**, 876–879.

Clancy, R.R. (2006a): Prolonged electroencephalogram monitoring for seizures and their treatment. *Clin. Perinatol.* **33**, 649–665.

Clancy, R.R. (2006b): Summary proceedings from the neurology group on neonatal seizures. *Pediatrics* **117**, S23–S27.

De Vries, L.S. & Hellstrom-Westas, L. (2005): Role of cerebral function monitoring in the newborn. *Arch. Dis. Child. Fetal Neonat. Ed.* **90**, F201–F207.

Dzhala, V.I, Talos, D.M., Sdrulla, D.A., Brumback, A.C., Mathews, G.C, Benke, T.A, Delpire, E., Jensen, F.E. & Staley, K.J. (2006): NKCC1 transporter facilitates seizures in the developing brain. *Nat. Med.* **11**, 1205–1213.

Evans, D. & Levene, M. (1998): Neonatal seizures. *Arch. Dis. Child. Fetal Neonat. Ed.* **78**, F70–F75.

Evans, D.J, Levene, M. & Tsakmakis, M (2007): Anticonvulsants for preventing mortality and morbidity in full term newborns with perinatal asphyxia. *Cochrane Database Syst. Rev.* **18**, CD001240.

Farwell, J.R., Lee, Y.J., Hirtz, D.G., Sulzbacher, S.I., Ellenberg, J.H. & Nelson, K.B. (1990): Phenobarbital for febrile seizures – effects on intelligence and on seizure recurrence. *N. Engl. J. Med.* **322**, 364–369.

Ferrari, F., Biagioni, E. & Cioni, G. (2001): Neonatal electroencephalography. In: *Fetal and neonatal neurology and neurosurgery*, 3rd edition, ed. M. Levene, F.A. Chervenak, M. Whittle, M.J. Bennett & J. Punt. Edinburgh: Churchill Livingstone.

Ferrari, F., Roversi, M.F., Guerra, M.P., Ori, L., Berardi, A., Bonvicini, F., Gargano, G. & Cavazzuti, G.B. (2002): Convulsioni neonatali da asfissia perinatale: quale terapia? *Riv. Ital. Med. Perinat.* **4**, 9–18.

Ferrari, F., Roversi, M.F., Guerra, M.P., Lugli, L. & Cavazzuti, G.B. (2006): Neonatal seizures and epileptic syndromes of neonatal onset. *Ital. J. Pediatr.* **32**, 19–27.

Ferriero, D.M. (2004): Neonatal brain injury. *N. Engl. J. Med.* **351**, 1985–1995.

Guillet, R. & Kwon, J. (2007): Seizure recurrence and developmental disabilities after neonatal seizures: outcomes are unrelated to use of phenobarbital prophylaxis. *J. Child Neurol.* **22**, 389–395.

Haglund, M.M. & Hochman, D.W. (2005): Furosemide and mannitol suppression of epileptic activity in the human brain. *J. Neurophysiol.* **94**, 907–918.

Hahn, C.D. & Riviello, J.J. (2004): Neonatal seizures and EEG: electroclinical dissociation and uncoupling. *NeoReviews* **5**, e350–e355.

Hall, R.T., Hall, F.K. & Daily, D.K. (1998): High-dose phenobarbital therapy in term newborn infants with severe perinatal asphyxia: a randomized, prospective study with three-year follow-up. *J. Pediatr.* **132,** 345–348.

Hoffmann, G.F., Schmitt, B., Windfuhr, M., Wagner, N., Strehl, H., Bagci, S., Franz, A.R., Mills, P.B., Clayton, P.T., Baumgartner, M.R., Steinmann, B., Bast, T., Wolf, N.I. & Zschocke, J. (2007): Pyridoxal 5(phosphate may be curative in early-onset epileptic encephalopathy. *J. Inherit. Metab. Dis.* **30,** 6–9.

Holmes, G.L. & Ben-Ari, Y. (2001): The neurobiology and consequences of epilepsy in the developing brain. *Pediatr. Res.* **49,** 320–325.

Holmes, G.L. (2004): Effects of early seizures on later behavior and epileptogenicity. *Ment. Retard. Dev. Disabil. Res. Rev.* **10,** 101–105.

Holmes, L.B., Harvey, E.A., Coull, B.A., Huntington, K.B., Khoshbin, S., Hayes, A.M. & Ryan, L.M. (2001): The teratogenicity of anticonvulsant drugs. *N. Engl. J. Med.* **344,** 1132–1138.

Holmes, L.B., Wyszynski, D.F. & Lieberman, E. (2004): The AED (antiepileptic drug) pregnancy registry: a 6-year experience. *Arch. Neurol.* **61,** 673–678.

Hunt, R.W. & Inder, T.E. (2005): Neonatal seizures: have we got the treatment right? *J. Paediatr. Child Health* **41,** 311–312.

Kuban, C.K. & Filiano, J. (1998): Neonatal seizures. In: *Manuel of neonatal case*, ed. P.J. Cloherty. Boston: Lippincott-Raven.

Levene, M. (2002): The clinical conundrum of neonatal seizures. *Arch. Dis. Child. Fetal Neonat. Ed.* **86,** F75–F77.

Malingré, M.M., Van Rooij, L.G., Rademaker, C.M., Toet, M.C., Ververs, T.F., Van Kesteren, C. & De Vries, L.S. (2006): Development of an optimal lidocaine infusion strategy for neonatal seizures. *Eur. J. Pediatr.* **165,** 598–604.

Marsh, E.D., Brooks-Kayal, A.R. & Porter, B.E. (2006): Seizures and antiepileptic drugs: does exposure alter normal brain development? *Epilepsia* **47,** 1999–2010.

McBride, M.C., Laroia, N. & Guillet, R. (2000): Electrographic seizures in neonates correlate with poor neurodevelopmental outcome. *Neurology* **55,** 506–514.

Meador, K.J. & Zupanc, M.L. (2004): Neurodevelopmental outcomes of children born to mothers with epilepsy. *Cleve. Clin. J. Med.* **71,** S38–S41.

Miller, S.P., Weiss, J., Barnwell, A., Ferriero, D.M., Latal-Hajnal, B., Ferrer-Rogers, A., Newton, N., Partridge, J.C., Glidden, D.V., Vigneron, D.B. & Barkovich, A.J. (2002): Seizure-associated brain injury in term newborns with perinatal asphyxia. *Neurology* **58,** 542–548.

Mizrahi, E.M. (1999): Acute and chronic effects of seizures in the developing brain: lesson from clinical experience. *Epilepsia* **40,** S42–S50.

Painter, M.I., Pippenger, C. & Wasterlain, C. (1981): Phenobarbitol and phenytoin in neonatal seizures: metabolism and tissue distribution. *Neurology* **31,** 110–117.

Painter, M.J., Scher, M.S., Stein, A.D., Armatti, S., Wang, Z., Gardiner, J.C., Paneth, N., Minnigh, B. & Alvin, J. (1999): Phenobarbitone compared with phenytoin for the treatment of neonatal seizures. *N. Engl. J. Med.* **341,** 485–489.

Rennie, J.M. & Boylan, G.B. (2003): Neonatal seizures and their treatment. *Curr. Opin. Neurol.* **16,** 177–181.

Rennie, J. & Boylan, G. (2007): Treatment of neonatal seizures. *Arch. Dis. Child. Fetal Neonat. Ed.* **92,** F148–F150.

Rennie, J.M., Chorley, G., Boylan, G.B., Pressler, R., Nguyen, Y. & Hooper, R. (2004): Non-expert use of the cerebral function monitor for neonatal seizure detection. *Arch. Dis. Child. Fetal Neonat. Ed.* **89,** F37–F40.

Riviello, J.J. (2004): Pharmacology review: drug therapy for neonatal seizures: part 1. *NeoReviews* **5,** e215–e220.

Sanchez, R.M., Dai, W., Levada, R.E., Lippman, J.J. & Jensen, F.E. (2005): AMPA/kainate receptor-mediated downregulation of GABAergic synaptic transmission by calcineurin after seizures in the developing rat brain. *J. Neurosci.* **25,** 3442–3451.

Sankar, R. (2004): Initial treatment of epilepsy with antiepileptic drugs: pediatric issues. *Neurology* **63,** S30-S39.

Sankar, R. & Painter, M.J. (2005): Neonatal seizures: after all these years we still love what doesn't work. *Neurology* **64,** 776–777.

Scher, M.S., Alvin, J., Gaus, L., Minnigh, B., Painter, P. & Painter, M.J. (2003): Uncoupling of EEG – clinical neonatal seizures after antiepileptic drug use. *Pediatr. Neurol.* **28,** 277–280.

Shany, E., Benzaqen, O. & Watemberg, N. (2007): Comparison of continuous drip of midazolam or lidocaine in the treatment of intractable neonatal seizures. *J. Child. Neurol.* **22,** 255–259.

Sheth, R.D., Buckley, D.J., Gutierrez, A.R., Gingold, M., Bodensteiner, J.B. & Penney, S. (1996): Midazolam in the treatment of refractory neonatal seizures. *Clin. Neuropharmacol.* **19,** 165–170.

Shoemaker, M.T. & Rotenberg, J.S. (2007): Levetiracetam for the treatment of neonatal seizures. *J. Child Neurol.* **22,** 95–98.

Silverstein, F.S. & Jensen, F.E. (2007): Neonatal seizures. *Ann. Neurol.* **62,** 112–120.

Tekgul, H., Gauvreau, K., Soul, J., Murphy, L., Robertson, R., Stewart, J., Volpe, J., Bourgeois, B. & Du Plessis, A.J. (2006): The current etiologic profile and neurodevelopmental outcome of seizures in term newborn infants. *Pediatrics* **117,** 1270–1280.

Volpe, J.J. (1989): Neonatal seizures: current concept and seizures classification. *Pediatrics* **84,** 422–428.

Volpe, J.J. (2000): *Neurology of the newborn*, 4th edition. Philadelphia: W.B. Saunders Co.

Wirrel, E.C. (2005): Neonatal seizures: to treat or not to treat? *Semin. Pediatr. Neurol.* **12,** 97–105.

Zupanc, M.L. (2004): Neonatal seizures. *Pediatr. Clin. North Am.* **51,** 961–978.

Chapter 24

Therapeutic approaches to psychomotor delay

Ermellina Fedrizzi and Elena Andreucci *

Fondazione Mariani ONLUS, viale Bianca Maria 28, 20129 Milan, Italy;
* *Division of Developmental Neurology, Istituto Neurologico C. Besta, via Celoria 11, 20133 Milan, Italy*
efedrizzi@libero.it

Summary

In the early years of life, psychomotor or developmental delay is a non-specific sign of conditions that are often undiagnosed at the time. Nevertheless, paediatricians and clinicians involved in neurorehabilitation emphasize the opportunity for early intervention, even without a diagnosis, because of the reorganizational capacity of the young nervous system. The key issue at present concerns the meaning of 'early intervention'. Since the 1970s, when facilitation techniques such as those of Bobath and Vojta were used, the theoretical framework underlying interventions has evolved and now the main objective of treatment is to improve the quality of life of the child and the child's family. This change of approach to early intervention has been related to two main factors. First, a review of outcome studies on early intervention in 2005 showed that physiotherapy is ineffective but that treatment based on educational programmes and family participation has positive effects both on cognitive and motor performance. Second, recent advances in neuroscience, both in neurobiology and in neuroradiology, have provided insight into the architecture of different brain functions and into the processes of neuronal reorganization after brain lesions. Neurobiological studies in animals have produced evidence that behavioural therapy is especially helpful in reversing some of the devastating consequences of brain damage. Studies on cognitive function in relation to the motor cortex and to the involvement of the motor cortex and the corticospinal tracts in motor imagery have emphasized the role of mental training in rehabilitation treatment. Finally, the chief clinical implications for the treatment of developmental delay are related to studies on the mirror neuron system and its functional role in action understanding and in action initiation.

Introduction

Psychomotor or developmental delay refers to a delay in the development of cognitive, motor, linguistic, and emotional competence in relation to what is appropriate for the child's chronological age. In the first two years of life psychomotor delay is a non-specific symptom, reflecting the early expression of several disorders, the diagnosis of which is often unknown at the time. It could be the first clinical sign of cerebral palsy or of genetic, metabolic, or degenerative syndromes. Nevertheless, paediatricians and clinicians involved in neurorehabilitation emphasize the opportunity for early intervention, even without a diagnosis, because of the reorganizational capacity of the young nervous system. However, there is controversy about which therapeutic approaches are most appropriate for a child with psychomotor delay, and about when the interventions should be initiated. At present, the key issue concerns the meaning of the term 'early intervention', which has been undergoing an evolution since the early 1970s.

Historical evolution of the concept of early intervention

During the decade from 1970 to 1980, early intervention was used as a preventive strategy for children at biological risk of developmental disorders, and specifically for low birth weight premature babies. The intervention programmes consisted mainly of facilitation techniques such as neurodevelopmental therapy (NDT), according to Bobath's principles (Bobath & Bobath, 1984) and the Vojta method (Vojta, 1984). Normal motor and behavioural development was interpreted for many years within the framework of neuromaturationist theory, based on the hypothesis that development is predetermined by gradual myelination and by increasing cortical control over lower reflexes (Gesell & Amatruda, 1947; Peiper, 1963). These assumptions formed the basis of the neurofacilitation techniques. Treatment was started very early in life, before the clinical expression of psychomotor delay or dysfunction, thus making the intervention superfluous in those at-risk children who would not have developed any disability.

Later, during the two ensuing decades (1980 to 2000), new knowledge from the neurosciences led to a change in the theoretical framework underlying the principles of intervention. Motor development and behaviour are now no longer explained in terms of reflex mechanisms; on the contrary they now are regarded as the result of the interaction of multiple systems and components, both intrinsic and extrinsic. For instance, in motor development the intrinsic factors are muscle strength, postural support and balance, motor control, and the level of brain development, while the extrinsic factors are the environmental conditions and the problems the child has to face. These new theoretical models have resulted in a shift to new therapeutic approaches based on motor control and on the motor learning model.

Furthermore, during the same period the first outcome studies on the effect of physiotherapy as NDT treatment began to be published (Palmer et al., 1988). None of the NDT studies showed a statistically significant effect of the intervention on motor development, while programmes consisting of general infant stimulation and including enhancement of parent-infant interaction showed a significantly positive effect on motor development. Consequently, the focus of early intervention programmes shifted from the improvement in motor development to broader outcomes on adaptive functions and the quality of life of the child and the child's family.

At present, 'early intervention' serves as an umbrella term covering the whole field of childhood intervention (Blauw-Hospers & Hadders-Algra, 2005), defined as follows: 'Early intervention consists of multidisciplinary services provided to children from birth to 5 years of age to promote child health and wellbeing, enhance emerging competencies, minimize developmental delays, remediate existing or emerging disabilities, prevent functional deterioration, and promote adaptive parenting and overall family functioning. These goals are accomplished by individualized developmental, educational, and therapeutic services for children provided in conjunction with mutually planned support for their family' (Shonkoff & Meisels, 2000). Recently, the evolution of the meaning of 'early intervention' towards a broader field of child development has been confirmed in several further studies.

Early intervention outcome studies

In 2005 a review was published of 34 studies on the effect of interventions starting between birth and a corrected age of 18 months in infants at high risk of impaired development (Blauw-Hospers & Hadders-Algra, 2005). Seventeen of these studies were undertaken within a neonatal intensive care unit (NICU). The results indicated that the Newborn Individualized Developmental Care and Assessment Program (NIDCAP) (Als et al., 1994) had a temporary positive effect (up to 9 months of age) on motor development in infants at high risk of developmental disability. The only NICU study showing that developmental intervention had a significant positive effect on motor and cognitive development was one carried out by Resnick and colleagues (Resnick et al., 1987; Resnick et al., 1988). In this programme, developmental intervention for low birth weight premature infants started in hospital and continued for 2 years at home, with the involvement of the parents, who had an important role in the interventions.

Twelve other randomized controlled studies on the effect of interventions in high risk infants were reviewed; these started between the time of discharge from the NICU and 18 months of age. The results indicated that intervention programmes in the early postnatal years, based on the principles of NDT or Vojta, did not have a beneficial effect on motor development in children at high risk of developmental disorders or in those with cerebral palsy or Down syndrome. However, there is now good evidence that specific developmental training and general development programmes in which parents learn how to promote infant development and active interaction can have a positive effect (Blauw-Hospers & Hadders-Algra, 2005).

Several other studies on the efficacy of early intervention to enhance the cognitive, behavioural, and health status of low birth weight premature infants have been carried out in the past decade. The Infant Health and Development Program (Ramey et al., 1992) was a randomized controlled trial conducted in the USA and involving 985 families of at-risk infants. The intervention began immediately after the infant's discharge from hospital and continued until 3 years of age. The intervention modes included:

- Paediatric follow-up with medical, developmental, and social assessment.
- Weekly home visits in the first year and every two weeks thereafter, focusing on providing emotional support for the parents and helping parents to learn specific ways to foster their child's intellectual, physical, and social development.
- Child development centres, attended daily by the children after 12 months of age, where a systematic educational programme was provided.
- Parent support groups, in which parents could share information and concerns about child rearing and learn about specific topics in child development.

The effect of the Infant Health and Development Program (IHDP) on cognitive development was studied during the first 3 years of life (Brooks-Gunn et al., 1992) and the results showed benefits across cognitive domains at 24 and 36 months, most pronounced for receptive language and visual-motor and spatial skills. The same IHDP population was reassessed at the age of 5 years (Brooks-Gunn et al., 1994) and at the age of 18 years (McCormick et al., 2006). Both the follow-up assessments documented greater cognitive competence in premature children of higher birth weight (2,000 to 2,500 g) who had undergone the intervention programme in the first 3 years of life.

The outcome of these studies supports the view that early educational intervention can result in long-term changes in children at developmental risk.

Recent knowledge from neuroscience

Recent advances in the neurosciences – neurobiology, neurophysiology, and neuroradiology – have provided new insights into the architecture of the different functions of the nervous system and on the process of neuronal reorganization after brain lesions. These advances may help clinicians to improve their current approaches and to develop new and innovative intervention strategies.

The neurobiological studies by Kolb and colleagues (Kolb et al., 2001) exemplify the recent research on plastic changes after lesions of the cerebral cortex in young and adult rats. These studies revealed that newborn rats with cortical lesions, placed for the first three months of life in a complex environment in which there where novel stimuli and ample opportunity for both sensory and motor stimulation, developed significant functional compensation over the postoperative period. Analysis of the brains showed a reversal of the atrophy with an increase in dendritic arborization and spine density, correlated with functional compensation. The investigators emphasized the role of experience in compensating for the injury-induced changes in cortical structure. This is encouraging as it suggests that behavioural therapy should be especially helpful in reversing some of the devastating consequences of brain damage in the later periods of prenatal development in human infants. Moreover, the experimental data showed that not all experiences are equally effective in changing behaviour after cortical injury. Training animals in specific and repeated motor patterns, such as skilled reaching, is not effective in facilitating recovery. In contrast, placing animals in complex environments in which they have varied social, sensory, and active motor experiences is effective in stimulating recovery. This implies that therapeutic programmes should be initiated early after cortical injury in infants, and that the therapy would include perceptual stimulation, novelty, social interaction, and motor activities.

Studies by Jeannerod (Jeannerod & Pacherie, 2004; Jeannerod, 2006) on the cognitive function of the motor cortex and on the involvement of the motor cortex and the corticospinal tracts in motor imagery have implications for the therapeutic approach. The assumption that representing an action and executing it are functionally equivalent – based on experimental studies with neuroimaging techniques (functional magnetic resonance imaging and trans magnetic stimulation, TMS) – provides a framework for the use of mental training in rehabilitation. Mental training is currently used by a wide range of motor performers, such as sports professionals and musicians; it has been shown to affect several aspects of motor performance, such as increasing the strength of muscular contraction, improving motor speed and accuracy, reducing variability, and increasing the temporal consistency of movements (Jeannerod, 2006). This approach to treatment could not be used with infants, but by the second year of life a therapist can help a child face a task by following a problem-solving approach, guiding the child to define an action plan and a spatial and temporal sequence before executing the plan.

Recently, the most relevant clinical implications for the treatment of developmental delay have been related to studies on the mirror neuron system and its functional role in action understanding and action imitation (Rizzolatti et al., 1996; Rizzolatti et al., 2001; Rizzolatti & Craighero, 2004). The functional properties of the system formed by mirror neurons have been studied in monkeys. The first basic property of these neurons, which are located in area F5 and which respond when the monkey sees object-directed action, is action understanding. Rizzolatti et al. (2001) showed that each time an individual sees an action done by another individual, neurons that represent that action are activated in the observer's premotor cortex. This motor representation of the observed action corresponds to what is spontaneously generated during an activity whose outcome is known to the acting individual. Thus the mirror neuron system transforms visual information into knowledge.

The property of making the meaning of other individuals' actions understandable is of great importance for child development, and is essential for communicative and interactive behaviour. Thus, in defining the intervention programme according to the problem-solving approach, the therapist needs to take into account the functional role of the mirror system and to show the child tasks and environmental situations whose meaning can be readily understood in relation to the child's age and cognitive level.

The mirror neuron system plays another fundamental role in action imitation: experimental data in humans, using neuroimaging and neurophysiological techniques, clearly show that the basic circuit underlying imitation coincides with that which is active during action observation. This property may explain the human capacity to learn by imitation. Rizzolatti & Craighero (2004) hypothesized that during the learning of new motor patterns by imitation, the observed actions are broken down into elementary motor acts that activate, through the mirror mechanism, the corresponding motor representations. Once these motor representations are activated, they are recombined by the prefrontal cortex according to the observed model.

Sequential learning by imitation plays an important role in motor, cognitive, communicative, and interactive behaviour through infancy and childhood. Knowledge of the mechanisms and processes underlying the human ability to learn will help clinicians and therapists to plan the treatment for children at developmental risk as well as for children with disabilities.

Conclusions

All data coming from outcome studies and from neuroscience research indicate that a therapeutic approach to psychomotor delay in the first years of life must be started as soon as possible. Programmes involving mostly passive handling techniques such as NDT or Vojta should be avoided, while general developmental and educational programmes, aimed at enhancing the child's exploration of active motor, communicative, and interactive behaviour during play and the activities of daily living, are recommended.

References

Als, H., Lawhon, G., Duffy, F.H., McAnulty, G.B., Gibes-Grossman, R. & Blickman, J.G. (1994): Individualized developmental care for the very low-birth-weight preterm infant. Medical and neurofunctional effects. *JAMA* **272**, 853–858.

Blauw-Hospers, C.H. & Hadders-Algra, M. (2005): A systematic review of the effects of early intervention on motor development. *Dev. Med. Child Neurol.* **47**, 421–432.

Bobath, K. & Bobath, B. (1984): The neurodevelopmental treatment. In: *Management of the motor disorders of children with cerebral palsy*, ed. D. Scrutton. London: Blackwell Science.

Brooks-Gunn, J., Liaw, F. & Klebanov, P.K. (1992): Effects of early intervention on cognitive function of low birth weight preterm infants. *J. Pediatr.* **120**, 350–359.

Brooks-Gunn, J., McCarton, C.M., Casey, P.H., McCormick, M.C., Bauer, C.R., Bernbaum, J.C., Tyson, J., Swanson, M., Bennett, F.C., Scott, D., Tonascia, J. & Meinert, C.L. (1994): Early intervention in low-birth-weight premature infants: results through age 5 years from the Infant Health and Development Program. *JAMA* **272**, 1257–1262.

Gesell, A.& Amatruda, C.S. (1947): *Developmental diagnosis. Normal and abnormal child development*, 2nd edition, p. 496. New York: Harper & Row.

Kolb, B., Brown, R., Witt-Lajeunesse, A. & Gibb, R. (2001): Neural compensation after lesion of the cerebral cortex. *Neural Plasticity* **8**, 1–16.

Jeannerod, M. (2006): *Motor cognition: what actions tell the self*. New York: Oxford University Press.

Jeannerod, M. & Pacherie, E. (2004): Agency, simulation and self-identification. *Mind Lang.* **19,** 113–146.

McCormick, M.C., Brooks-Gunn, J., Buka, S.L., Goldman, J., Yu, J., Salganik, M., Scott, D.T., Bennett, F.C., Kay, L.L., Bernbaum, J.C., Bauer, C.R., Martin, C., Woods, E.R., Martin, A. & Casey, P.K. (2006): Early intervention in low birth premature infants: results at 18 years of age for the Infant Health Development Program. *Pediatrics* **117,** 771–780.

Palmer, F.B., Shapiro, B.K., Wachtel, R.C., Allen, M.C., Hiller, J.E., Harryman, S.E., Mosher, B.S., Meinert, C.L. & Capute, A.J. (1988): The effect of physical therapy on cerebral palsy. A controlled trial in infants with spastic diplegia. *N. Engl. J. Med.* **318,** 803–808.

Peiper, A. (1963): *Cerebral function in infancy and childhood*, 3rd edition, p. 683. New York: Consultant Bureau.

Ramey, C.T., Bryant, D.M., Wasik, B.H., Sparling, J.J., Fendt, K.H. & LaVange, L.M. (1992): Infant Health and Development Program for low birth weight, premature infants: program elements, family participation, and child intelligence. *Pediatrics* **89,** 454–465.

Resnick, M.B., Eyler, F.D., Nelson, R.M., Eitzman, D.V. & Bucciarelli, R.L. (1987): Developmental intervention for low birth weight infants: improved early developmental outcome. *Pediatrics* **80,** 68–74.

Resnick, M.B., Armstrong, S. & Carter, R.L. (1988): Developmental intervention program for high-risk premature infants: effects on development and parent-infant interaction. *J. Dev. Behav. Pediatr.* **9,** 73–78.

Rizzolatti, G. & Craighero, L. (2004): The mirror-neuron system. *Annu. Rev. Neurosci.* **27,** 169–192.

Rizzolatti, G., Fadiga, L., Fogassi, L. & Gallese, V. (1996): Premotor cortex and the recognition of motor actions. *Cogn. Brain Res.* **111,** 246–252.

Rizzolatti, G., Fogassi, L. & Gallese, V. (2001): Neurophysiological mechanisms underlying the understanding and imitation of action. *Nat. Rev. Neurosci.* **2,** 661–670.

Shonkoff, J.P. & Meisels, S.J., eds. (2000): *Handbook of early childhood intervention*, pp. XVII-XVIII. Cambridge, UK: Cambridge University Press.

Vojta, V. (1984): The basic elements of treatment according to Vojta. In: *Management of the motor disorders of children with cerebral palsy*, ed. D. Scrutton. London: Blackwell Science.